Management
of Hospitals

Management of Hospitals

Rockwell Schulz, Ph.D.
Alton C. Johnson, Ph.D.

University of Wisconsin, Madison

McGraw-Hill Book Company

A Blakiston Publication

New York   St. Louis   San Francisco   Auckland
Düsseldorf   Johannesburg   Kuala Lumpur   London
Mexico   Montreal   New Delhi   Panama   Paris
São Paulo   Singapore   Sydney   Tokyo   Toronto

Library of Congress Cataloging in Publication Data

Schulz, Rockwell.
    Management of hospitals.

    "A Blakiston publication."
    Includes index.
      1. Hospitals—Administration. I. Johnson, Alton
Cornelius, date, joint author II. Title.
    [DNLM: 1. Hospital administration. WX150 S389m]
    RA971.S36   658'.91'36211   75-4799
    ISBN 0-07-055651-2

MANAGEMENT
OF HOSPITALS

1 2 3 4 5 6 7 8 9 0 K P K P 7 9 8 7 6 5

This book was set in Press Roman by Allen Wayne Technical Corp.
The editor was Cathy Dilworth; the designer was Allen Wayne Technical Corp.;
the production supervisor was Judi Allen.
The cover was designed by Weschler & Waters Design, Inc.
Kingsport Press, Inc., was printer and binder.

Dedicated to Carol, Virginia, and our children

Contents

PART THREE ADMINISTRATIVE FUNCTIONS
Transformation of Inputs to Outputs

PART FOUR ENVIRONMENTAL INFLUENCES AND
            CONSTRAINTS

Preface

Hospitals are among the more complex and dynamic institutions in our society. There are many issues surrounding the management of hospitals, and in recent years considerable research has been done in relation to these issues. This book is designed as a text and reference focusing on issues and related research.

The book is designed not just for hospital administrators but also for the many other individuals involved with the administration of hospitals such as medical, nursing, and other professionals, staff specialists, and other department heads. It provides an overview for students who will be in administrative roles, students in related disciplines such as health economics and medical sociology, and practicing hospital administrators, trustees, chiefs of staff, department heads, planners, and others who are involved in or have dealings with the community general hospital. The community general hospital is an appropriate basic model from which applications can be made to other health institutions such as group practices, health maintenance organizations (HMOs), mental hospitals, and extended care facilities.

There is a need for an organized resource book that collates the thinking and research of a large number of experts in diverse but related fields. Research in the administration of health institutions has expanded rapidly in recent years. Whenever appropriate, we have attempted to relate these findings to the many issues (e.g., consumerism, cost and quality control, and collective bargaining) facing administrators, trustees, chiefs of staff and medical departments, other department heads, and planners. We have also applied research from other industries where it seems appropriate. However, the scope of this book constrains us from describing extensively theoretical approaches to management from such basic disciplines as social psychology and operations research.

Our focus may at times make hospitals appear to be in a state of chaos. Such is not the case, but misconceptions may arise out of our emphasis on problem areas rather than on all the positive elements of today's hospitals. Indeed, we have attempted to be provocative in our conclusions. The reader is encouraged not to patently accept our conclusions, but to examine them against his or her own experience and thinking. We hope this will help to stimulate a continuing pattern of learning, one that includes seeking new evidence and revising opinions as changes continue to occur in health care and management.

The systems approach is an appropriate way of examining the community hospital with its complex external and internal relationships. Part 1 begins by introducing a framework for examining system objectives and the prevalent models of health delivery systems within which hospitals and other health institutions function as components. In this context the hospital is described as an open system. Part 2 considers internal hospital systems from the perspective of governance, medical staff, nursing and other programs, and administration. Part 3 is concerned with the transformation of inputs to outputs and the administrative functions of achieving high-quality services, cost containment, and other institutional objectives. Part 4 explores collective bargaining and other pressures on hospitals as well as the management of health institutions in the future.

The organization of this book in the systems context outlined above can be portrayed as follows:

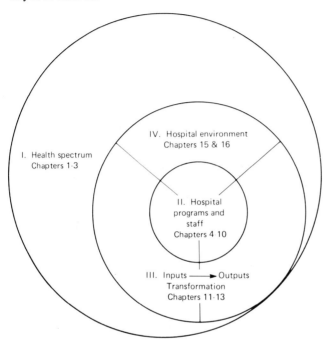

We want to express our appreciation to the faculty members of the University of Wisconsin Program in Health Services Administration who provided considerable assistance, especially John Bracken, Andre Delbecq, Don Detmer, M.D., David Gustafson, and Jerry Rose. We also thank Edward Connors, Irwin Schulz, M.D., Kent Peterson, M.D., and Kevin McMullan for their critical reviews and suggestions. Those who provided help with specific chapters include Jeff Kunz for the chapter on medical staff, Sue Kern, R.N., Marie Zimmer, R.N., and Joy Calkin, R.N., for the chapters on nursing and other professionals, Charles Perrow and Gordon Johnsen for the chapter on roles of administrators, David Zilz for help with the chapter on other professionals, Werner Frank for the chapter on functional specialists, Joseph Morreale on cost controls, and Sarah Dean for the chapter on external relationships. We of course do not hold any of them responsible for the material and conclusions presented in this book, nor do we mean to imply that they necessarily always agreed with us or with one another.

Rockwell Schulz
Alton C. Johnson

Part One

The Hospital as a Subsystem of the Health Care System

The hospital is generally thought to be the center of the health care system. The hospital may be the center for treatment of the sick and injured, but we suggest that in most communities the hospital could play a larger role in improving health. Factors other than treatment of the sick and injured have at least as much and probably more impact on the health of a community and of individuals.

Chapter 1 looks at the hospital as just one component in a macro system whose overall objective is to provide optimum health for populations and individuals. This chapter concludes that there is a great deal more to health care than the diagnosis and treatment of disease. Environment, behavior, heredity, and their interactions have a major influence on health. Moreover, although medical treatment receives the greatest emphasis, promotion of health, prevention of disease, rehabilitation, and custodial services are also important in the delivery of personal health services.

Chapter 2 considers the organization of personal health care services from the perspective of desirable objectives. We suggest that most personal health care services in the United States fall within five general models all of which have advantages and disadvantages. Roles of hospitals will vary somewhat within these models.

Chapter 3 examines hospital systems and the community general hospital as complex components of the total health system. Hospitals have complex and inter-related external and internal systems. Moreover, the patient is considerably more than a biological being. We conclude that hospitals have multiple and sometimes conflicting functions and objectives.

Chapter 1

The Health System

Health care is one of the largest and most complex industries in the United States. For the fiscal year 1974, health care expenditures amounted to $104 billion, or $485 per capita, and made up 7.7 percent of the gross national product. There are approximately 4.4 million individuals involved in providing health services to the American public (DHEW, 1975). The Department of Labor lists 225 job titles that have a direct relationship to the rendering of personal health services. Health is considered one of the largest industries in the country, if not the largest, in terms of employment and expenditures. Yet when one examines the impact of the rapid advances in the health service industry on the health of our society, one is faced with serious questions about the cost and benefits of traditional medical services. Haggerty (1972) for example, notes "... we are forced to look very long and hard to find evidence that medical care makes much difference to mortality and morbidity (i.e., presence of disease)." However, it is important to note that medical care has helped humans to cope with disease.

Inputs to Health

The World Health Organization (WHO) defines health as a state of "complete physical, mental, and social well-being and not merely the absence of disease."

While there is some disagreement as to whether this is a useful definition because it presents an unattainable and unmeasurable ideal, it is unquestionably a desirable objective for the health industry. It is clear that health is indeed a comprehensive concept and that hospital care is but a small component in the provision of complete physical, mental, and social well-being.

An alternative approach to defining health is the ecological one, which considers health to be a state of optimal physical, mental, and social adaptation to one's environment. For example, an individual with a chronic disease condition, e.g., arthritis or chronic heart disease, can never return to complete well-being, but can adjust and adapt quite adequately. A more direct example would be patients with terminal illness. Facilitating adaptation in this case would mean helping to prepare for and adjust to the realities of death.

Blum (1974) suggests that the ultimate needs and goals for the health system are:

Prolongation of life through prevention of premature death

Minimization of departures from physiologic or functional norms for optimal health (Such nouns have yet to be defined.)

Minimization of discomfort (illness)

Minimization of disability (incapacity)

Promotion of high-level "wellness" or self-fulfillment (internal satisfaction)

Promotion of high-level satisfaction with the environment (external satisfaction)

Extension of resistance to ill health and creation of reserve capacity (positive health)

Increasing capacity for the underprivileged to participate in health matters

In Figure 1-1 Blum (1974) presents the health spectrum showing environment, behavior, heredity, and health care services as inputs to psychosocial (emotional and mental) and somatic (physical) health or well-being. These four inputs relate and affect one another through ecological balance, natural resources, population characteristics, cultural systems, and mental health.

Environment

Natural physical characteristics of the environment such as climate, soil conditions, and topography relate to health directly as well as interacting to affect the economy, the culture, and other forces that contribute to a state of healthfulness. Moreover, man-made aspects of the environment have an increasing influence on health. Inadequate housing, for example, contributes to disease. The (Wisconsin) Governor's Health Policy and Planning Task Force (1972) identified inadequacies in transportation and communication as major barriers to the adequate delivery of health services. Since accidents are the fourth leading cause of death in the United States, safety in work and leisure is another major factor. Sanitation in its broadest sense i.e., the control of air, water, and noise and aesthetic pollution, obviously contributes to good health. While advances in technology have had a major impact on improving health, they sometimes lead to new hazards e.g., the noise pollution associated with airplanes.

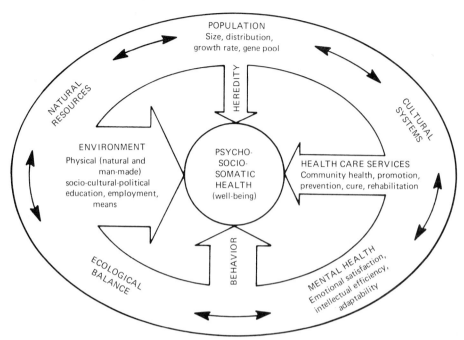

The width of the four huge input-to-health arrows indicates assumptions about the relative importance of the inputs to health. The four inputs are shown as relating to and affecting one another by means of an encompassing matrix which could be called the "environment" of the health system.

Figure 1-1 Inputs to Health (Adapted from Henrik L. Blum, *Planning for Health: Development and Application of Social Change Theory*, Human Sciences Press, New York, 1974, p. 3.)

Sociocultural factors are inputs to health. Cultural patterns affect nutrition, exercise, personal habits, and other factors related to health. Social stress and the responses of cardiovascular, respiratory, gastrointestinal and other systems have been widely researched and relationships detected (Graham and Reeder, 1972). Fuchs (1974) suggests that lifestyle contributes in a major way to health status in developed countries—more so than income or medical care. He suggests that lifestyle may account for otherwise unexplained differences in health between males and females, races, middle-aged adults in Sweden and the United States, those with differing marital status, people with varied occupations, and the populations of Nevada and Utah. Politics as reflected in laws on alcohol and safety, for example, contribute to health. The reduction in deaths on the road as a result of the reduction in speed limits is a recent example.

There is increasing evidence that individuals' educational levels are correlated with their health (Lefcowitz 1973; Richardson, 1972). While a number of researchers have found that family income is not directly correlated with health, the capacity of an individual to obtain an education, live in a healthful area, and purchase other services contribute to a high quality of life and health. Occupations have an important

Table 1-1 Chronic Conditions and Limitation of Major Activity, by Occupation of Currently Employed Persons over 44 Years of Age

Occupation	Of all occupations percent with chronic conditions	Of all with 1+ chronic conditions percent with limitation of major activity
Professional, technical	68	7
clerical	68	9
Operative	66	13
Craftsmen and Foremen	67	14
Sales	72	15
Managers, officials proprietors (nonfarm)	69	15
Service, except private household	69	15
Laborers, except farm and mine	69	24
Private household	77	24
Farm laborers and foremen	72	33
Farmers and farm managers	77	33

Source: "Limitation of Activity and Mobility Due to Chronic Conditions," *Vital and Health Statistics,* PHS Pub. No. 1000, Series 10, No. 45, pp. 48–49, Public Health Service, Washington, D.C., 1968.

relationship to health, as shown in Table 1-1. For example, the table indicates that 33 percent of farmers over 44 years of age have work-limiting chronic conditions as compared with only 7 percent of professional workers.

Behavior

Personal behavior and habits such as smoking, drinking, dangerous driving, over-eating, abuse of drugs, neglect of personal hygiene, and delay in seeking medical care are major influences on health and well-being. The physiological responses to personal emotions such as a face flushed with anger or loss of energy and desire due to sadness have been observed by all of us. The effect of personal behavior on an individual's health reflects the way in which he or she reacts to environmental, hereditary, and health care services influences.

Heredity

Heredity or genetic endowment, that is, the intrinsic nature of the individual, is recognized as having a primary influence on susceptibility to disease as well as inheritance of disease. Genetic endowment interacts with both environmental and behavioral factors. Cultural considerations such as ethnic or racial proclivities limit the choice of marital partners and so influence the genetic potential of offspring and their susceptibility to certain diseases. An example would be sickle cell anemia, which occurs almost exclusively among blacks. However, this disease can be diagnosed and treated through personal behavior and health care services. Problems arising from genetic factors can be controlled through screening, increasingly through genetic counseling, and potentially through genetic engineering.

Health Care Services

Health care services include the community health services delivered by environmental and public health agencies. These services can intervene on environmental problems of pollution, occupational safety, housing conditions, etc. Health promotion delivered by public and personal health services is another major input to health. Health promotion activities are directed at behaviors such as exercise, rest, attitudes, and good nutrition. For example, the results of the widely recognized Framingham, Massachusetts studies, among others, have shown a positive relationship between physical inactivity and the risk of heart disease (National Heart Institute, 1966). Scrimshaw (1974) and others have reported on the importance of nutrition on health and on the outcomes of contracted disease.

The prevention of disease includes health screening and early diagnosis, and good personal habits. For example, smoking has been shown to increase the risk of death from cancer, bronchitis, and chronic heart disease. The cancer of the lung death rate for persons smoking 21 to 30 cigarettes a day was found to be about 17 times greater than for those who never smoked.

Cure or diagnosis and treatment factors, i.e., physician and hospital services, receive primary attention when health is studied. Of the $104 billion expended for health care in 1974 over $99 billion went for personal health services and supplies, primarily for hospital and physicians' services. The balance—only $4.8 billion or less than 5 percent—was spent on public health services and research (Social Security Administration, 1974). A large part of the $99 billion was spent to correct the problems caused by demographic, behavioral, physical, and genetic factors, and health promotion and prevention deficiencies. Medical and hospital services are usually crisis care, sometimes referred to as "heroic medicine" or "too late medicine"; they are concerned with illness, not health. This is partly due to health insurance that encourages crisis care, and the lack of promotion and prevention services; it is also due to personal attitudes—people respond only when they have to. Moreover, as Scrimshaw (1974) notes, "No matter what is done most patients get well most of the time. Therefore, anything done in the name of health [cure] will be successful most of the time. This includes prayer, incantations, copper bracelets, manipulations of joints, special foods, prescription drugs, anything at all!"

Rehabilitation or restorative services designed to return patients to their maximum state of health are being provided through hospitals, extended care facilities, and rehabilitation centers. Custodial care delivered by institutions and home health services also provide inputs to health.

To complete the picture of health inputs it is important to note that individuals' health is also affected by environmental factors such as their employment, housing, etc. It is also important to point out that we are not suggesting there is always a cause and effect relationship between inputs and health. Although there is good evidence of correlation, because the inputs are intricately interwoven it is difficult in most cases to determine the relative influence of each factor.

In summary, we want to stress that although this book, like the health care system in the United States, focuses on diagnosis and treatment services, many other important factors affect health in addition to hospital and physician services. A dramatic example of this was given when Jack Gieger, M.D., then chairman of Preventive Medicine at Tufts University, opened a modern neighborhood health center in the poverty-stricken community of Mound Bayou, Mississippi, in the late 1960s. For the first time, modern medicine was brought to the area. However, it was not the modern medical miracles that improved health in the community, but the effects of improved diets, housing, jobs, education, and other nonmedical factors. Initially, physicians treated infants for pneumonia or diarrhea, but found that they would quickly return to the health center. The doctors discovered that their most effective prescriptions were for food, improved housing, education, and so forth, rather than for medicine. The People's Republic of China has also demonstrated the effectiveness of concentrating on nonmedical factors to improve health (Challenor, 1975; Horn, 1969; Quinn, 1972; Sidel, 1972).

Increasingly, questions are being raised regarding the emphasis on treatment services in the United States. Winkelstein et al. (1970) suggest that ". . . medical care is largely unrelated to health status of the population . . . that ecology is the primary determinant of the health status . . . ." Lewis Thomas (1972), former Dean of Yale School of Medicine and currently President of Memorial Sloan Kettering Cancer Center suggests not only that our medical services are extremely costly, but also that they are not significantly improving the health of our citizens. (He argues for more basic research to develop immunizations and chemotherapy that can prevent or alter disease.) Fuchs (1974) and many others suggest that since the introduction and use of antibiotics between the 1930s and 1950s there has been little advance in medical care that has influenced the health of populations. White (1973) in his article on "Life and Death and Medicine" notes the statistical ambiguity at the root of the problem of trying to establish priorities for the allocation of health care resources in the United States. In Figure 1-2 he ranks 12 principal disease categories (as defined by the World Health Organization) according to three different measures of ill health. The three measures, all of which are expressed in terms of the number of people affected per year in the United States, are limitations of activity, hospital admissions, and estimated deaths. The lack of correlation between the respective rank orders is evident.

Who Has Responsibility for Delivering Health Services?

The responsibility for delivering health services in the total health spectrum or health industry has been fragmented among environmental, public, and personal health groups. Other services that relate to health but are outside the health service

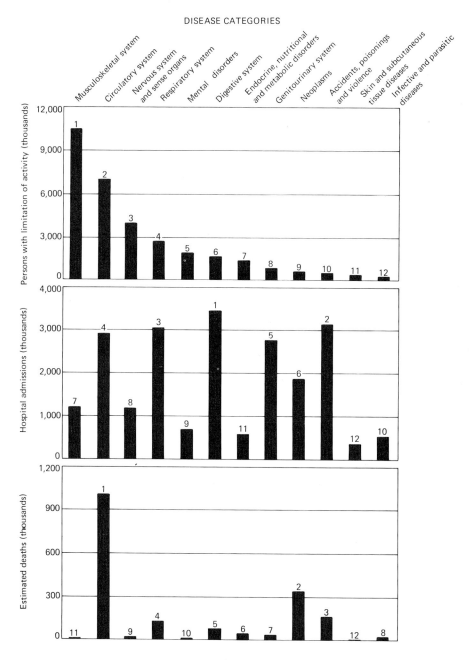

Figure 1-2 Relationships of disease categories with persons with limitation of
activities, hospital admissions, and deaths. (*Source:* Kerr L. White, "Life and
Death and Medicine," *Scientific American,* vol. 229, no. 3, p. 24, Sept. 1973.
The data on which the illustration is based are for 1971, the latest year for
which usable figures for the 12 WHO categories were available from the U.S.
National Center for Health Statistics in Bethesda, Md.)

system are social services and educational systems. There have been attempts to integrate these delivery systems, for example, in the Department of Health, Education and Welfare at the governmental level, but without much demonstrable success. *Public health* has traditionally been the responsibility of the government in the United States, *personal health* the responsibility of the individual and of practicing physicians, and almost everyone has at least a piece of the responsibility for *environmental health.*

Public health services are concerned with populations and have traditionally included:

Communicable (infectious) disease control
Sanitation
Maternal and child health
Public health nursing
Public health education
Vital statistics

These programs have been administered through state, county, and local health districts.

Increasingly, public health services provided by government go beyond the basic six services listed above. They now include programs and activities for:

Health planning and policy determination
Health maintenance
Continuous assessment of community ecology and resources
Reduction of health hazards
Research

Environmental health programs relate to public health and are carried out through a number of governmental and private organizations. They include more than public health services, and frequently there is overlap and conflict among public health agencies, industry, labor, conservation, and other governmental and private agencies. This has handicapped the development of effective and efficient programs. Environmental health programs include the following:

Water supply and pollution control
Solid waste disposal
Insect and rodent control
Milk and food sanitation
Air pollution control
Noise pollution control
Control of radiological hazards
Housing and land use
Occupational health

Personal health care is usually provided by private physicians, hospitals, nursing homes, and so forth. As suggested in Figure 1-1, it can be classified as: (1) promotion of health, (2) prevention of accidents and disease (both of which overlap with public health), (3) cure or diagnostic and treatment services, and (4) rehabilitation or restorative care and custodial care. Personal health care systems will be considered in some depth in the rest of this chapter and in the next, for it is in this area of responsibility that hospitals function.

Promotion of Health[1]   Promotion of health is usually considered the responsibility of the individual. It includes such factors as diet, exercise, and rest. In most cases information and prescriptions regarding these important aspects of health are provided by the individual's cultural environment, family, and schools, and through the mass media. Management is usually by the individual. Pediatricians concerned with well-baby care and dentists are among the few providers of personal health service that appear actively concerned with the promotion of health. Others who are concerned with the promotion of health are usually outside the health system; they include physical and mental health educators. One would expect that employers would be more concerned, and indeed, they may be the locus for health promotion efforts in the future.

It is also apparent that improved health is an insufficient incentive for many individuals to adopt good personal health practices. As a society we are concerned about placing incentives on members of the health team, but do little to place incentives on the individual. In the important area of promoting health, health insurance companies and other funding agents could insist that the health potential of every individual be professionally assessed, a proper promotional program of exercise, rest, diet, and personal habits prescribed, and goals established. Those who did not follow prescriptions or preferred to continue habits such as smoking would be required to pay higher prepaid or indemnity health care premiums. Similar procedures are followed for life and automobile insurance. Incentives could also be established to encourage individual health education in preventive and treatment methods. We need to find ways for the health team, including the individual consumer, to work together more effectively.

There has been little professional success in defining an optimum state of health, let alone professional prescriptions on how individuals might best achieve their maximum potential. One can speculate, however, that such efforts might have at least as important an influence on an individual's health as the kind of medical treatment services he receives. Moreover it is conceivable that more emphasis on the promotion of health would result in significant improvement in the joys of living

---

[1] A draft paper for the National Conference on Preventive Medicine in Washington, D.C., June 1975 takes a much broader view of health promotion. It states that the term *health promotion* applies to a set of policies adopted by government at various levels and other public and private institutions and agencies, and designed to promote individual, community, and national health by various means or strategies. These include research, education for the health professions, public health, environmental protection, occupational health, consumer health education, and the diagnosis and treatment of disease. According to this definition, individual consumer health education is only one of the various strategies aimed at health promotion. (*Source:* Anne R. Somers, Associate Professor, Department of Community Medicine, College of Medicine and Dentistry of New Jersey–Rutgers Medical School and Chairman, Task Force on Consumer Health Education, National Conference on Preventive Medicine, personal communication, February 27, 1975.)

and in individual and national productivity (Hoke, 1968). A hopeful sign is that healthful behavior itself tends to promote more healthful behavior.

Prevention Cooperation between professional health services and the individual for the prevention and early detection of disease is more common than for promotional health purposes. All diagnostic and therapeutic activity has a preventive component in that it seeks to forestall or prevent further deterioration of an individual's health. Here again, the individual has a responsibility to be alert to hazards and to emotional and physiological changes, and to seek professional assistance.

Early detection of disease through mass screening services among higher-risk populations is another component of preventive medicine. It is favored by some and may have potential for greater application. However, others question this approach from an economic standpoint noting that the cost of detecting pathology through multiphasic health screening units is high, particularly when it is considered that most individuals with pathology detect changes in themselves (Felch, 1973; Forst, 1972). However, other studies have shown that selective screening could save both lives and dollars (Collen, 1970).

Prevention of disease by controlling personal habits, e.g., refraining from smoking, is usually an individual matter.

Primary prevention is a direct and specific service designed to protect against a specific disease, and its prototype is immunization, for example, against polio or tetanus. Leavell and Clark (1965) also include health promotion as a part of primary prevention. Early disease detection is considered to be secondary prevention. Health screening by multiphasic clinics or an annual physical examination, and surveillance of individuals with a suspected proclivity toward certain diseases all fall into this category. Rehabilitation is considered tertiary prevention by Leavell and Clark (1965).

Cure Services Cure, i.e., diagnoses and treatment services, can be categorized as ambulatory outpatient care or inpatient hospital care. Outpatient services are usually provided in physicians' offices or clinics, although hospitals increasingly provide them. Specialized diagnostic and treatment services have also attracted ambulatory patients such as alcoholics and drug abusers to hospitals. Inpatient services are usually provided by hospitals. Home care services offer an alternative that has a potential for more development among hospitals.

Treatment services are also categorized as primary, secondary, and tertiary care (White, 1973; Hansen, 1970). Primary care can be defined as the site of entry into the health system and coordination through it. It is usually obtained through the family physician who may be a family or general practitioner, internist, pediatrician, or general surgeon. Primary care services are usually provided on an ambulatory or office visit basis. Secondary care services are consultant services that are intermediate in generality. The services of a classically educated internist or general surgeon would fit in this category.[2] Tertiary care refers to subspecialty or categorical referral services provided in a regional medical center.

---

[2]This is but one of the many examples of the difficulty in classifying the health services delivery systems. In this case a single physician could fit into all three categories at various times.

Mental health ambulatory treatment services such as those offered by community mental health centers are frequently organized quite independently of physical health services. Mental health inpatient services are increasingly organized within community hospitals. Dental health is another important but frequently segregated component of health care.

Restorative and Long-Term or Custodial Care Services Restorative services are organized in a variety of institutions such as hospitals, convalescent centers, group practice clinics, separate rehabilitation centers, and public agencies. Convalescent long-term, extended custodial care services are provided primarily by private and governmental institutions. In recent years increasing numbers of hospitals established long-term care units.

Each of the above components of personal health services involves a wide variety of independent individuals and governmental, proprietary, voluntary, and church institutions. The financing of such services is just as diverse. Because of the diversity in health service delivery in the United States, some refer to it as a nonsystem. Certainly it is a pluralistic one. Traditionally, it has been fragmented within and between environmental, public health, and personal health delivery services. Frequently there has been considerable overlap and duplication as well as substantial gaps in services. In recent years however, efforts have been made to provide comprehensive services in a continuum through neighborhood health centers, health maintenance organizations (see Chapter 2), and regionalization of health services (see Chapter 15).

CONCLUSIONS

Although physician and hospital services have been and still are by far the largest, most expensive, and most glamorous component of the health industry, the medical care component represents only one of many input factors. Considerably more emphasis should be placed on other components. Hospitals could have a much larger role in improving the health of the population. Indeed, we suggest that with increasingly scarce resources, more centralized planning and funding, and the application of cost-benefit analytical techniques, there will be a reordering of priorities away from treatment services and toward environmental, promotion, and preventive health services. A number of hospitals are beginning to expand their roles by meeting the broad health needs of the community through outreach services such as home care, meals on wheels, and health education services. More can be done if hospitals will take the leadership in helping to identify community health needs, in seeing that these needs are met, and in serving as a catalyst for social, environmental, public, and medical health services. We will expand on some of these opportunities for hospitals to be true centers of the health system in future chapters, and suggest that a broader community role will necessitate reordering objectives away from institutional expectations and toward community expectations.

In the next chapter we examine the personal health delivery components of health care services, the objectives of personal delivery services, alternative models of delivery, and the role of the hospital within these models; we also assess the models in relation to delivery objectives.

REFERENCES

Anderson, James G.: "Demographic Factors Affecting Health Services Utilization: A Causal Model," *Medical Care,* vol. 11, no. 2, pp. 104–120, March-April, 1973.

Blum, Henrik L.: *Planning for Health: Development and Application of Social Change Theory,* Human Sciences Press, New York, 1974.

Challenor, Bernard: "Health and Economics Development: the Example of China and Cuba," *Medical Care,* vol. 13, no. 1, pp. 79–84, Jan. 1975.

Collen, Morris, Robert Feldman, Abraham Siegelaub, and Derek Crawford: "Dollar Cost per Positive Test for Automated Multiphasic Screening," *New England Journal of Medicine,* vol. 283, no. 9, pp. 459–463, Aug. 27, 1970.

DHEW: *Forward Plan for Health,* U.S. Department of Health, Education and Welfare, 1975.

Felch, William: "Does Preventive Medicine Really Work?" *Prism,* October 1973, pp. 26 ff.

Forst, B.E.: *An Economic Analysis of Periodic Health Examination Programs,* Institute of Naval Studies, Arlington, Va., AD-735-949.

Fuchs, Victor (Professor of Economics and Community Medicine, Mount Sinai School of Medicine of the City University of New York): seminar presentation, University of Wisconsin, July 22, 1974.

Graham, Saxon and Leo G. Reeder: "Social Factors in Chronic Diseases," in Howard Freeman, Sol Levine and Leo G. Reeder (eds.), *Handbook of Medical Sociology,* 2d ed., Prentice-Hall. Englewood Cliffs, N.J. 1972, pp. 63–107.

Haggerty, Robert J.: "The Boundaries of Health Care," *The Pharos of Alpha Omega Alpha,* vol. 35, no. 3, pp. 106–111, July 1972.

Hansen, Marc: "An Educational Program for Primary Care," *Journal of Medical Education,* vol. 45, pp. 1001–1006, Dec. 1970.

Hoke, Bob: "Promotive Medicine and the Phenomenon of Health," *Archives of Environmental Health,* vol. 16, pp. 269–78, Feb. 1968.

Horn, J.S.: *Away with all Pests, an English Surgeon in the People's Republic of China, 1954-1969,* Monthly Review Press, New York, 1969.

Leavell, H.R. and E.G. Clark: *Preventive Medicine for the Doctor in His Community,* 3d ed., McGraw-Hill, New York, 1965.

Lefcowitz, Myron L.: "Poverty and Health: A Re-Examination," *Inquiry,* vol. 10, no. 1, pp. 3–13, Mar. 1973.

National Heart Institute: U.S. Public Health Service Bulletin No. 1515, Washington, D.C., 1966.

Quinn, Joseph R. (ed.): *Medicine and Public Health in the People's Republic of China,* DHEW Publication no. 72-67, National Institutes of Health, June 1972.

Richardson, William: *Ambulatory Use of Physicians' Services in Response to Illness Episodes in a Low-Income Neighborhood,* Center for Health Administration Studies, University of Chicago, 1972.

Scrimshaw, Nevin: "Myths and Realities in International Health Planning," *American Journal of Public Health,* vol. 64, no. 8, pp. 792–797, Aug. 1974.

Sidel, Victor W.: "Some Observations on Health Services in the People's Republic of China," *International Journal of Health Services,* vol. 2, no. 3, pp. 385–393, 1972.

Social Security Administration: *Research and Statistics Note,* DHEW, Publication no. SSA 74-11701, Nov. 29, 1974.

Thomas, Lewis: "Guessing and Knowing: Reflections on the Science and Technology of Medicine," *Saturday Review,* Dec. 23, 1972, pp. 52–57.

White, Kerr L.: "Life and Death and Medicine," *Scientific American,* vol. 229, no. 3, pp. 23–33, Sept. 1973.

Winkelstein, Warran and Fern E. French: "The Role of Ecology in the Design of a Health Care System," *California Medicine,* vol. 113, no. 5, pp. 7-12, Nov. 1970.

Wisconsin Governor's Health Planning and Policy Task Force: Final Report, Nov. 1972, Wisconsin Department of Administration, 1 West Wilson Street, Madison, Wis., 1972.

Chapter 2

Personal Health Care Delivery Models

Anne Somers (1971), the particularly perceptive author of a number of publications related to hospitals, and others have described the transition of the hospital from a workshop for physicians to a center for the delivery of personal health services. However, it is important to remind readers that the hospital is not the only component in the delivery of personal health services; nor is it always the professional center of the health care world. There are a number of different organizational models for the delivery of personal health service in the United States, and considerable national debate is taking place regarding the strengths and weaknesses of each. To put these models in an evaluative perspective, we suggest desirable objectives for delivery services, and then assess the models against these objectives. It is important to note that comments on the strengths and weaknesses of each represent the authors' opinions, which are often but not always supported by references or data.

OBJECTIVES FOR ORGANIZING PERSONAL HEALTH CARE

Organizational arrangements for personal delivery services should be designed to function within the overall objectives for the health spectrum described in Chapter 1. Donabedian (1973, pp. 39-43) suggests that objectives for delivery of health services can be defined from several perspectives. A *client-oriented* perspective would include: (1) access to service; (b) use of service; (c) quality of care; (d) maintenance of direct autonomy and dignity; (e) responsiveness to client needs, wishes, and convenience; and (f) freedom of choice. A *provider-oriented* perspective (i.e., that of physicians, hospitals, nurses, etc.) would include: (a) freedom of professional judgment and activities; (b) maintenance of professional proficiency and quality of care; (c) adequate compensation; (d) control over conditions and term of practice; and (e) maintenance of professional norms. *Organization-oriented* objectives would include: (a) cost control; (b) control of quality; (c) efficiency; (d) ability to attract clients; (e) ability to recruit employees and staff; and (f) mobilization of community support. Other objectives that he calls *collectively-oriented* include: (a) proper allocation of resources among competing needs; (b) nonpartisanship; (c) political representation; (d) representation of interests affected by the organization; and (e) coordination with other agencies.

It is clear that the objectives for the delivery of health services are not as self-evident as one might expect, and a number of scholars have devoted considerable effort to the issues involved.[1] Nevertheless, in order to evaluate the goals of the various models for delivery of health services in a systematic way, we suggest seven major objectives:

1 *High-quality technical services* Knowledge related to science has advanced and with it have come increasingly complex skills and technology. The full scope of such knowledge and skills should be available through comprehensive services in a continuum to meet the requirements of individuals. It is important to note that quality (which is very difficult to measure), is not an ideal measure of effectiveness, but this represents the state of the art and the best we have to go on.

2 *Accessibility and availability of comprehensive services* Individuals should have access to a broad scope of required services through adequate transportation, communication, and financial mechanisms. Services should be readily available when required. Individuals and health team members should know when and how to obtain required services or information. The barriers created by fear, discrimination, or perceived impersonality of service should be minimized.

3 *Efficiency*[2] Organization of personal health services should promote maximum effectiveness while conserving limited national resources.

4 *Satisfaction of individuals* Beyond providing them with technical quality, services should take account of the needs of individuals. Such needs would include self-respect, comfort, and convenience.

5 *Efficiency to individuals* The individual should obtain maximum effectiveness from services while conserving his or her limited resources of funds and time. This is a difficult objective to measure because the relationship of costs to both the quality and the value of service eludes satisfactory measurement. It is also important to note that what may be efficient for the individual may be less so for the system. For example,

---

[1] For example, see "Medical Cure and Medical Care," *Milbank Memorial Fund Quarterly,* vol. L, no. 4, part 2, Oct. 1972.

[2] The World Health Organization defines efficiency as the effects or end results achieved in relation to the effort expended in terms of money, resources and time (WHO, 1971).

home kidney dialysis is efficient for the individual who needs it, but from the point of view of allocating national resources to health, it may be neither as efficient nor as effective as other services.

6 *Satisfaction of health professionals* Expectations of members of the health team should be served. Satisfaction relates to the distribution and the quality of service in addition to being a desired objective in itself.

7 *Accountability* Health professionals and institutions should be accountable to appropriate bodies to ensure that services are effectively directed toward achieving appropriate goals.

Analysis of the objectives cited above will show that some are in conflict with others; therefore, priorities among objectives should be established. However, since priorities vary according to the changing health needs of society as well as with local situations, it is impossible to arrive at a universal listing of priorities that would be applicable to all situations and time periods.

BASIC MODELS OF CURRENT ORGANIZATIONAL ARRANGEMENTS

Figure 2-1 lists several existing alternative organization models for delivering personal health services. It relates them to components of comprehensive health

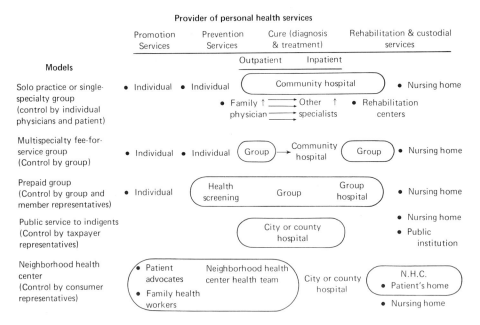

Note: The circled provider components suggest the unifying core for comprehensive services in a continuum. In the case of the solo or single-specialty practice model the individual physician and patient have been the core, but increasingly it is the hospital. See discussions in the text.

Figure 2-1 Models for delivering personal health services related to components of comprehensive service in a continuum.

services in a continuum—promotion of health, prevention of disease, treatment, and restorative and custodial services. You will note we have not included community (i.e., environmental and public health) services. They will be referred to in later chapters. Figure 2-1 also identifies those who have primary control in these models, e.g., individual physicians and patients, and group practices.

There are, of course, variations on each of these models, as well as other models such as free clinics sponsored by neighborhood groups; however, the vast majority of citizens in the United States receive their personal health services through one of these general models or some combination of them.

Solo Practice

Although increasing numbers of physicians are going into group practice, solo practice (i.e., the physician who practices alone or with others, but does not pool his income or expenses) is still predominant. It was estimated that in 1968 only 7 percent of nationwide visits to physicians were made by ambulatory patients to all group offices (a formal organization of three or more physicians) and only 3 percent to prepaid group practices (McNamara and Todd, 1970).

In many respects solo practice is a misnomer today. Much of a physician's practice centers around the hospital where he practices in association with other health professionals. Moreover, the autonomy of the individual practitioner in the hospital has diminished significantly, for he is subjected to formal review of the quality of his work by other physicians on the medical staff (peer review). He is also subjected to scrutiny by lay groups such as the hospital governing board and administrative staff. Many solo practitioners provide their outpatient services in a professional building where they are in physical association with other physicians; frequently the building is adjacent to a hospital.

Figure 2-1 suggests that the community hospital serves as the unifying core for solo and single-specialty group practice. Most hospitals provide outpatient diagnostic and treatment services, and rehabilitation services, and some even provide long-term care, in addition to traditional inpatient acute services. Increasing numbers of community hospitals also provide dental and mental health treatment services.

In evaluating solo practice against the organizational objectives presented earlier, we propose the following:

The technical quality of solo practitioners may vary more than that of physicians practicing in groups. Except for peer review in hospitals and through Professional Standards Review Organizations (PSROs) (see Chapter 10), the care rendered by solo practitioners is less subject to the scrutiny of other physicians. The quality not only varies with regard to the training of the physicians but also concerns how willing they are to refer patients, and to whom they are referred. Patients are usually unable to evaluate technical competency. However, the solo practitioner as family physician (groups can also have family physicians) has a better opportunity to understand and be responsive to the whole person and his family.

Accessibility to comprehensive services is potentially greater under solo practice systems if these are in urban areas with a broad range of specialists. Physicians in multispecialty groups are under some pressure to keep referrals within the group. Solo practice can provide a broader geographic availability of physicians. However, with the increase in knowledge and specialization, solo practitioners are beginning to centralize their offices. The fee-for-service mechanism under which patients pay physicians for each service rendered promote good physician-patient relationships, but it also presents a barrier to seeking services at an early stage. Solo practitioner services are usually less available than those of groups in which physicians share services more extensively. However, hospitals provide emergency services for solo practitioners, and other physicians are usually designated to cover for them when they are unavailable.

The efficiency of various forms of delivering personal health services has received relatively little study. Contrary to most expectations, and regardless of the promotion given to group practice, solo practice may be more economical than group practice in most urban settings. Bailey (1970) found in his studies that solo practitioner internists reported significantly higher productivity on a monthly output basis than internists in groups. Yankauer (1970) found higher productivity and more patient care task delegation to allied health workers among solo practice pediatricians than among pediatricians in larger groups. On the other hand, after reviewing a number of studies, Donabedian (1973) suggests that solo practice physicians are less productive. However, he, like others who share his view, includes ancillary services such as laboratory and x-ray in the productivity of group practice physicians. Solo practitioners usually refer their ancillary services to hospitals, and outpatient diagnostic and treatment services performed in hospitals for solo practitioners usually result in economies of scale over similar services performed in group facilities, unless the groups are very large.

Satisfaction to individuals will be influenced by many variables. Moreover, studies comparing satisfaction among various forms of practice are limited. In a New York study, Freidson (1961) concluded that patients generally believed that solo practitioners took more personal interest in them and found care to be more convenient than in group practice. In solo practice physicians are more directly dependent on the satisfaction of their patients; consequently, it is logical to assume they will be more responsive to patients' expectations. Becker (1974) and Becker and Maiman (1975) found that the practice of patients seeing the same physician was correlated with satisfaction of patients, appointments kept, compliance with physician recommendations, and other factors beneficial to effective and efficient care.

Efficiency to individuals must be considered in relation to the quality of service, as is true of the other objectives listed here. Nevertheless, in his study of internists, Bailey (1970) found physician fees per hour and per visit to be lower for solo practitioners than for practitioners in smaller-sized groups. Solo practitioners, who do not benefit financially from ancillary services such as laboratory and x-ray services, have less incentive to order such services. However, busy individual practitioners may also have less incentive to keep patients out of the hospital. Hospitalizing patients helps to increase the productivity of physicians in addition to minimizing the risks to the patients.

Satisfaction to physicians will probably be affected more by personal characteristics than by organization models. The solo practitioner generally has more independence, which is an important professional expectation. However, he probably has less independence in scheduling time for recreation and professional study.[3] Mechanic (1974), in his study of general practitioners and pediatricians in solo, fee-for-service group, and prepaid group settings, found more dissatisfaction among pediatricians in solo practice settings, while more general practitioners were dissatisfied in prepaid group settings (see Table 2-1).

The accountability of the solo practitioner to peers and consumer groups is lower than that of physicians in group practice, although with the development of PSROs the accountability of the solo practitioner is increasing. The solo practitioner is directly accountable to the individual patient, but the individual is seldom able to evalute anything beyond his or her personal relations with the physician.

Solo practice as a means of meeting personal health demands is under scrutiny at present. Physicians and medical students do not appear to favor it (Freidson, 1972). Changes in the organization of physician's practices could either stimulate or retard the development of hospitals as centers of health delivery services. These implications are discussed at the end of this chapter.

Single-Specialty Group Practice

Single-specialty group practice, i.e., physicians in the same specialty, e.g., pediatrics or orthopedic surgery, who pool their expenses, income, and offices, is the fastest growing model of physicians' organization. In 1959, single-specialty groups represented about 25 percent of all groups; by 1969, this increased to nearly 53 percent (McNamara and Todd, 1970). The average size of the single-specialty group is 3.4 physicians.

The single-specialty group model resembles the solo practice model more than the multispecialty group model in its impact on delivery systems and the hospital. Differences between solo practice and the single-specialty group as they relate to the objectives presented earlier are noted on the following page.

Table 2-1 Self-rating of Satisfaction among General Practitioners and Pediatricians in Solo Practice and Group Settings

Physicians' overall self-rating	Solo Practitioners		Fee-for-service group		Prepaid group	
	G.P.s (N=606)	Peds. (N=136)	G.P.s (N=113)	Peds. (N=43)	G.P.s (N=108)	Peds. (N=154)
Very satisfied	52%	39%	56%	47%	42%	44%
Fairly satisfied	44	53	42	49	51	53
Not very satisfied/ dissatisfied	4	8	3	5	7	3

[3] It is usually assumed that the physician in group practice will spend more time in professional study. Peterson (1965) found no relationship between organization of practice and physician continuing education practices. Freidson (1964) also found that over half the physicians in multispecialty groups received their intellectual stimulation outside the group.

Quality-control measures are likely to be higher in a group than in individual practice. Groups will attempt to recruit doctors of equal or better skills. Because they frequently share patients, physicians are not likely to tolerate less than continuing high-quality service. Moreover, the mistakes and poor practices of a particular physician are easily exposed to a partner.

Physicians in single-specialty groups may have somewhat less independence than solo practitioners. However, they can provide better coverage for their patients, they are able to schedule their time better, and they have more security and professional stimulation through their colleagues in practice. They are also able to share the burdens and rewards of certain facilities and services.

The group physician may be somewhat less responsive to the expectations of each individual patient and have less personal knowledge of him and his family. Physicians in single-specialty groups tend to have less of a family practice and more of a referral practice. At times the patients of single-specialty groups become their own diagnosticians by choosing which group of physicians to call for a certain complaint; at times they may also have to be the arbiter when physicians in different specialties make conflicting recommendations.

Single-specialty groups, like solo practitioners, tend to center around the hospital for ancillary services and referrals to other specialists. The hospital therefore serves as a unifying core for comprehensive services.

Multispecialty Fee-for-Service Group Practice

The Mayo Clinic in Rochester, Minnesota, is a widely known example of a multispecialty fee-for-service group. The Mayo Clinic has hundreds of physicians; however, the average size of multispecialty groups is about 10 physicians. About 38 percent of all groups are multispecialty,[4] and about 60 percent, or over 24,000, of the 40,000 physicians in groups in the nation are in multispecialty groups.

Figure 2-1 showed the group as the unifying core in the multispecialty group model. In this model the hospital is limited mainly to providing inpatient services. Multispecialty fee-for-service group practice is evaluated below in relation to our objectives for delivery systems:

High-quality technical services are fostered by multispecialty group practice because it represents a physician team approach. Increased association and communication among specialists make a broader perspective of knowledge available to patients. Solo and single-specialty group physicians also have this advantage through their hospital associations, but usually to a more limited extent.

Accessibility to comprehensive specialty services is a distinct advantage of multispecialty groups; it explains why they tend to be developed in medium-sized communities more frequently than in larger cities. A group can provide professional attractions that would not otherwise be available in smaller communities. However, incentives to keep referrals within the group may prevent a patient from gaining

[4] General-practice groups are not considered in this section. They represented 9 percent of all group practice.

access to the most competent physician in a specific field. Also, solo practitioners frequently prefer not to refer patients to group specialists for fear they may lose the patient. Availability of services in groups is fostered by multiple coverage in a variety of specialties. Multiple coverage aids the scheduling and evening of loads resulting in more prompt appointments and emergency service.

Efficiency through economies of scale is an often-stated benefit of multispecialty groups, and indeed this may exist in very large groups and groups directly associated with hospitals.[5] However, most studies that lend support to this view include laboratory, x-ray, and other ancillary services in physician productivity. When physicians' services are considered alone as in Bailey's and Yankauer's studies, and group ancillary services are compared with hospitals, it becomes questionable whether groups are a more economic model. Newhouse (1971) suggests productivity is lower in groups unless financial incentives are built into methods of distributing group income.

Satisfaction to the physicians in multispecialty groups is fostered by professional to convenience of referrals and the existence of ancillary services in one location. Groups may be less responsive to patients' expectations than solo practitioners.

Efficiency to individuals served by multispecialty groups in terms of costs to the patient is open to question. On the one hand, groups have more incentives to keep patients out of the hospital. For example, one widely known and highly competent California group performs most of its tonsillectomies on an outpatient basis in its clinic. On the other hand, ancillary services comprise a significant portion of group income so there are financial rewards as well as the possibility of aiding a diagnosis or uncovering unexpected pathology involved in ordering extensive ancillary services in groups.

Satisfaction to the physicians in multispecialty groups is fostered by professional stimulation from an interdisciplinary team, more free time for study and recreation without financial sacrifice (due to income from ancillary services), and greater ability to concentrate on their specialty. However, there are often serious conflicts among group physicians. Causes of conflict can be attributed to a variety of sources, among them the different approaches of specialties to treating an illness and, more importantly, problems with distribution of income. Well-established groups have been known to have serious problems in distributing income between the high-earning, low-cost surgical-specialty practice and the low-earning, high-cost but referring medical and pediatric practice.

Professional accountability in multispecialty groups can be accomplished formally or informally through frequent referrals and sharing coverage. Groups will seldom tolerate substandard practices. Groups, however, are not subjected to accrediting surveys and some have been known to permit physicians to perform services beyond their training to keep patient services within the group. For example, an internist and/or surgeon may read the group's x-rays because volume is not large enough to employ a radiologist and the group wishes to keep x-ray income for itself.

---

[5] Among the studies that suggest economies of scale in group practice are: Harris (1965), Roemer (1969), Yett (1967), Kovner (1968), Fein (1967), and Boan (1966).

Prepaid Multispecialty Group and Hospital Plan

The prepaid multispecialty group plan, shown as the prepaid group plan in Figure 2-1, is a health care financing plan tied to physician (and in this model also hospital) services. The Kaiser Health Plan is a well-known example of this type of plan and one that has been a model for the health maintenance organization (HMO), which has been widely promoted in recent years. The prepaid mechanism has also been applied to solo and single-specialty practices currently referred to as foundation plans or health maintenance plans patterned after the San Joaquin, California Foundation Plan (Harrington, 1970). The individual, or in most cases a group of individuals, such as a company employee group, pays a specified premium for designated health services. Providers of health services are reimbursed on a per capita basis rather than through a fee-for-service mechanism. Physicians and hospitals are therefore rewarded financially if they prevent or avoid costly services to patients. Under the traditional financing mechanism, physicians and hospitals receive more income when patients receive more service—just the opposite of prepaid plans.

Prepaid or HMO programs hold promise for combating rapidly rising health care costs, and therefore have been widely promoted by federal agencies and consumer groups such as cooperatives and labor unions.

Figure 2-1 shows the Kaiser-type plan with both the group and hospital serving as the unifying core for personal health services. The model comes close to providing truly comprehensive services in a continuum. A single patient record for all health services is an important advantage of this system (although an impersonal one as far as the patient is concerned) since services among specialties are coordinated. Control is by the group, which may be provider-dominated as in the Kaiser Plan, or consumer-dominated as in Group Health Associates of Puget Sound, Washington, which is influenced by those to whom the plan is sold.

Prepaid group plans are evaluated below in reference to objectives for personal health care delivery:

Technical quality in prepaid groups has most of the advantages and disadvantages found in other multispecialty groups. The single patient record also fosters better care. Some may say, however, that the incentives to minimize costly services could compromise quality. Studies of prepaid practice also report that consumers are more likely than those of fee-for-service practice to feel that practitioners are less responsive to their needs and seem less interested in them (Freidson, 1961; Donabedian, 1965).

Accessibility to comprehensive services is increased by removing the barrier of cost considerations to seeking service. However, prepaid group plan facilities are more widely dispersed than individual practitioners, and therefore currently inconvenient to some subscribers. Availability of services is improved if the group itself offers comprehensive services. Comprehensive services offered in a continuum from preventive to restorative services also promote availability.

Efficiency of the prepaid group and hospital model appears to be fostered through economies of scale and by minimizing duplications. This model also has incentives for efficiencies that are lacking in other models. A reduction in the use of expensive inpatient services of up to 40 percent is a widely publicized claim for prepaid plans. However, an initial review of such savings indicates that a 10 percent reduction is probably more accurate, though still a significant saving (Klarman, 1969). The prepaid mechanism also provides consumers with an opportunity to compare prices for personal health services. However, some individuals or groups with major health problems are not accepted for coverage by prepaid plans since they are heavy utilizers of services and could raise costs for the rest of the enrolled population.

Satisfaction to individuals appears to present a serious problem of prepaid plans. Studies show that many prepaid plan subscribers who have paid up health services go outside the plan for private services at additional personal expense (Bashur, 1967; Wolfman, 1961). Freidson (1961) found over 48 percent of Montefiore Health Insurance Plan (HIP) prepaid plan members used physician services outside the plan. In a review of studies on choice and utilization of prepaid group practice plans, Weinerman (1964) suggested "fee-for-service plans still attract a majority of workers in dual choice situations, especially when their benefits are broad in scope." He states in reference to those who select prepaid groups that "most significant is the repeated observation that enrollees respond primarily to the prospect of comprehensive benefits, and seem less concerned with the alternative of group versus solo practice." Roemer et al. (1972), however, found less dissatisfaction with prepaid group insurance programs than with commercial or provider (Blue Cross, etc.) programs. While consumers as a collective body may have a greater voice in prepaid plans, the individual has less direct control.

Efficiency to individuals may be greater in prepaid plans in terms of quality services at lowest cost. However, if a sufficient number of patients prefer to pay additionally for services outside the system, the end economies relative to money and time expended may be subject to question.

Satisfaction to the health professional is presumably comparable to that of physicians in other multispecialty practices. Mechanic (1974) found general practitioners to be less satisfied in prepaid groups, but pediatricians somewhat more satisfied. Close group and hospital relations reportedly results in better physician-hospital relations; however, this has not been tested to our knowledge. A physician in a prepaid program probably has even less independence than one in a nonprepaid plan multispecialty group due to greater consumer involvement in the former. Physician incomes appear to be generally comparable. Mechanic (1973) reports that general practitioners and pediatricians in prepaid group practices are more than three times as likely as nongroup fee-for-service physicians to indicate that 50 percent or more of their patients' visits are trivial or inappropriate. He suggests this reflects the attitude of the physicians toward their patient loads rather than the type of patients involved. The number of physicians reported to have quit the Kaiser or Group Health Cooperative plans does not appear to be high compared with the number leaving fee-for-service groups.

Accountability in prepaid plans is to consumer groups in addition to professionals as in other multispecialty groups.

Public Service to Indigents

The traditional public service to the indigent consumer model as provided by the large "charity" hospitals will not be reviewed. Control is usually by taxpayer representatives whose primary objectives are to hold down taxes. This model usually achieves the objectives listed in this chapter to a lesser degree than other models. For example, this model seldom provides for health promotion and preventive services (although some are establishing such services) even though consumers of these public hospitals are not as well prepared as consumers of private services to provide them for themselves. The large teaching outpatient clinics do not foster patient satisfaction.

Improvements are being made in these institutions and many do provide outstanding technical services to critically ill patients.

Neighborhood Health Center

The neighborhood health center model, funded primarily from federal sources, has been applied to services for the disadvantaged in inner city and rural locations. While such centers provide truly comprehensive ambulatory personal health care services to families, many have had to rely on the large public indigent care hospital for inpatient services, thereby interrupting comprehensive services in a continuum. The centers maximize a health team approach that includes neighborhood residents as family health workers and legal advisors as patient care advocates, as well as nurses, dentists, medical specialists, and other health workers. The promotion of personal health and environmental standards is a major goal. Individuals served by the center seldom have the education or the economic resources to carry out health promotion activities on their own. Neighborhood health centers have also addressed themselves to the broader environmental health care issues such as education, housing, jobs, and behavior.

The neighborhood health center concept is evaluated below in relation to our objectives:

Technical quality is served quite effectively by attracting well-qualified interdisciplinary health team members to areas that have previously been almost without personal medical services. Continuity of service is broken in some of the centers where unconnected hospitals are used for inpatient services and emergency services when the center is closed.

Accessibility to comprehensive care is increased by locating centers in the neighborhoods served, following up on patients in their homes, and lowering financial barriers to patients through federal funding. Availability of appropriate services is aided by patient advocates and family health workers. Lack of inpatient and night emergency services in some centers is a handicap.

It is difficult to compare the efficiency of this model with other models. The programs are expensive, but cover broad activities to meet the almost overwhelming needs of the poor. Other attempts to bring the poor into the mainstream of health care services, for example, through Medicare and Medicaid, have not been as successful.

Satisfaction to the individual can be measured by the marked improvement this represents over no service at all or mass service in large, frequently inconvenient, hospital and medical school outpatient clinics. While consumers as a group are supposed to have ultimate control over the centers, it is unlikely that individuals have much control.

Professional satisfaction to health team members is probably great in terms of rewards inherent in meeting the needs of the society. The working hours in the centers are reportedly attractive to physicians, but the locations and lack of independence are not. Consumer control over the centers diminishes the independence of professionals such as physicians.

Ultimate control of the center is designed to be in the hands of consumer representatives but in reality seldom is. Additional controls are provided by multi-disciplinary peer review and critical patient advocates. Accountability is to both consumers and professionals as collectives, less directly to the individual.

CONCLUSIONS

A review of existing models for delivering health services in the United States shows that there are unique strengths and weaknesses in each. In terms of providing comprehensive services in a continuum, the neighborhood health center comes closest to offering community, promotion, prevention, cure, and rehabilitation services. Prepaid group HMO services also approach the goal of comprehensive services in a continuum. In other models, individuals take the primary responsibility for improving their environment and behavior, and obtaining health care services. This is not an unreasonable expectation for most middle- and upper-income families. We also conclude that no single model necessarily provides the highest quality or is necessarily the most efficient. Given the diverse needs and expectations of the nation one model could not be the best for everyone. Our pluralistic system has a great deal going for it. However, there is room for substantial improvement, and administrators, governing board members, and others in the hospital can influence the efficiency and effectiveness of health care services input to communities as well as the psycho-socio-somatic health of individuals.

Models for delivery of personal health services do affect the roles of hospitals. There is increasing concern for comprehensive services in a continuum, which implies the integration of community and personal health care services. There are good reasons for organizing these services around hospitals:

Hospitals can provide the broad scope of services, from promotion to custodial, which are required for comprehensive care. They could also influence some environmental health inputs.

Hospitals can provide economies of scale for the ancillary and administrative services required for health and medical care.

Peer review programs can be expanded from the hospital.

It saves time for the physician to be located within short walking distance to the hospital.

Hospitals are looked upon as health centers today.

Integration of services can provide for a single patient record and other benefits.

Too often questions concerning the organization of health services center upon who has control—consumers or providers—the physicians or the hospitals. This is not the point. Quality, accessibility and availability, efficiency, satisfaction of individuals, efficiency to individuals, satisfaction of health professionals, and accountability are the most important objectives. Moreover, the integration of health services requires an atmosphere of trust among those involved and/or special incentives or regulations. This is discussed further in later chapters.

REFERENCES

Bashur, Rashid L., et al.: "Consumer Satisfaction with Group Practice, the CHA Case," *American Journal of Public Health,* vol. 57, no. 11, p. 1994, Nov. 1967.

Bailey, Richard M.: "A Comparison of Internists in Solo and Fee-for-Service Group Practice in San Francisco Bay Area," *Bulletin New York Academy of Medicine,* Nov. 1968; and "Philosophy, Faith, Fact, and Fiction in the Production of Medical Services," *Inquiry,* vol. 3, no. 1, 1970.

Becker, Marshall (Associate Professor, The Johns Hopkins University, Baltimore): Presentation at University of Wisconsin Seminar Dec. 2, 1974.

Becker, Marshall and Lois Maiman: "Sociobehavioral Determinants of Compliance with Health and Medical Care Recommendations," *Medical Care,* vol. 13, no. 1, pp. 10-24, Jan. 1975.

Boan, J.A.: *Group Practice,* Royal Commission on Health Services, Queens Printer, 1966, pp. 5 and 27.

Donabedian, Avedis: "A Review of Some Experiences with Prepaid Group Practice," *Bureau of Health Economics Research,* no. 12, School of Public Health, University of Michigan, Ann Arbor, 1965.

Donabedian, Avedis: *Aspects of Medical Care Administration,* Harvard University Press, Cambridge, Mass., 1973.

Fein, Rashi: *The Doctor Shortage: An Economic Diagnosis,* Brookings Institution, Washington, D.C., 1967, pp. 90-130.

Freidson, Eliot: *Patients' Views of Medical Practice,* Russell Sage Foundation, New York, 1961.

Freidson, Eliot: "Physicians in Large Medical Groups," *Journal of Chronic Diseases,* vol. 17, pp. 827-836, 1964.

Harrington, Donald C.: "System of Medical Administration and Health Care Delivery Based on Individual Practice System," Paper delivered at 1970 National Health Forum, Washington, D.C. National Health Council, New York.

Harris, Seymour, *Economics of American Medicine,* Macmillan, New York, 1965.

Klarman, Herbert E.: "Approaches to Moderating the Increases in Medical Care Costs," *Medical Care,* May-June 1969.

Kovner, Joel: "Production Function for Outpatient Medical Facilities," University Microfilms, Ann Arbor, Mich., 1968.

McNamara, Mary and Clifford Todd: "A Survey of Group Practice in the United States, 1969," *Journal of Public Health,* vol. 60, no. 7, pp. 1303–1312, July 1970.

Mechanic, David: "Patient Behavior and the Organization of Medical Care," (Monograph) University of Wisconsin, Madison, 1973.

Mechanic, David: "The Organization of Medical Practice and Practice Orientations Among Physicians in Prepaid and Non-Prepaid Primary Care Settings," (Monograph) University of Wisconsin, Madison, 1974.

Medical Economics: "Solo vs. Group Practice," Oct. 29, 1973, pp. 40ff.

Newhouse, Joseph: "The Economics of Group Practice," (Monograph) Rand Corporation, Santa Monica, Calif., 1971.

Peterson, O.L., et al.: "An Analytic Study of North Carolina General Practice 1953-54," *Journal of Medical Education,* part 2, Dec. 1965.

Roemer, Milton I. and D.M. DuBois: "Medical Costs in Relation to the Organization of Ambulatory Care," *New England Journal of Medicine,* May 1, 1969.

Roemer, Milton I., Robert W. Hetherington, Carl E. Hopkins, et al.: *Health Insurance Effects,* Bureau of Public Health Economics Research, Series No. 16, Ann Arbor, Mich., 1972.

Somers, Anne: *Health Care in Transition: Directions for the Future,* Hospital Research and Education Trust, Chicago, 1971.

Weinerman, E.R.: "Patients' Perceptions of Group Medical Practice," *American Journal of Public Health,* vol. 54, no. 6, pp. 880-889, June 1964.

Wolfman, B.I.: "Comparison of Blue Cross and Kaiser Family Medical Expenditures Under a Dual Choice," *Monthly Labor Review,* pp. 1186-1190, Nov. 1961.

WHO: Information in Health and Medical Services: Report on the Third European Conference on Health Statistics, Copenhagen, May 24-28, 1971.

Yankauer, Alfred et al.: "Physicians' Productivity in the Delivery of Ambulatory Care: Some Findings from a Survey of Pediatricians," *Medical Care,* Jan.-Feb., 1970.

Yett, Donald E.: "An Evaluation of Alternative Methods of Estimating Physicians' Expenses Relative to Output," *Inquiry,* pp. 3-27, Mar. 1967.

Chapter 3

Hospital Systems
and Functions

The hospital is one of the most complex organizations in our society. In this chapter, we do not attempt to present the hospital in simplistic terms, but to show it as it is with its complex interrelated systems. In the first part of this chapter we describe a number of hospital ownership patterns in the United States. The second part briefly describes ways of looking at hospital organizations from an administrative viewpoint and suggests that the most realistic approach is as an open complex system. Finally, we consider the functions of hospital systems looking especially at patient systems.

THE HOSPITAL INDUSTRY AND SYSTEMS OF OWNERSHIP

In Chapters 1 and 2 we pointed out that diagnostic and treatment services were not the only inputs into the very large health care system, even though they represent the largest component. In 1974 hospital care was the largest component of the health care industry and represented nearly 40 percent of health services expenditures or $40 billion of the $104 billion spent by the health industry. Moreover, AHA-registered hospitals employed over 3 million workers in 1973. These employees represented most of the 225 health vocations listed by the U.S. Department of Labor (1970).

Table 3-1 U.S. AHA-Registered Hospitals by Type of Ownership, and Characteristics of Each

Ownership	No. of Hospitals	No. of beds	Av'g length of stay	Av'g beds per hospital ‡	Total expense/ patient-day
Short-term (General, excludes T.B., and psychiatric, and all other)*					
Federal (Veterans Admin., Dept of Defense, Pub. Health Service, Indian Health Service, Dept. of Justice)	335	81,932	15.7	244.5	$94.35
State (Univ. and other short-term general)	147	30,085	9.6	204.6	$137.63
Local government (Hospital district, county, and/ or city)	1,618	176,886	7.8	109.3	$101.99
Nongovernment, not for profit (volunteer) (Church affiliated, community hospitals, co-operative hospitals operated by fraternal societies)	3,244	610,553	8.0	188.2	$104.88
Profit (Individual, partnership, corporation)	702	55,576	6.6	79.1	$98.38
Long-term (General, psychiatric, T.B., and all other)†					
Federal	65	60,374	133.7	928.8	$54.75
State	398	447,683	369.0	1,124.8	$21.44
Local government	101	40,098	396.9	207.4	$36.90
Nongovernment, not for profit	154	20,476	107.9	132.9	$56.12
Profit	57	4,896	55.1	85.8	$63.26

*Short-term: Over 50% of the patients admitted have a stay of less than 30 days.
†Long-term: Over 50% of the patients admitted have a stay of more than 30 days.
‡Average size computed by dividing total hospitals into total beds.

Source: Hospital Statistics, 1973 Edition, American Hospital Association, Chicago.

The hospital industry consists of a number of different hospital systems. Table 3-1 categorizes the 7,020 AHA-listed hospitals in the United States in 1972 by type of ownership, and relates ownership to number of hospitals, number of beds, average length of stay, average beds per hospital, and total expenses per patient day.

Federal hospitals include those operated under the Department of Defense for the armed services and their dependents; those operated by the Veterans Administration that treat illness related to service in the armed forces (also nonservice-connected disabilities of medically indigent veterans and some university hospital patients on an available bed basis); and Indian Health Hospitals and Public Health Service hospitals. State hospitals are predominantly for psychiatric illness. Hospitals operated by local government include a large number of short-stay general hospitals, which are similar to nongovernmental community hospitals. Local governmental hospitals also include the large charity hospitals for the poor such as Los Angeles County and Cook County in Chicago.

Voluntary or nongovernmental, not-for-profit community hospitals include church-operated or church-affiliated hospitals. However, they do not include Jewish hospitals that have their origin in the Jewish community rather than in the synagogue. Other voluntary hospitals include those operated by independent not-for-profit corporations, nonprofit industrial hospitals such as railroad hospitals, and hospitals sponsored by other groups such as the Shriners or the Kaiser Foundation Plan. A rather new development is the growth of the for-profit corporate chains, which operate a series of hospitals and have their stock traded publicly. They are located primarily in the South.

It is evident from Table 3-1 that the nongovernmental nonprofit short-term (or general acute) hospital is the largest component in the hospital system in relation to number of beds and national expenditures.

Figure 3-1 portrays graphically the size of various hospital service systems in terms of numbers of patients per day in each. It also shows changes in a ten-year period from 1963 to 1973. The nongovernmental not-for-profit short-term community hospital on which we focus in this book has grown more than any other type and is currently the largest system. Both psychiatric and TB hospitals have declined substantially due to advances in treatment which have reduced needs for inpatient services.

The hospital system has been as fragmented as other parts of the delivery system with separate mental, children's, extended care, and competing general hospitals sponsored by religious and other community and public groups. Some progress has been made in recent years toward rationalizing hospital services by integrating mental, dental, extended, and ambulatory services with general hospitals. Mergers, shared services, and satellite operations are other examples of integrated hospital systems. Chapter 15 discusses multihospital systems further.

Having examined the health system in the first chapter, and briefly looked at the personal health delivery industry and hospital systems within that industry, we now consider the hospital itself. In the following section we review ways of studying an organization, suggesting that it is most appropriate to examine the hospital as a complex system.

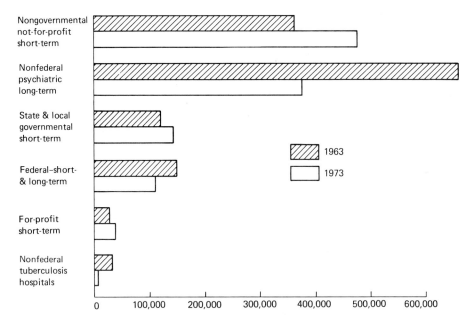

Figure 3-1 Total average daily census in various types of U.S. hospitals. (*Source: Hospital Statistics, Hospitals, J.A.H.A.*, 1974 ed., p. 19-21. Reprinted with permission, from *Hospitals, Journal of the American Hospital Association.*)

THE HOSPITAL AS A COMPLEX OPEN SYSTEM

The vast literature on administration shows us that organizations have been pictured in a variety of ways. Whether or not administrators recognize it, they too have theories about the nature of the organization they administer. The theory may not be articulated; it may be biased or incomplete, and may never be examined or revised in the light of new knowledge. If administrators were to examine their theories along with others, this should provide them with new insights and knowledge.

In the early decades of the twentieth century we tended to view enterprises as formal organizations that provided a structure or cradle within which the various employees performed their tasks. The major concern was the formal design of the structure, which should let each person know his position and function. Rationality was emphasized and an unemotional state was desired even to the extent of viewing the employee as a predictable self-motivated being who was given specific assignments. This has been referred to as the traditional or classical approach to organization. Because of the emphasis by hospitals on people, hospital administrators have not accepted this approach to the same degree as industrial managers in past years. However, there have been and still are autocratic administrators, administrators who adhere to Max Weber's (1946) seven rules of bureaucracy, and a general tendency toward the proliferation of rules and regulations.

A second general theory views the employee as the key to the organization to the extent of believing that a happy, well-satisfied employee is a productive one. Hence, why not contribute to (manipulate) an employee's satisfaction and happiness in order to increase productivity? The relationship between job satisfaction and productivity has been questioned in a number of studies, and the possibility has been advanced that productivity itself causes job satisfaction. No one likes to be manipulated, and those administrators who continue to use this method are generally suspect, so that productivity or effectiveness is hardly achieved.

More recently the behavioral model of the organization developed, with emphasis upon interactions between employees, the behavior of the employees individually and as group members, and the behavior of the total organization. Emphasis is on organizational development and change to bring about a better working environment in order to achieve sought-after synergy of $2 + 2 = 5$.

Attention has also been directed toward decision-making models, communication networks, and mathematical models in studying the organization. However, the important point is that all these approaches stressed the internal operations or relationships in the hospitals. In the 1960s, it became increasingly apparent that the hospital, like other manmade organizations, had external relationships. A systems theory or model was necessary to incorporate this development.

Two conclusions from this review of organizational theories require emphasis. The first is that a more comprehensive and accurate theory or explanation becomes possible as more is learned about administration and organizations. However, despite the fact that much knowledge has been developed, we do not want to imply that a complete, widely held explanation is available to us. The second is that the administrator or manager is a creature of the period in which he lives. When production was praised as the worthwhile goal via the assembly lines of the automobile industry, emphasis was upon efficiency, specialization, and hierarchical arrangements. During the depression of the 1930s when business and productivity appeared to have failed, emphasis was placed upon the individual. Now, with increased concern for the patient, consumer, client, customer, or recipient of goods or services, attention is being directed outside the organization toward external relationships.

General Systems Theory

A more encompassing and useful approach to organization is general systems theory (see Von Bertalanffy 1968; Churchman 1968; Miller 1972; Kast and Rosenzweig 1970; Katz and Kahn 1966). *Webster's New International Dictionary of the English Language* (Second Edition Unabridged) defines a system as "an aggregation or assemblage of objects limited by some form of regular interaction or interdependence" and "a formal scheme or method governing organization, arrangement, etc. of objects or material, or a mode of procedure."

General systems theory may be seen as analogous to tossing a stone into a pool of water and noting the shock waves moving outward in ever increasingly larger circles. The hospital is at the center of the focal point (see Fig. 3-2). When a patient enters a

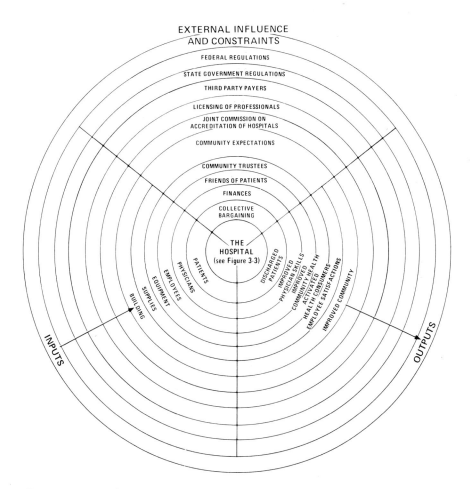

Figure 3-2 A systems view of the hospital showing that external systems affect the hospital's inputs and outputs.

hospital a great many groups are involved, both inside and outside the hospital. Inside, the patient is concerned with admissions, doctors, nurses, dietetics, the business office, and housekeeping, to name only a very few of the numerous internal relationships. Externally, the patient is involved with relatives, friends, and a third-party payer, and is influenced by government regulations, accreditation, and the community, to name a few.

What is most significant, however, is that the shock waves also work in reverse as far as the hospital is concerned. When the federal government changes its Medicare policies and procedures these eventually reduce in concentric circles through various agencies to impinge directly upon hospitals. Closer to home, the community, through a planning agency and fund raising, may or may not encourage a hospital to build an addition. The reader can no doubt supply additional evidence concerning forces which converge or impinge upon the hospital.

Basically, a system converts inputs into outputs. In a hospital, the patient is the key input, but the skills and knowledge of the doctors, the equipment utilized, the nurses, support people, etc., are all a part of the total input. Revans (1966) suggests that there are five steps that mark the progress of a patient through the hospital.

First the patient, on sufficiently convincing evidence, is admitted to the hospital. Secondly, on a detailed and specific examination, a diagnosis is made of his condition. Thirdly, based on this diagnosis, he is launched upon a program of treatment. Fourthly, his response to this treatment is continuously observed and compared with the response anticipated when the treatment was selected. Finally, in accordance with the results of this comparison, the patient is either discharged, his treatment amended or prolonged or his condition rediagnosed. To simplify the model still further, the five patient-stages may be listed as: (1) admission, (2) diagnosis, (3) treatment, (4) inspection and (5) control. These stages are locked together in two dimensions: by the availability and capacity of the physical resources themselves; and, by the network of power and communications through which are generated and transmitted the decisions that, in effect, control the experiences of the patient in any one stage and his transfer to the next.

This suggests that the administrator would do well to consider the patient flow, or treatments to the patient, as his key or basic system. Consider, however, the many subsystems which affect the patient. Depending upon hospital size and the needs of the patient these include: admitting, the medical staff, nursing services, laboratory, x-ray, surgery, central supply, dietary, purchasing, medical records, respiratory services, occupational or physical therapy, housekeeping, patient accounts, computer services, and volunteer services to identify only a part of the many subsystems in the modern hospitals which relate to the basic patient system.

Figure 3-3 fits inside the previous figure, which portrayed the hospital's external systems. Figure 3-3 shows the internal systems of the hospital with the patient at the core. It identifies the three major components of the internal hospital system:

1   The medical staff who diagnose, admit, and treat patients and perform quality control procedures through their medical staff organization.
2   Programs for the direct care and cure of patients such as nursing, x-ray, and laboratory.
3   Support and administrative services such as governance, administration, and business services.

It is important to note again that these concentric circles move both inward and outward, and affect each other as if a handful of pebbles were thrown into the water. Patient program departments such as nursing take orders from physicians and have line responsibility to administration, but all focus on patient needs. There are multiple lines of communication in hospitals; consequently, the traditional hierarchical organization chart is basically inappropriate for understanding relationships and influences in hospitals.

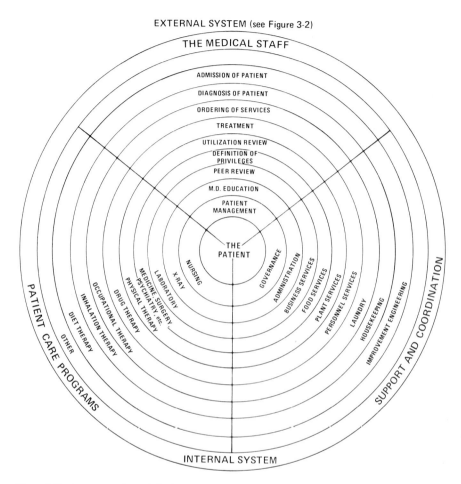

Figure 3-3 A systems view of the internal organization of the hospital showing medical staff, patient care programs, and support and coordination services.

Thus, we begin to see the advantage of the systems approach in the total picture aspect as well as the complications of the maze of subsystem activities and internal and external relationships.

HOSPITAL FUNCTIONS AND THE PATIENT CARE SYSTEMS

Systems exist to serve a function or functions.[1] While the function of the hospital may appear to be obvious, in reality hospitals have multiple functions that are not only changing over time, but are in some respects conflicting. In this section, we will

[1] Functions are essentially synonymous with objectives. In systems terminology they are frequently called *objective* functions.

explore hospital functions. We will then look more specifically at the patient for whom the hospital really exists to serve and then at some of the other functions or objectives that hospitals appear to be pursuing.

Changes in the functions of hospitals become evident from a historical review of their roles. The word *hospital* was derived from the Latin *hospitalis* referring to a guest. Originally, hospitals were a place for the shelter or entertainment of guests or strangers. Historically, the functions of hospitals reflected their mission as charitable institutions for refuge, maintenance, or education of the needy, aged, or infirm, or of young persons. They had little to offer beyond custodial and comfort nursing care services. In fact, they provided a public health service to isolate the infirmed from the rest of society as a nursing care service.

These functions or objectives persisted into the early years of the twentieth century. McDermott (1969) suggests that decisive medicine was not introduced until the 1930s when antimicrobial drugs became available. Although effective surgical intervention existed earlier, decisive medical intervention and surgical progress can be traced to that time. The principal function of most voluntary hospitals from the 1930s through the 1950s was to provide a workshop for physicians to practice decisive medicine.

During this period knowledge expanded at an accelerating rate as did diagnostic and treatment services, and specialization proliferated. Beginning in the 1960s and continuing into the early 1970s the community hospital has emerged as a community diagnostic and treatment health center with a team of health professionals; it is no longer just a workshop for individual physicians. In the following sections the various functions of the hospital are considered.

Patient Care Function and Systems

At present, the primary function of the hospital is to treat the ill patient. (For purposes of this discussion, we will exclude obstetrical patients and worried well patients who may not be physically ill.) Just as the hospital is a complex system so is the patient. Human behavior involves interactions between the individual's biological, psychological, environmental, social, cultural, and temporal systems. Table 3-3 lists human systems as categorized by Straus (1972) and shows their relationships to illness behavior and treatment behavior.

In years past a lack of biological knowledge resulted in hospitals concentrating on psychological and other nontechnical systems of care. Today biological systems and cure have become the focus of attention as the understanding and technological treatment of patients as biological beings have improved. Indeed, there is increasing concern that hospital and medical services are largely ignoring the other systems of man that also have an influence on treatment outcomes.

The importance of the psychological systems of man and the relationships of anxieties and stress to physical and mental health are well documented (King 1972). Moreover, the attitudes and behavior of health professionals are known to have an important influence on patient care (Rosengren and DeVault, 1963) and quality of care (Mechanic, 1970).

Table 3-3   Human Systems Affecting Illness and Treatment Behavior

Human Systems	Relationships to illness behavior	Relationships to treatment behavior
Biological: Man the organism	Genetic, chemical, nutritional, functional adequacy	Organic responses to technical treatment
Psychological: Man the personality	Intelligence, anxiety level, stress	Responses to anxieties, stress, and other interpretation of behaviors of hospital staff
Environmental: Man in his physical milieu	Demographic, behavioral, and physical environment	Response to noise, aesthetics, comfort of the hospital environment
Social: Man's roles as a member of his society and various social systems	Relationships within his family, occupation, friends and so forth	Response to dependency role, visitors, anticipated attitudes of his social system, relationships with the hospital staff
Cultural: Man responding to his normative and material culture	Customs, attitudes, values, expected way of behavior as developed from his religious, family, neighborhood and other associations.	Response to the hospital culture, culture of the hospital staff, and material culture of hospital equipment and supplies
Temporal: Man's orientation to dimensions of time	Time tables of age, rest, activity, eating, and so forth	Response to hospital schedules

Source: Robert Straus, "Hospital Organization from the Viewpoint of Patient-Centered Goals" in Basil Georgopoulos (ed.), *Organization Research on Health Institutions,* The Institute for Social Research, Ann Arbor, Mich., 1972, pp. 203-222.

Environmental systems such as air, water and noise pollution, and demographic and physical factors were discussed in Chapter 1. The physical environment of the hospitals also affects patients' response to treatment. Jaco (1972) reported that patients and nurses were more satisfied with circular-designed nursing units for the more seriously ill patients, but preferred traditional rectangular units for more mobile patients. Sommer and Dewar (1963) reported on the effects on patients of arranging furnishings in a mental hospital, suggesting that patients will passively adapt to the environment while visitors are more likely to change it, in this case rearranging furniture to suit them.

Social systems also affect illness behavior. Gonda (1962), for example, found a relationship between age and family size and persistent complaints, with older people and those from large families more likely to be persistent complainers. Scheff (1966) found social and demographic factors to be better predictors of the use of a college psychiatric clinic than the seriousness of the patients' illness. The social climate in the hospital such as the attitude of the staff toward the patient has an obvious influence on patient care and progress. The change in status from an independent individual in normal life to a passive, partially clothed dependent hospital patient is obvious to anyone who has been hospitalized.

Cultural relationships to illness behavior have been documented in studies by Zborowski (1952) and Croog (1961), who demonstrated the relationships between ethnic background and pain and symptoms of illness. Italian and Jewish patients, for example, tended to exaggerate pain and to report more symptoms than others. Within the hospital, cultural differences have been shown to affect patient care; for example, lower-income persons have problems communicating with higher-socio-economic-status physicians (Roth, 1969).

The effects of temporal differences are reflected in the higher hospital occupancy rates in January through March, the higher incidence of disease among the elderly, and the cyclical differences in mental illness, births, and other factors requiring hospitalization. Within the hospital, the common complaints of patients about being awakened much earlier than they are accustomed, and of having meals at the convenience of the hospital rather than at their own are evidence of the effects of time changes on patients.

While the primary function of the hospital is to serve patient needs, seldom do we consider the patient as a whole person with complex needs; rather, the patient is treated as a biological system that must conform to effective and efficient medical and hospital technical services. Treating the patient as a whole person is a major challenge to physicians, nurses, and other professionals and to trustees and administrators who have ultimate responsibility to ensure that patient needs are met. Some hospitals have established patient advocacy—ombudsman or patient-care counselor positions. Clergy, social workers, and consultant behavioralists might be utilized more effectively to help identify complex patient care needs and to propose improved patient care systems. Administrators, physicians, trustees, and others often gain new insights into and empathy for the broad scope of patient care needs after they have had to be patients. The complexities of human systems also underscore the importance of a team approach for identifying and meeting patient needs.

Other Functions of the Hospital

Providing a workshop for physicians is still a function of the hospital even though most hospitals look upon their role in the broader sense of providing care to patients. The traditional patient-physician relationship is still sacred and subject only to the surveillance of fellow physicians on the medical staff through peer review procedures. Even in government-controlled health systems such as that of the U.S.S.R., the physician's right and obligation to treat patients according to what he sees as their best interests is inviolate. As Freidson (1970, p. 115) suggests, "In circumstances most commonly studied *in the United States, the physician is not so much a part of the hospital as the hospital is part (and only one part) of the physician's practice.*" (Emphasis is his.) It is the physician who practices medicine; the hospital provides the resources to help the physician to diagnose and treat patients.

An emerging function for the hospital is that of a *community health center* taking a proactive role to improve the health of the populations it serves, not just a reactive role of crisis care. As major community health centers, hospitals can sponsor programs of environmental and occupational health, home care services, and so forth.

A seldom mentioned but nevertheless primary objective, and probably a marginal function of hospitals, is to *serve the institution itself* by achieving perpetuation, growth, and prestige for the institution, its staff, and its community. In a number of communities, hospitals have been established to enhance the status of the community or of a particular sponsoring group. Moreover, it is not unusual for institutional objectives to take priority over community service objectives. A major problem facing health planning agencies concerned with duplications and surpluses in hospital services in many communities is that of motivating hospitals to combine unnecessarily duplicated services. The objectives that hospitals are actually pursuing do not appear to have been studied. However, in a study of perceived and preferred objectives of universities, Gross and Grambsch (1968) found that institutional objectives such as prestige, academic freedom, and other personal objectives took priority over student and research output objectives. It is not impossible that similar results might be found if operative hospital objectives were studied.

Functions and their priorities will also vary by type of hospital. For example, the functions of local governmental hospitals providing charity service to the poor will differ from those of the voluntary community hospital. Originally some of the former were founded to provide public health services to minimize contamination from the sick poor to the rest of the community. Today, most of the large public charity hospitals furnish "clinical material" for medical education, and teaching is an important objective of the medical staff in addition to service.

CONCLUSIONS

Objectives, inputs, outputs, and external influences and constraints are broader and more complicated for hospitals than they are for most production-oriented industrial enterprises. Moreover, hospital governing board members and administrators have less control over these elements than does management in other industries. In such a setting and without easily defined goals for output quality, sales, and profits, those governing and managing hospitals face unusual challenges. Because it is an open rather than a closed system, the classical hierarchically oriented organization that is still appropriate for many large batch production industries may not be as well suited for hospitals. For this and other reasons, we disagree with those who propose a hierarchical corporate form of organization for hospital management. This is discussed in more depth in the balance of the book, particularly in Chapters 8 and 15.

REFERENCES

Churchman, C. West: *The Systems Approach,* Dell Publishing, New York, 1968.
Croog, S.H.: "Ethnic Origins, Educational Level and Responses to a Health Questionnaire," *Human Organization,* vol. 20, pp. 65-89, 1961.
Donabedian, Avedis, S.J. Axelrod, C. Swearungen, and J. Jameson: *Medical Care Chart Book,* 5th ed., School of Public Health, University of Michigan, Ann Arbor, 1972.
Freidson, Eliot: *Profession of Medicine,* Dodd, Mead and Co., New York, 1972.
Gonda, T.A.: "The Relation Between Complaints of Persistent Pain and Family Size," *Journal of Neurology and Neurosurgery, and Psychiatry,* vol. 25, pp. 277-281, 1962.
Gross, Edward and Paul U. Grambsch: *University Goals and Academic Power,* American Council on Education, Washington, D.C., 1968.
Jaco, E. Gartly: "Ecological Aspects of Patient Care and Hospital Organization," in Basil Georgopoulos (ed.), *Organization Research on Health Institutions,* Institute on Social Research, Ann Arbor, Mich., 1972, pp. 223-254.
Kast, Fremont E. and James E. Rosenzweig: *Organization and Management: A Systems Approach,* McGraw-Hill, New York, 1970.
Katz, Daniel and Robert L. Kahn: *Organizations and the Systems Concept,* John Wiley & Sons, New York, 1966.
King, Stanley H.: "Social Psychological Factors in Illness," in Howard Freeman et al. (eds.), *Handbook of Medical Sociology,* 2d ed., Prentice-Hall, Englewood Cliffs, N.J., 1972, pp. 129-147.
McDermott, Walsh: "Demography, Culture and Economics and the Evolutionary Stages of Medicine," in Edwin Kilbourne (ed.), *Human Ecology and Public Health,* Macmillan, 1969.
Mechanic, David: "Correlates of Frustration Among British General Practitioners," *Journal of Health and Social Behavior,* vols. 1 and 2, pp. 87-104, June 1970.
Miller, James G. "Living Systems: The Organization," *Behavioral Science,* vol. 17, no. 1, Jan. 1972.
Revans, Reginald W.: "Research into Hospital Management and Organization," *Milbank Memorial Fund Quarterly,* vol. 44, no. 3, p. 2, July 1966.
Rosengren, W.R. and S. DeVault: "The Sociology of Time and Space in an Obstetrical Hospital," in Eliot Freidson (ed.), *The Hospital in Modern Society,* Free Press, New York, 1963.
Roth, Julius: "The Treatment of the Sick," in Kosa et al., *Poverty and Health: A Social Analysis,* Harvard University Press, Cambridge, Mass., 1969, pp. 214-243.

Scheff, T.: "Users and Non-Users of a Student Psychiatric Clinic," *Journal of Health and Human Behavior,* vol. 7, pp. 114-121, 1966.

Sommer, R. and R. Dewar: "The Physical Environment of the Ward," in Eliot Freidson (ed.), *The Hospital in Modern Society,* Free Press, New York, 1963.

Straus, Robert: "Hospital Organization from the Viewpoint of Patient-Centered Goals," in Basil Georgopoulos (ed.), *Organization Research on Health Institutions,* The Institute for Social Research, Ann Arbor, Mich., 1972, pp. 203-222.

U.S. Department of Labor: *Job Descriptions and Organizational Analysis for Hospitals,* rev. ed., Washington, D.C., 1970.

Von Bertalanffy, Ludwig: *General System Theory,* George Braziller, New York, 1968.

Weber, Max: *From Max Weber; Essays in Sociology,* translated by H.H. Gerth and C. Wright Mills, Oxford University Press, New York, 1946.

Zborowski, M.: "Cultural Components in Responses to Pain," *Journal of Social Issues,* vol. 8, pp. 16-30, 1952.

Part Two

The Hospital

Part One presented an overview of the health system within which the hospital functions, the patient, and other hospital outputs. In Part Two, we discuss the internal system of the governing board, which has ultimate authority for the hospital and serves as a link between the hospital and its environment (Chapter 4), physicians and the medical staff organization who are in many respects outside the hospital organization (Chapter 5), issues associated with nursing and other major patient care programs (Chapters 6 and 7), and the administrator whose role has been and still is changing (Chapters 8 and 9), and functional specialists (Chapter 10).

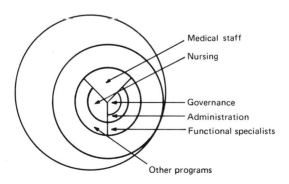

Chapter 4

Hospital Governance

The governing board is the formal link between the internal hospital system and the external system of which the hospital is a part. It is because of its unique position that we deal with hospital governance first in our detailed analysis of the hospital system and its subsystems.

Chapter 4 begins with a general description of governing boards. The second section explores some of the issues in governance. Finally, our conclusions suggest that the primary function of the governing board is to set objectives for the hospital based on the needs it exists to serve, and to continually evaluate operations and objectives in reference to changing needs and changes in the hospital environment.

THE NATURE OF HOSPITAL GOVERNING BOARDS

This section describes hospital governing boards, examining questions such as what their functions are, who their members are, how members are selected and what are found to be common organizational arrangements.

What Are the Functions of the Hospital Governing Board?

The governing board (board of directors or board of trustees) has three primary functions: (1) it has formal and legal responsibility for controlling and maintaining organizational effectiveness (Lattin, 1959); (2) it helps to gain support for the hospital from its environment; and (3) it represents, and should be accountable to, the region and/or subgroups from its environment. The importance of each of these functions varies by institution. We consider the varying emphasis of these functions in later sections of this chapter.

The American Hospital Association (AHA) (1965) in a pamphlet currently used for public distribution describes the hospital governing board as follows:

> The hospital governing board represents every individual in the community. It is the policymaking arm of the hospital which charts the hospital's present and future course.
>
>   . . . Members of the board serve without pay—out of a sense of civic service—to make better hospital care available to you and your family. Board members are selected for their demonstrated leadership in the community and their willingness to devote skill, time and thought to the hospital. The governing board is the very essence of the voluntary hospital system.
>
> . . . THE BOARD SETS POLICY
> Hospital trustees set the board policies under which medical staff and administrative procedures are developed. The governing board has the final responsibility for:
>   quality of medical care provided in the hospital
>   appointment of medical staff members
>   appointment of the hospital administrator, who in turn is responsible for the
>   effective day-to-day operation of the hospital
>   extent of the services provided by the hospital
>   protection of the community investment in the hospital, and prudent use of hospital assets and income.
>   The board meets regularly to review the reports of the medical staff and the administration. Based on careful study, it recommends policy and action on planning, specific aspects of hospital operation, and efficient use of facilities and services.
>   The board decides when new or expanded services should be provided to meet a community need.
>   Trustees seek ways to extend prepayment of hospital care in order to ensure sound hospital financing and to lessen the burden of unexpected hospital bills for patients. They also encourage adequate payment by government for care of welfare patients.
>   The governing board keeps posted on community changes that affect health care needs and works with community agencies for coordinated and comprehensive health services. It fosters community understanding and support for the hospital's program.
>   "Progress with purpose" is the objective of the hospital governing board. Through the guidance and leadership of this concerned group of citizens, your hospital moves progressively forward to meet community health needs.

A commonly used phrase in describing the role of the board is that it is the bridge between the hospital and the community. The internal and external role of the board is certainly evident in the AHA statement.

In their book, *The Give and Take in Hospitals*, Burling, Lentz, and Wilson (1956, p. 41) noted that "The [governing] board holds the hospital in trust. A private voluntary hospital is a gift of private donors to serve a community need. It is the responsibility of the board to provide and maintain an institution which will serve these needs according to the wishes of the donors." Hence, governing board members are commonly referred to as trustees. Today, most of the financing of hospital operations and capital emanates from patients and their third-party payers such as Blue Cross, commercial insurers, or Medicare; consequently the hospital should be held in trust for consumers and the community, not just for private donors. The term *trustee* appears to be used less frequently today.

Most of the literature related to functions of hospital governing boards is prescriptive (what functions should be), rather than descriptive or predictive (what actually the functions are). We will attempt to utilize the available research in describing the functions of the hospital governing board.

In summarizing the literature on the functions of hospital governing boards, Hickey (1972) lists the functions as follows:

1 Establish institutional objectives
2 Organize the board of directors to perform the work of the board
3 Review and approve major plans and programs
4 Review and approve major institutional policies
5 Select, appoint, and evaluate the chief executive officer
6 Maintain qualified medical staff
7 Perform an advisory role to operating management
8 Review and approve major institutional decisions
9 Evaluate institutional performance
10 Trusteeship

Hickey also surveyed administrators and governing board members of 206 hospitals with over 100 beds in five southern and southwestern states. The 527 governing board members who responded (out of 1,024 total governing members in the 105 hospitals that agreed to participate in the survey) ranked the importance of these functions as shown in Table 4-1.

While this does not describe specifically what boards actually do, it does suggest that those responding to this survey see as their most important function appointing an administrator as chief executive to operate the hospital and then reviewing and approving what he does and recommends. Establishing institutional objectives ranked second in importance, yet Schulz (1971) found evidence to suggest that few hospitals have attempted to formally define objectives.

Kaluzny and Veney (1972) surveyed 373 governing board members, and 135 administrators, including associate and assistant administrators, in 49 general acute community hospitals in New York State, excluding New York City, for their

Table 4-1 Directors' Ranking of the Importance of the Functions of the Hospital Board of Directors by Percentage of Respondents

Function	High	Medium	Low
Select, appoint and evaluate chief executive officer	93.21	5.52	1.27
Establish institutional objectives	90.96	7.11	1.93
Review/approve major plans and programs	90.32	8.47	1.21
Review/approve major hospital policies	87.24	11.52	1.24
Trusteeship	84.36	12.85	2.79
Maintain qualified medical staff	82.07	15.49	2.44
Evaluate institutional performance	78.08	19.40	2.52
Organize board of directors	77.70	17.88	4.42
Review/approve major institutional decisions	76.07	21.55	2.38
General advisory role to management	63.78	29.44	6.78

Source: W. J. Hickey, "The Functions of the Hospital Board of Directors," *Hospital Administration*, Summer 1972, p. 49. Reprinted with permission from the quarterly journal of the American College of Hospital Administrators.

study of trustee participation in hospital decision activities. Table 4-2 shows that the administrators perceive greater participation by trustees than do the trustees themselves.

On the other hand, Kovner (1974), in a survey of 506 trustees in 38 general acute hospitals with about 200 beds in the Greater Philadelphia-South New Jersey area, found that 92 percent of the board members perceived that the board exclusively or primarily established hospital objectives, strategies, and broad policies. However, in this same survey 97 percent of the trustees said that the hospital executive director (administrator) determined to at least some extent which policy issues the board discussed.

Laur (1969) studied the internal versus external orientation of board members in 11 metropolitan Minneapolis hospitals. He found that 52 percent of the governing board members studied were primarily interested in internal affairs, 15 percent in external affairs; 29 percent were equally interested in both, and 4 percent had little interest in either. Concerning their interest in governing the relationships between their hospitals and other community health organizations, 26 percent of the trustees had a high degree of interest, 35 percent a moderate degree and 38 percent low interest. One can conclude that the trustees in these hospitals were oriented more toward internal than external hospital functions.

On the other hand, it appears from Pfeffer's (1973) survey of 27 private non-profit-nonreligious hospitals that obtaining support and resources from the hospital's environment is the primary function of the board in those hospitals. Research on functions of governing boards in settings other than hospitals suggests boards may be *used* to manage the organization's environment as if they were *instruments* of corporation executives (Pfeffer, 1972; Selznick, 1949; Price, 1963; Vance, 1964; Lanser, 1969; Zald, 1967, 1969). That is, board members may be used primarily to aid fund raising and/or to influence planning bodies or other sources of regulation or support for the hospital.

Table 4-2 Trustee Participation as Viewed by Trustees and Administrators

Areas of trustee participation	Amount of trustee participation as viewed by:	
	Administrators	Trustees
Allocation of total hospital income	Considerable	Some
Adoption and implementation of new hospitalwide programs and services	Considerable	Some
Development of formal affiliation with other organizations	Considerable	Some or none
Appointment and promotion of administrative personnel	Some	Some
Appointment of medical staff members	Considerable	Some or none
Long-range planning for new hospital-wide services	Considerable	Considerable or none

Source: Arnold D. Kaluzny and James Veney, "Who Influences Decisions in the Hospital? Not Even the Administrator Really Knows," Modern Hospital, Dec. 1972, p. 52.

The results of these studies of the perceptions of board functions and influence are conflicting. However, it should be noted that, while Kovner reported a rather dominant role for the board in setting hospital policies, he also found that administrators had control over much of the information used by the board in setting policies. Moreover, Kovner (1975) notes a lack of empirical verification of what trustees and administrators said are the functions of the board. More research is needed on the functions of the board and on hospital effectiveness. Our experiences have been more in keeping with the findings of Kaluzny and Veney and of Pfeffer's. It appears to us that boards have an increasingly passive role and are used to manage the hospital's environment.

Who Are Governing Board Members?

Governing board members appear to represent community leadership. In a survey of 48 not-for-profit hospitals in the Detroit, Michigan area, Goldberg and Hemmelgard (1971) found that hospital governing boards were dominated by business executives, members of the legal and accounting professions, and spokesmen for medicine and hospitals. Berger and Earsy (1973) reported similar findings in Boston. These authors concluded that hospital boards are not representative of, nor do they reflect the composition of, the community generally. Goldberg and Hemmelgard did find that hospitals controlled by local government had boards somewhat more representative of the community at large, presumably reflecting the political composition of the local government.

Historically, boards of hospitals owned by religious groups have been dominated by ministers or Catholic sisters. Many of the Catholic hospitals had what might be considered internal governing boards similar to many industrial corporations in which the majority of board members were officials within the organization. Most Protestant hospitals changed to include external members many years ago although a number still have several ministers on the board and require that some trustees be of the same religious faith. Catholic hospital boards are changing rapidly with many including or even having a majority of community leaders who may or may not be Catholic (Goldberg and Hemmelgard, 1971).

A national survey of 632 governmental, not-for-profit, and proprietary (for-profit) hospitals conducted in 1971 for the AHA tended to support the findings of Goldberg and Hemmelgard that trustees represent community leaders rather than consumers (Gilmore and Wheeler, 1972). A more recent study by the editors of *Trustee* magazine also tends to corroborate this (*Hospitals*, 1975). Table 4-3 identifies the careers of nearly 10,000 board members in the 632 hospitals in the Gilmore and Wheeler study. The sampling procedures for the national survey were designed to be representative of the number of beds in the nation rather than of the hospitals; consequently the sample includes disproportionately more hospitals of larger bed size. Note that blue-collar workers and minority-group representatives total only 3.2 percent of the board members in the survey. This chart tends to support the criticism in recent years that hospital boards represent the community establishment rather than the consumers whom hospitals serve.

Ewell (1974) concluded from his study that there appeared to be a significant relationship between hospital program innovation and boards with a more mixed occupational membership, and those that included more women, more minority groups, more members whose places of residence were closer to their hospitals, and more members from younger age groups. He also concluded that boards with a more diverse membership appeared to have a higher level of concern for external environmental issues relating to community needs and cooperative health programs.

Table 4-3   Career Identification of Board Members

	Number	Percent
Medicine	689	7.1
Other health professions	342	3.5
Other professional groups	1,311	13.6
Clergy	604	6.2
Executives, managers, white-collar supervisory	3,489	36.1
Proprietors, self-employed	1,779	18.4
Blue-collar workers	224	2.3
Member of hospital women's auxiliary	194	2.0
Housewife	416	4.3
Other	531	5.5
Minority-group representatives	86	0.9
Total	9,665	100.0

Source: Kay Gilmore and John R. Wheeler, "A National Profile of Governing Boards," *Hospitals, J.A.H.A.*, vol. 46, pp. 105–108, Nov. 1972. Reprinted, with permission, from *Hospitals, Journal of the American Hospital Association.*

How Are Governing Board Members Selected?

In voluntary hospitals sponsored by churches or fraternal organizations, board members are usually selected by the sponsoring organization. In Catholic hospitals, the religious community usually selects board members. Nonchurch voluntary hospitals frequently have a corporate organization that selects the board. While the board is responsible to the corporation, as pictured below, the corporation has little influence over the board in most situations.

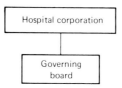

Corporate members are like a stockholder group in a large corporation. Membership is usually large, consisting of everyone who may have contributed to the hospital. The corporate members usually meet only once a year at a public relations type of gathering in which they elect governing board members nominated by a nominating committee, which is frequently appointed by the board itself.

Table 4-4 shows that in one-third of the hospitals surveyed the governing board selected their own members (Gilmore and Wheeler, 1972). It should be pointed out that the by-laws of many boards limit the number of successive terms a director may serve.

In for-profit industries, Thompson and Walsh (1965) found that present directors and senior executives usually suggest candidates for board vacancies. One might also conclude, although there is no reported data, that the backgrounds of hospital corporate members are similar to those of hospital governing board members. This is

Table 4-4   Membership Selection Procedures in 632 Hospitals

Selection Procedure	Type of Hospital			
	Government (163 total)	Not-for-profit (448 total)	For-profit (21 total)	Percent of total
Board elected	8.6%	42.2%	28.6%	33.1
Corporate elected	2.4	35.7	47.6	27.5
Elected by other group	25.8	7.1	9.5	12.0
Appointed	62.0	12.0	14.3	25.0
Other	1.2	2.9	0	2.4

Source: Kay Gilmore and John R. Wheeler, "A National Profile of Governing Boards," *Hospitals, J.A.H.A.*, vol. 46, pp. 105–108, Nov. 1972. Reprinted, with permission, from *Hospitals, Journal of the American Hospital Association.*

usually because a contribution fee is required in order to become a corporate member; moreover, the average consumer does not know he can become a member of the corporation.

Many hospitals were founded as proprietory hospitals by physicians who needed facilities for their patients. During the depression of the 1930s, most converted to nonprofit status. Many of these hospitals continued to have physicians on the governing board. Goldberg and Hemmelgard (1971) found that in the Detroit area hospitals with under 100 beds had a higher proportion of physicians on the board, which may reflect their origins as proprietary institutions.

A primary function of the board is to provide a linkage with its environment (Pfeffer 1973). Consequently, selection of board members would be expected to relate to the importance of influencing a specific hospital environment. For example, the private nonprofit hospital is dependent upon community support and funds: thus the function of the board, with the help of its members, is to gain this support for the hospital. One would expect therefore that the ability of a board member to raise money and a board member's influence in the community would be important criteria in the selection of board members in private not-for-profit hospitals. Results of a survey by Pfeffer (1973) among 57 hospitals tend to suggest that indeed ability to raise money and influence in the community were important criteria in the *selection* of board members in the private nonprofit hospitals he surveyed. Moreover fund raising was also perceived as an important *function* of boards in private nonprofit hospitals.

Catholic hospitals' major area of influence, at least in the past, has been the religious community of the order, many of whose members work in the hospitals. The primary link with this environment is, of course, provided by the sisters in the religious community. Pfeffer found evidence that hospital administration was an important function of board members in hospitals classified as religious whereas it was not an important function for private nonprofit hospitals. The environmental influences over Catholic hospitals are changing as in other hospitals, and increasingly they must depend upon support from their clients. Pfeffer found a correlation between religious hospitals and the importance of selecting board members for their regional or subgroup representation; he also found that selecting board members for their ability to raise money was not important. Catholic hospitals are appointing more lay members to their boards and Pfeffer's findings suggest that religious hospitals may be developing boards that are more broadly representative of the communities they serve than the boards of nonreligious hospitals.

It is logical to assume that the most important environment for governmental hospitals is the political environment. It is not surprising therefore that Pfeffer found that the selection of board members for their political connections was important in hospitals that were more dependent upon operating funds from the government. Governing boards of governmental hospitals seem to be more involved in administration than boards of other types of hospitals. One might attribute this to a concern about controlling tax-generated expenditures. Pfeffer found that the more a hospital was dependent upon the government for its resources, and the more the government influenced hospital decisions, the more important administration was as a board *function*.

If, as some authors suggest, boards are instruments designed to link organizations to their environments, we might be able to predict changes in the selection of board members by examining environmental changes. For example, with increasing emphasis on consumer interests, one might predict that hospitals will continue to select more individuals from labor groups, more women, and more representatives from minority groups in order to provide a cross-section of consumer interests. Moreover, as governmental environmental influence over community hospitals increases, we might expect to see more nongovernmental hospitals select board members with political connections.

How Are Boards Organized and What Are Their Organizational Relationships?

A traditional community hospital organization chart is shown in Figure 4-1.

Boards typically delegated responsibility for medical affairs to the medical staff. The medical staff has functioned as essentially an autonomous self-governing body. A joint conference committee with representatives from the medical staff and the board exists in most hospitals with the purpose of providing liaison between the two

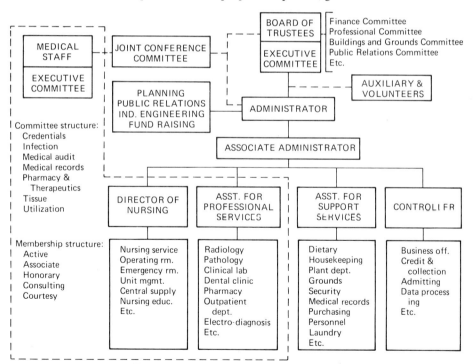

Figure 4-1 Prototype hospital organization chart. *Source: A Primer for Hospital Trustees*, Chamber of Commerce of the United States, Washington, D.C., 1974, p. 31.

bodies. In essence, hospitals are a duopoly in organizational arrangement, with the board and administrative organization on one hand and medical staff on the other (Smith, 1955). The administrator usually functions in a coordinative role with the medical staff. This is discussed further in future chapters.

Governing boards generally meet monthly. In some hospitals the board meets quarterly with an executive committee of board officers, board committee chairmen, and the administrator meeting monthly. Boards are usually organized into committees such as finance, endowment, personnel, planning, and/or building committees in addition to the executive committee. In the past, administrators would frequently complain about governing board members usurping responsibilities. Even today one hears of an occasional hospital in which a board chairman has an office in the hospital and tends to become involved in day-to-day operations, thus undermining the role of the administrator.

Pfeffer (1973) also found that board size varies by hospital ownership and board function. He found a correlation between private nonprofit hospitals that depended upon community support and large boards. Governmental hospitals that had more board concern for administration tended to have small boards. Frequently, larger boards with over 20 or so members meet only quarterly and smaller executive committees perform board functions on a regular monthly basis. On some boards the chairmen of board committees are members of the executive committee. The hospital administrator usually is ex-officio without vote on all committees and on the board itself. The research literature on group size contains insights which are of interest in studying the dynamics of trustee groups, although the primary emphasis has been on smaller groups (Ewell 1974). In general, the findings appear to show that group cohesiveness tends to decrease as size begins to exceed ten to twelve members (Hare, 1952); consensus is more likely in groups of between five and seven (Rath and Misra, 1963); group size is negatively correlated to participation (Hare, 1952); member satisfaction is greater in smaller groups (Forehand and Gilmer, 1965); performance is more effective in small groups (Hare, 1952); leadership behavior becomes more complicated as group size increases (Whyte, 1949); and members become more tolerant of highly structured leadership styles as size increases (Hemphill, 1957).

Group decision making may be a key concept in viewing the role and function of the hospital trustee, particularly with regard to the committee structure, where major decisions most often originate. At the committee level, where decisions must often satisfy measures of both quality and acceptability, the wide variety of decisions required makes a flexible strategy essential. Delbecq (1967) suggests a multiple-strategy conceptualization that allows for flexibility in group decision making. The approach would vary according to the characteristics of the decision setting. Delbecq specifies strategies for:

1 *Routine decision making*—where the group is in agreement on goals, means are available, objectives are shared by members, and members are homogenous.

2 *Creative decision making*—where there is agreement on goals but means are unclear, membership is heterogenous, and the group is free-wheeling, loosely structured, and more creative.

3 *Negotiated decision making*—where the group may disagree on both goals and means, procedures are formalized, and compromise is sought. A problem-solving mood is emphasized and conflict is seen as helpful and natural. Membership is generally divided between two factions who express differing norms, values, and orientation.

The function of the hospital board under this source of direction might be to appraise the nature of the problem, determine which structural arrangement was called for, and then appoint committees.

Relationships between the president or chairman of the board and the hospital administrator are usually very close. It is common for the head of the board to meet formally once a week with the administrator, and informally more often when there are important issues pending. In keeping with a doctrine of "no surprises" (and to influence the board) most administrators want their board chairman to be fully informed—particularly of any pending problems. The administrator will usually prepare agenda for board meetings and discuss items, reports, and strategy for board action with the board chairman or president.

In summary, research findings would imply that if a link to the external environment, and creative programs, are most important, a relatively large heterogenous board would be helpful. If, on the other hand, a cohesive, internally concerned board is most important, a smaller group of less than 10 members would be preferable.

ISSUES IN HOSPITAL GOVERNANCE

Some of the current issues in governance concern who really controls hospitals, internal versus external boards, and consumerism.

Who Really Controls the Hospital?

Governance is defined in *Webster's New World Dictionary* as ". . . to direct, control, rule, manage . . ." The hospital governing board has been charged legally, such as in the Darling case,[1] and traditionally as having ultimate responsibility and control. However, evidence on who actually controls or is the dominating influence in the hospital is contradictory. Brown (1970) suggests that the hospital is an "organization model with no avowed head, but with three proclaimed legs—trustees, administrator and medical staff."

Perrow, in a case study of one hospital, traced dominance over a period of years from the board to the medical staff to the administrator and finally to a sharing among the three (Perrow, 1963). In the early period of the hospital, when there was a substantial amount of free care and annual donations to hospitals, the governing board funded and dominated much of the operations. In the 1930s and 1940s, the technological knowledge of the medical staff gave them the greatest influence. Moreover, in that period the source of funding emanated from the patients that physicians brought to the hospitals. In the 1950s and into the 1960s, the coordination of complex

[1] *Darling v. Charleston Community Memorial Hospital,* 211 N.E. 2d 253 (1965) cert. denied 383 U.S. 946 (1966).

services and the negotiations with third-party payers (Blue Cross, etc.) that fell to the administrator gave him or her increasing influence.

Increasingly, administrators are being given the title of president and being elected to hospital governing boards much like chief executives in for-profit industries. The increasing dominance of administrators has been reported by a number of authors, among them Georgopoulos and Mann (1962). On the other hand, a survey sponsored by the American College of Hospital Administrators (ACHA) reported that "trustees and medical staffs do not view the administrator as a leader, but as a generally passive influence caught between the board and the doctors . . ." (Modern Hospital, 1968).

Holloway et al. (1963), in a case study of one 345-bed community general hospital in a middle-sized midwestern community, found that individuals who they defined as "economic influentials (EIs)" had more control over other board members and the administrator. Non-EIs on the board had control over the administrator although less than the EIs. However, their study was based on interactions during board meetings using sociometric techniques, and therefore measured attempted rather than actual control.

Toomey (1970) suggests that the influence of the board has been eroded by comprehensive planning agencies who control facilities, Social Security Administration and rate review boards, which control utilization and costs, unions, which control wages, and other groups external to the hospital.

Again, it is evident that the traditional hierarchical organization chart with the governing board on top does not really describe relationships appropriately, that is, the varying amounts of influence wielded by the governing board, the administrator, the medical staff and the employees. In Chapter 3 (Figure 3-2) we showed the environmental factors and constraints that affect the entire hospital, factors such as laws, licensure, and accreditation. Filley and House (1969), in summarizing Simon (1957) and French and Raven (1959) among others, suggest there is substantial agreement that ability to influence is derived primarily from: (1) legitimacy; (2) control of rewards and sanctions including money; (3) expertise; (4) personal liking; and (5) coercion. Clearly, the administrator and medical staff have some legitimate authority, although the trustees have the ultimate authority. Each group in the hospital has some base of influence over the others (see Figure 4-2). Trustees and the administrator control money and facilities. Physicians also exert some control over money by deciding when and where patients are admitted, particularly in communities where there are multiple hospitals and a surplus of beds. Physicians have used "heal-ins" in public charity hospitals and boycotts in private hospitals. Employees also have power through scarcities of labor (primarily in the recent past), expertise, and their attitudes in handling patients (Mechanic, 1962). Moreover, employees can apply sanctions through collective bargaining or at least threats of it. Medical staff members, administrators, and employees have expertise in their profession and/or control of information.

We suggest therefore that external forces, the board, the administration, the medical staff, and the employees all have some influence or power. The traditional hierarchy, with a manager who hires, fires, and supervises, does not appropriately describe a hospital organization. Administration should be a team effort.

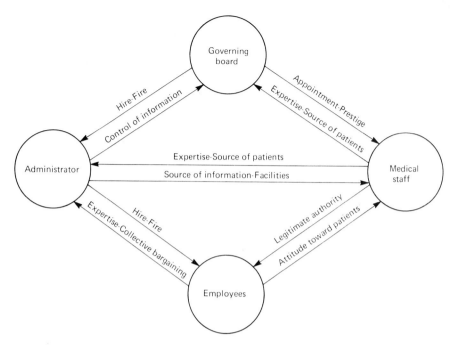

Figure 4-2 Internal sources of influence

We suggest that accountability rather than control is the important issue; accountability to consumers, individual patients, those who provide funds and other resources, regulatory agencies, sponsoring groups, and other members of the hospital family. Accountability should help provide justification for taking community resources, to improve effectiveness and efficiency, and to provide incentives for improved performance. Bowen (1973) suggests the following ingredients for a system of accountability:

A clear statement of goals and objectives with an ordering of priorities
Allocation of resources toward maximum returns in relation to goals and objectives
Cost and benefit analysis including allocation of costs and benefits to particular programs within the institution
Evaluation of actual results
Reporting on evaluation to all concerned

If hospitals followed these guidelines and publicized results, it is unlikely that questions of who controls hospitals, consumer representation, and so forth would be of as much concern as they are today.

Should Board Membership Be Internally or Externally Dominated?

Internally dominated governing boards are those in which most members are from within the organization; for example, in some Catholic hospitals most members are sisters who also work in the hospital in varying capacities. Externally dominated governing boards are those in which most members are neither hospital employees nor medical staff members. The vast majority of community nonprofit, nonchurch hospitals have what would be considered external boards dominated by community leadership (Gilmore and Wheeler, 1972; Pfeffer, 1973). The majority do not appear to have any voting members from the hospital such as medical staff members, although in almost all hospitals the administrator will at least attend board meetings.

Schulz (1972) found in his study of hospitals in Illinois and Wisconsin that in over half the hospitals at least one medical staff member attended board meetings. Increasing numbers of hospitals appear to be moving toward more of a mixture of internal and external members. As noted previously, Catholic hospitals appear to be selecting more members from the community. Schulz (1971) found a trend toward more hospitals having at least one member of the medical staff as voting members of the governing board. However, he found that 76 percent of these hospitals had *no* medical staff member participating actively in major board decisions related to income and expenses. Vance (1973) sees an emerging trend toward appointing administrators to voting membership on governing boards.

The American Medical Association and physicians in many hospitals have been actively promoting medical staff membership on governing boards (Blasingame, 1970). The AHA does not necessarily deny the value of having physicians as board members, but believes it should not be compulsory and that they should not be selected by the medical staff as argued by the AMA (Hahn and Bornemeir, 1970). Arguments against having physicians on the hospital board stem from the position taken by the late Malcolm T. MacEachern, M.D., one of the pioneers in professionalizing the field of hospital administration in the 1930s. His arguments, which are still used today, are (MacEachern, 1946, pp. 75-76):

1 Membership on the governing board gives undue publicity to the individual physician, thereby placing him in a position which he may not have earned by his professional efficiency and favorably affecting his private practice.

2 Members of the governing board who are physicians may readily use their position to promote themselves on the medical staff of the hospital.

3 Physicians appointed to the governing board are often not elected by the medical staff and therefore are not regarded by the other physicians as their chosen representatives.

4 Placing a physician on the governing board not only tends to create jealousy among his confreres on the medical staff, but blights the interest of other staff members who have no connection with the governing board.

5 The physician-member of the governing board may be regarded by the medical staff as an inspector who is unduly critical of their work, his position thus becoming a barrier to cooperation between the medical staff and the governing board.

6 When the legal responsibility imposed upon a hospital trustee is considered, it is realized that a physician who is also a trustee might be subjected under certain circumstances to a double liability.

7 There is a tendency occasionally on the part of the medical representative to express his own personal judgment rather than the collective or group opinion of the medical staff which he represents.

8 The hospital may encounter difficulty in adopting the commendable practice of making medical staff appointments annually if preferred physicians are retained on the governing board.

9 A physician on the governing board may exert his authority in the employment of hospital personnel, which eventually may lead to charges of favoritism, thereby disturbing the morale of the institution. . . .

Ainsworth (1970) and many others argue for broad physician participation in hospital management, not just physician membership on governing boards. Ainsworth suggests a number of benefits, paraphrased below, for the physician, administrator, trustee and patient from medical staff participation:

The physician:
  gains upward mobility within the institution.
  develops a sense of security and stability.
  achieves a role in formulating policy, not only in long-range planning, but on a day-to-day basis.

The administrator:
  gains shared responsibility for his budget to help control costs.
  gains support from the medical staff.
  has less interference from trustees in administrative affairs, because participation helps keep trustees in a policy-making role.

The trustee:
  no longer needs to play a day-to-day administrative role because administrator-medical staff conflicts of interest are minimized.
  achieves shared medical staff warranty for the quality of care and better control over the practice of individual staff members by a management team.

The patient:
  receives higher-quality care through better control over quality and costs.
  benefits from more orientation to patient needs because the physician and hospital are one.

As one authority bluntly stated, "The average practicing physician mistrusts the hospital."

In reference to the controversy over who should select physicians for board membership, Schulz (1972) found that physicians selected primarily by the board participated more actively in hospital decision activities than those selected primarily by the medical staff. This finding raises a number of questions. Are those selected by the board the ones who have greater interest in decision activities; or are those selected by the medical staff ones who sit in as observers to ensure medical staff interests are not compromised; or is the board unwilling to involve persons for whose selection they were not mainly responsible?

In suggesting there is a trend for hospital administrators to have voting membership on boards, Vance (1973) argues: (1) There has been a significant improvement in the role of the administrator; (2) there is considerable dissatisfaction with present trustee structure; (3) changes are needed because of public pressures for more representative boards; and (4) cost-benefit squeeze requires stronger management.

We suggest that arguments regarding medical staff and administrator memberships on the governing board are only manifestations of more fundamental issues. Physicians appear to want membership on boards because they mistrust the administration or other board members to represent them appropriately. They want their own representation. We see no harm and some benefits to communications in having physicians on the board. In his two state surveys, Schulz (1972) found that administrators who had physicians on the board reported benefits in communication and no particular problems. However, medical staff membership on boards will not in itself meet expectations for physician involvement and accountability for hospital costs. Moreover, there are other ways to improve communications and achieve physician participation in decision activities.

We also see no particular harm in administrators having voting membership on the governing board. However, this appears to be primarily a manifestation of attempts to make the administrator a chief executive officer in fact, with authority and titles similar to the president of an industrial corporation. Our experience shows that board membership and the title of president do not necessarily make a chief executive officer. Moreover, we suggest there may be other effective roles for an administrator than just the role of a chief executive officer (see Chapter 8).

The more important issue seems to be the internal versus external board. The effectiveness of internal versus external boards would logically be related to the organization's environment. Research in for-profit corporations found that internal boards were associated with organizational success more than external boards (Vance, 1964; Lanser, 1969). Linkage with the internal environment is of primary importance to most corporations. If the hospital's ability to influence its environment in order to obtain more resources continues to deteriorate as controls and regulation increase, an internal board may prove to be a better link to the environment. At that time, management of the internal organization within established outside constraints will be most important. An internal board should include other members of top administration such as the director of nursing services, the financial officer, and possibly others in addition to medical staff and chief administrator membership. The management team in the reorganized British National Health Service functions as an internal board and is a case in point (Schulz and Chester, forthcoming).

How Does Consumerism Relate to Hospital Governance?

In recent years consumer advocates have criticized hospitals for being unresponsive to their needs. Most of the criticisms stemmed from the fact that the urban poor had not received appropriate services particularly in comparison to the services and amenities available to the middle and upper classes. The only services available to many of the poor were the large public-charity hospitals. These public institutions were (and many still are) governed by individuals appointed by local governmental groups. In essence, they served the taxpayers of the community, and their implicit goals were to hold down costs rather than to provide superior service, the implicit goal of most community nongovernmental hospitals. However, as the urban poor attain more political power, board members are becoming more responsive to the needs of consumers rather than just those of taxpayers.

The original intentions of Medicaid and Medicare were to provide the poor with health care funds so they could enter the mainstream (i.e., the private sector) of health care. This goal has never been achieved for a number of reasons, although progress has been made.

As an alternative, the Office of Economic Opportunity (OEO) funded a number of neighborhood health centers to provide comprehensive health services to the poor with strong consumer involvement in governance. However, consumer representation or dominance in governance has not met expectations in many of these centers. For example, dominance by consumers who had no previous experience in governing a complex health service reportedly contributed to the problems of the Mound Bayou, Mississippi Delta Health Center. On the other hand consumer representatives can frequently be coopted so they no longer appropriately represent or appear to represent their constituency (Shostak, 1969). Studies in other settings show that group representatives play a rather passive role as board members and their communication and legitimacy with the group they represent gradually become weaker (Thorsrud, 1970). Wise (1971) argues that in the ghettoes community participation in health governance is not relevant because of the mobility of the population (about 50 percent turnover of residents every five years) and the lack of client participation in organized groups of any kind.

It is not only difficult to find what might be considered broadly based consumer representation, but in our opinion it is also a fallacy to assume that consumers are the best judges of what are the best interests of the community. We have seen a number of situations where citizen groups have demanded construction of unnecessary facilities over the strong objections of physicians and/or administrators.

Group Health Cooperative in Seattle, Washington, has a consumer-dominated governing board that successfully employs physicians and other health services personnel. However, it has leadership in its governance that is aware of the requirements for institutional success in an environment where there is considerable competition from traditional fee-for-service independent health services. It is also interesting to note that the highly successful Kaiser Health Plan is essentially provider-dominated in its governance.

To date, consumerism has not been an issue with middle- and upper-class segments of the population. Under the prevailing system of largely independent, fee-for-service medical and hospital services, hospital providers must be responsive to individual paying consumers if they are to succeed. In most communities, therefore, individual consumers exercise control by selecting the physicians and hospitals that please them most.

It is important not to associate consumer controls only with the governance of health services. Other possible alternatives for consumer controls over medical services are as follows:

1 Market controls with consumers and providers having freedom of choice and each having resources needed by the other. This has worked quite well for the middle and upper classes. However, Medicaid, which was intended to accomplish this for the poor, has not worked as well as some had hoped primarily because of uninformed consumers and the inaccessibility of private health services for the poor. The publication of physician and hospital charges and of utilization and quality indicators, and suggestions on how to avoid unnecessary surgery are among the current recommendations and practices aimed at developing informed consumers.

2 Consumer dominance in the governance of health institutions. Lack of education and/or cooperation of the poor limits the effectiveness of this alternative.

3 Bargaining by groups of consumers with providers. This alternative may hold some promise if it can be made attractive to providers and if the consuming poor as well as the providers hold some sanctions.

4 Establishment of a nationalized system. Few are ready to overturn a traditionally private system that has been successful for most consumers simply because the minority are not reaping the same benefits. Moreover, there are no assurances that a nationalized system will meet consumer expectations more effectively.

5 Utilizing group process techniques to get consumer inputs into the governance and management of hospitals (Delbecq, 1972).

Some of these alternatives are discussed further in later chapters. (Also see Duke University 1973 National Forum on the *Citizenry and the Hospital,* available from Duke University Program in Health Administration.)

CONCLUSIONS

We have suggested that the primary functions of the governing boards are: (1) to control and maintain organizational effectiveness, (2) to represent and be accountable to the region and its subgroups in order to ensure that community needs are met, and (3) to obtain support and resources from (or coopt) the hospital's environment. These three functions are not mutually exclusive, however. We suggest that a governing board can more effectively fulfill all three functions by carefully *defining hospital objectives* in explicit terms and then *evaluating* hospital operations.

Establishing objectives is not a simple task. An effective statement of objectives requires that a number of criteria be met:

1 Objectives should be based on a careful study of needs the hospital should exist to serve. Health planners, policy-makers, researchers, and consumers need to be consulted in order to determine needs objectively and knowledgeably.

2 In addition to the administrator, medical staff members and key employees should be involved in formulating objectives.

3 Objectives should be explicit. Better patient care at lowest cost is a meaningless statement. Quality, cost, and other objectives should be defined in explicit, measurable terms so it can be determined whether or not they have been achieved.

4 Priorities should be identified, since objectives will often conflict.

5 Objectives should include explicit targets and time frames.

6 Objectives should be operational. Perrow (1967) suggests that the actual objectives pursued by individuals in an organization (operational objectives) may be quite different from official or stated institutional objectives. It is essential that official and operational objectives be the same.

The governing board must periodically evaluate operations against objectives and the needs that objectives should be defined to meet. (Drucker [1973] elaborates on the importance of objectives in managing public service institutions in his book *Management: Tasks; Responsibilities; Practices.*) Information systems in hospitals must be based on the measurements of achieving objectives. Finally, the bylaws as well as the actual activities of the board need to be constantly reexamined in order to achieve the objectives of the hospital.

REFERENCES

American Hospital Association: *The Hospital Governing Board,* Chicago, 1965.

Ainsworth, Thomas H.: "The Physician as a Manager," *Hospitals, J.A.H.A.,* vol. 44, pp. 53-55, 1970.

Berger, Ian and Robert Earsy: "Occupations of Boston Hospital Board Members," *Inquiry,* vol. 10, no. 1, pp. 42-46, 1973.

Blasingame, F.J.L.: "Governance of Hospitals: The Cases for Physicians as Board Members," *Trustee,* vol. 23, pp. 21-25, 1970.

Bowen, Howard R.: "Holding Colleges Accountable," *Chronicle of Higher Education,* March 12, 1973.

Brown, Ray: "Strictures and Structures," *Hospitals, J.A.H.A.,* vol. 44, no. 16, pp. 79-81, 1970.

Burling, Temple, Edith Lentz, and Robert N. Wilson: *The Give and Take in Hospitals,* Putnam's Sons, New York, 1956, p. 41.

Delbecq, Andre L.: "The Management of Decision-Making with the Firm: Three Strategies for Three Types of Decision-Making," *Academy of Management Journal,* vol. 10, no. 4, pp. 329-339, Dec. 1967.

Delbecq, Andre L.: "Critical Problems in Health Planning," paper presented at 32nd Annual Meeting of Academy of Management, Cleveland, Aug. 13-16, 1972.

Drucker, Peter: *Management: Tasks, Responsibilities, Practices,* Harper & Row, New York, 1973.

Duke University Graduate Program in Health Administration, Report on the 1973 National Forum on Citizenry and the Hospital, Department of Health Administration, Duke University, Durham, North Carolina, 1974.

Ewell, Charles: "Relationships Between Program Innovation and Hospital Governance," Ph.D. dissertation, University of Wisconsin, Madison, 1974.

Filley, Alan C. and Robert J. House: *Managerial Process and Organizational Behavior,* Scott Foresman and Company, Glenview, Ill., 1969, pp. 60-64.

Forehand, G.A. and B. Gilmer: "Environmental Variation in Studies of Organizational Behavior," *Psychological Bulletin,* vol. 62, pp. 361-382, 1965.

French, J.R.P. and B. Raven: "The Basis of Social Power," in D. Cartwright (ed.), *Studies in Social Power,* University of Michigan, Ann Arbor, 1959.

Georgopoulos, Basil S. and Floyd C. Mann: *The Community General Hospital,* Macmillan, New York, 1962, p. 567.

Gilmore, Kay and John R. Wheeler: "A National Profile of Governing Boards," *Hospitals, J.A.H.A.,* vol. 46, pp. 105–108, 1972.

Goldberg, Theodore and Ronald Hemmelgard: "Who Governs Hospitals?" *Hospitals, J.A.H.A.,* pp. 72-79, Aug. 1, 1971.

Hahn, J.A.L. and W.C. Bornemeir: "Views on Physician Board Membership," *Hospital Topics,* vol. 48, pp. 24-25, 1970.

Hare, A.P.: "A Study of Interaction and Consensus in Different Sized Groups," *American Sociological Review,* vol. 17, pp. 261-267, 1952.

Hare, A.P.: *Handbook of Small Group Research,* Free Press, New York, 1962.

Hemphill, J.K.: "Leader Behavior Associated with Administrative Reputations of College Departments," in R. M. Stodgill and A. E. Coons (eds.), *Leader Behavior, Its Description and Measurement,* Monograph 88 Bureau of Business Research, Ohio State University, Columbus, 1957.

Hickey, W.J.: "The Functions of the Hospital Board of Directors," *Hospital Administration,* pp. 43–52, Summer 1972.

Holloway, R.G., J.W. Artis, and W.E. Freeman: "The Participation Patterns of Economic Influentials and Their Control of a Hospital Board of Trustees," *Journal of Health and Human Behavior,* vol. 4, pp. 88-89, 1963.

Hospitals, J.A.H.A.: "Profile of a Hospital Trustee," vol. 49, p. 51, Jan. 16, 1975.

Kaluzny, Arnold D. and James Veney: "Who Influences Decisions in the Hospital? Not Even the Administrator Really Knows," *Modern Hospital,* pp. 52–53, Dec. 1972.

Kovner, Anthony R.: "Hospital Board Members as Policy-Makers: Role, Priorities, and Qualifications," *Medical Care,* vol. 12, no. 12, pp. 971-982, Dec. 1974.

Kovner, Anthony R.: "Governing Boards," *Hospital Administration,* vol. 20, no. 1, pp. 65-72, Winter 1975.

Lanser, Ross E.: "Visible Traits of Boards of Directors," Ph.D. dissertation, Stanford University, 1969.

Lattin, Norman D.: *The Law of Corporations,* Foundation Press, Brooklyn, N.Y., 1959, pp. 211-278.

Laur, Robert: "A Study of the Extramural Sector of Governing Board Responsibilities in Non-Profit General Hospitals: Trustee Interest in Inter-Organizational Relations," Ph.D. dissertation, University of Minnesota, 1969 (available from University Microfilms, Ann Arbor, 1970).

MacEachern, Malcolm T.: *Hospital Organization and Management,* Physicians Record Co., Chicago, 1946.

Mechanic, David: "Sources of Power of Lower Participants in Complex Organizations," *Administrative Sciences Quarterly,* vol. 7, pp. 349-364, 1962.

Modern Hospital: "Trustees' View of Administrators Told," *Modern Hospital,* p. 29, Oct. 1968.

Perrow, Charles: "The Analysis of Goals in Complex Organizations," in W.A. Hill and D.M. Egan (eds.), *Readings in Organization Theory,* Allyn and Bacon, Boston, Mass., 1967, p. 130.

Perrow, Charles: "Goals and Power Structure: A Historical Case Study," in Eliot Friedson, *The Hospital in Modern Society,* The Free Press, New York, 1963.

Pfeffer, Jeffrey: "Size and Composition of Corporate Boards of Directors: The

Organization and Environment," *Administrative Sciences Quarterly,* vol. 17, no. 2, pp. 218-228, 1972.

Pfeffer, Jeffrey: "Size Composition and Function of Hospital Boards of Directors: A Study of Organization-Environment Linkage," *Administrative Sciences Quarterly,* vol. 18, no. 3, pp. 349-363, 1973.

Price, James L.: "The Impact of Governing Boards on Organizational Effectiveness and Morale," *Administrative Sciences Quarterly,* vol. 8, pp. 361-378, 1963.

Roth, R. and S.K. Misra: "Changed Attitudes as a Function of Size of Discussion Groups," *Journal of Social Psychology,* vol. 59, no. 2, pp. 247-257, 1963.

Schulz, Rockwell: "Relationship Between Medical Staff Participation in Hospital Management and Factors of Cost of Hospital Care," Ph.D. dissertation, University of Wisconsin, 1971 (available from University Microfilms).

Schulz, Rockwell: "Does Staff Representation Equal Active Participation?" *Hospitals, J.A.H.A.,* vol. 46, pp. 31–55, 1972.

Schulz, Rockwell and T.E. Chester: "Physician Participation in Hospital Management Decisions: Expectations in the United States and Experiences in England" (forthcoming).

Selznick, Phillip: *TVA and the Grass Roots,* University of California Press, Berkeley, 1949.

Shostak, Arthur B.: "The Future of Poverty," in John Kosa (ed.), *Poverty and Health,* Harvard University Press, Cambridge, Mass., 1969, pp. 264-291.

Simon, H.A.: "Authority," in C. M. Arensberg (ed.), *Research in Industrial Human Relations,* Harper & Row, New York, 1957.

Smith, Harvey L.: "Two Lines of Authority Are One Too Many," *Modern Hospital,* Mar. 1955.

Thompson, G.C. and F.J. Walsh, Jr.: "Selection of Corporate Directors," Conference Board Record 2, pp. 8-16, 1965.

Thorsrud, Einar: "Participation—Industrial Democracy," speech before International (IUC) 17th Annual Conference, Bergen, Norway, Aug. 23, 1970 (unpublished). Author's address is Work Research Institutes, Oslo, Norway.

Toomey, Robert E.: "Governance of the Hospital: Place of the Trustee," in *The Governance of Hospital,* A Report of the 1970 National Forum on Hospital and Health Affairs, Duke University Graduate Program in Hospital Administration, pp. 39-49, 1970.

Vance, Stanley C.: "Administrators on Hospital Governing Boards: A Growing Trend," *Trustee,* pp. 18–26, January 1973.

Vance, Stanley C.: *Boards of Directors: Structure and Performance,* University of Oregon Press, Eugene, 1964.

Whyte, W.F.: "The Social Structure of the Restaurant," *American Journal of Sociology,* vol. 54, pp. 302-310, 1949.

Wise, Harold: "A Closer Look at Community Control," *4th Annual Report: Martin Luther King Health Center,* Bronx, New York, 1971, pp. 32-44.

Zald, Mayer N.: "The Power and Function of Boards of Directors: A Theoretical Synthesis," *American Journal of Sociology,* vol. 75, pp. 97-111, 1969.

Zald, Mayer N.: "The Social Control of General Hospitals," in Basil Georgopoulos (ed.), *Organization Research on Health Institutions,* Institute for Social Research, Ann Arbor, Mich., 1972, pp. 51-81.

Zald, Mayer N.: "Urban Differentation, Characteristics of Boards of Directors and Organizational Effectiveness," *American Journal of Sociology,* vol. 73, pp. 261-272, 1967.

Chapter 5

The Medical Staff

"The physician's attitude toward the hospital is that it is an instrument designed to serve him and his patient, and that, within reasonable bounds he has the right to demand the resources he deems essential for the optimal care of his patient" (Pellegrino, 1972, p. 302). "Most hospitals are in fact run by the doctors" (Knowles, 1970, p. 58). "The doctor was and is officially a guest of the hospital (he is outside the formal organization)" (Guest, 1972, p. 294). These quotations suggest just some of the issues and dilemmas related to the medical staff in the community general hospital.

The medical staff is the organization of physicians who have appointments to admit and treat patients in the hospital. It is important therefore that we have some understanding of the physicians who make up the medical staff—where they come from, their education, and their resulting behavior patterns. In this chapter we also examine the organizational arrangement of physicians in the hospital, as well as their activities, responsibilities, and relationships as a collective body. Finally, some of the issues arising from physician-hospital relationships are considered.

PHYSICIANS WHO MAKE UP THE MEDICAL STAFF

This section describes the kinds of individuals who are selected for medical school, medical education and its influences on physician behavior, the profession of medicine, and some of the behavioral characteristics and impressions of physicians as identified in behavioral research.

Who Become Physicians?

Career choices for the professions are frequently determined early in life. Medicine is a field in which an individual can contribute in a major way toward meeting social needs in addition to receiving other intrinsic rewards. Freidson (1972), however, suggests that there is little evidence that individuals aspiring to become physicians have a stronger service orientation than those aspiring to other occupations.

Competition for entry into medical school is severe. For the medical class entering during the 1975-76 school year, there were approximately 350,000 applications filled by 45,000 applicants for 14,800 actual positions. Furthermore, those that apply usually have substantial qualifications, for it is well known that only those students with a strong academic preparation and high grades stand a chance of being admitted. Despite this fact, the number of applicants has substantially increased every year for the past several years. It is also estimated that there were approximately 6,000 Americans enrolled in foreign medical schools in the 1973-74 academic year. Moreover, almost every medical school in the United States in 1974 could probably have filled its first-year class with applicants who were already armed with a Ph.D. The University of Miami Medical School, for example, which has a special program for the conversion of scientists with a Ph.D. into physicians within two years, had over 649 applicants for its 28 positions in 1974.

The "average" medical student represents less than 5 percent of American college graduates. About 90 percent of his colleagues will graduate with an M.D. degree while some 10 percent will drop out, not completing their training for a variety of reasons. Today's medical student has a median IQ of 126.

In the past, over half of all medical students were children of physicians, but in 1968 only 15 percent were children of physicians (Smith, 1971). In 1971 only 11 percent of the entering class of future physicians were women. By 1974-1975 they increased to 22.2 percent. Indeed, it is interesting that the United States has one of the lowest percentages of women medical students and practicing physicians in the Western world. Over 88 percent of the students in public medical schools are state residents, while the percentage is increasing at private medical schools, reflecting increasing state financial support.

While black Americans constituted over 11 percent of our nation's population, in 1974-1975, 7.5 percent of the nation's medical students were black. The number of black and other minority group medical students is increasing yearly.

In a review of research related to attitudes of entering medical students, Freidson (1972, p. 174) suggests there is a trend toward an increasingly scientific orientation. However, at the same time we hear of increasing concern with behavioral problems in the treatment of patients. In his study of the ideology of physicians, Colombotos (1969) found that physicians from lower-class backgrounds were much more likely than those from upper-class backgrounds to emphasize the success values of social prestige and economic opportunity as their original reasons for going into medicine. However, when it comes to present concern with these values the differences according to socioeconomic backgrounds almost disappears; the more success-oriented become less so and the less success-oriented become more so according to Colombotos.

Beginning in the late 1960s entering medical students appeared to be more socially concerned and active, as were students generally. While only a very few of these students have entered practice at the time of this writing, a number of medical faculties report that today's students are more humanistically oriented, and more interested in primary care and less in superspecialization than were their predecessors (*Medical Economics,* 1973).

What Is the Conditioning Process of Medical Education?

From the first day of medical school through residency training, both their favorable and unfavorable experiences mold the future attitudes and behavior of the developing physicians.

It has been suggested that medical education tends to reinforce the values of aggressiveness, impersonality, and distance—complaints that are very frequently directed against physicians. Rezler (1974) suggests from a review of the literature that the medical school environment fosters cynicism.

One impression particularly relevant to the management of health institutions was stated in an address by James Dennis, M.D. (1967) when he was Dean of the University of Oklahoma School of Medicine:

As medical students, interns and house staff officers, we are exposed to a rigidly organized and structured discipline that provides no real opportunity to participate in or learn the democratic process. After six to eight years of professional conditioning as the lowest man in a feudal (futile?) system, the M.D. is trained to quickly assemble some facts, promptly make his decision and to stick to it. He learns to make a decision then to think in terms of right and wrong and not to compromise. Once in practice he must gain acceptance from his peers so he identifies with them and communicates with them almost to the exclusion of others—a process that guarantees the reinforcement of his own prejudices and fosters group bias, which is usually expressed in some form of "motherhood."

The actions and reactions of organized professional groups, including medical school departments, usually reflect these ingrained characteristics by assuming a positive posture of being "right"—frequently with dedication. Since it is wrong to compromise on what is "right," we tend to deal from a position of all or none.

Freidson (1972), in summarizing data on the values of physicians, concludes that:

. . . while physicians do not lack a service or collectivity orientation, it does not seem to be a very prominent value compared to others. Furthermore, the value is addressed to concern for helping individuals rather than serving society or mankind. Second, physicians have some intellectual investment in their work, everyday practitioners having less than others emphasizing instead practical knowledge and action. Third, physicians emphasize the value of the income and prestige connected with their occupation. And, finally everyday practitioners more than others emphasize the value of independence and autonomy. These values, I believe, stem from the social background of the practitioner more than from his work reflecting both the values of this bourgeois origins and special intent or career choice (p. 178).

Training to be a physician is a long and rigorous process. In the recent past—the 1950s and 1960s—it has meant four years to obtain a bachelor's degree, four years of medical school, and then another eight years for internship, residency, military service, and some practice time before becoming certified as a specialist. Of course, physicians are delivering medical care at least from the time of their internship. It is interesting to note, however, that of the physicians who graduated from medical school in 1960 and 1964 only about 45 percent obtained their license to practice medicine one year after graduation and approximately 30 percent were not licensed until five or more years after graduation from medical school (National Board of Medical Examiners, 1973). Moreover, the essentials of medical education policy statement endorsed by the Liaison Committee on Medical Education of the Association of American Medical Colleges (AAMC) and the American Medical Association, affirms that "undergraduate medical education prepares the student for further education in a graduate program and not for the independent practice of medicine" (Levit, 1974). Recently however there have been steps to shorten formal training periods. Some schools accept students after only two years of college, there is a strong trend toward a three- rather than four-year medical curriculum, the internship requirement has been eliminated by almost all specialty boards, and some boards have eliminated the practice requirement for certification.

Almost all graduates of United States medical schools pass state licensing exams on their first try and few doctors ever have their licenses revoked. Moreover, once a physician is licensed, he generally does not have to submit evidence of continuing education, unless he practices in one of the few forward-looking states that require this as a condition for reregistration of the license to practice.

Nearly 90 percent of medical school graduates in 1960 and 1964 went on to residency training. Only about 25 percent of those in family and general practice went on to residency training, but opportunities for family practice residences and certification have only really developed since 1969 (Janeway, 1974). Both the number of residencies offered and those filled have increased over the years. Unfortunately, the number of residency positions vacant has also risen and almost one-third of all residents are graduates of foreign medical schools. The large number of foreign medical graduates from non-Western nations in the United States has been called scandalous by many because of the less rigorous education standards of some foreign schools and the great need for physicians in other countries.

Internship and residency training presents unique opportunities and problems for teaching hospitals. By and large a teaching program is recognized as fostering higher quality care and enhancing the prestige of a hospital. An affiliation with a medical school is believed by most to be essential to a successful teaching program. Unique problems in teaching and medical school affiliations include: service versus educational responsibilities by and for house staff (i.e., interns and residents), the high costs of a teaching program, and aspects of the medical school affiliation agreement such as who pays what, how quality controls over patient care and teaching responsibilities are administered, and who are teaching patients.

A physician's choice of a specialty is very important, for it defines his contribution to health care. The increasing proportion of physicians training for subspecialties such as cardiology or gastroenterology continues to reduce the number of physicians involved in primary health care, e.g., family medicine, general pediatrics, and general internal medicine. This specialization has been an important factor in producing today's doctor shortage. In recent years, the American Medical Association, long regarded as a proponent of professional birth control, advocated expansion of the number of medical school students and a doubling of doctor output. The National Institute of Health estimates that there is a doctor shortage of almost 70,000 and the medical profession predicts there will be over 22,000 annual employment openings for physicians through 1980. However, it should be pointed out that while only 12,000 medical graduates are being produced annually, there is evidence that by the 1980s the number of graduates may exceed the need.

Every year the proportion of physicians providing general medical care decreases and patients find it more and more difficult to find a doctor who will serve as their family physician. During the Depression, 120,000 general practitioners provided primary health care, but by 1970 that number had dropped to 79,000. Although the ratio of all doctors to the population has increased from 140/100,000 to 158/100,000 over the past decade, the number of patient visits has doubled. Moreover, there has been a drain of physicians into residencies, teaching, research, administration, and retirement so that only 90/100,000 physicians remain in private practice with many of these in subspecialties. It is generally agreed that residency programs are training too many general surgeons. The tragic implication of having too many surgeons is that they may be overutilized—that is, perform unnecessary operations (Wolfe, 1972; Lewis, 1969; Knowles, 1972). Moreover, overpopulation in surgery contributes to the deprivation of those who need help from primary care physicians. It is interesting to note that the Province of Quebec in Canada reportedly is permitting only the top half (as measured by grades) of medical graduates to pursue specialty training. Similar practices occur in other countries, and have many important implications in addition to training more family practitioners, not the least of which is elitism.

Organized Medicine

The American Medical Association has long been the traditional voice for American physicians. In addition to its efforts to improve the quality of physicians' services, which it still pursues actively today, the AMA has worked toward reforms in the delivery of health services. For example, in 1917, it endorsed the concept of compulsory health insurance. This resolution was based on an AMA report that included the following prophetic statement (Somers and Somers, 1967, p. 2):

> The time is present when the profession should study earnestly to solve the questions of medical care that will arise under various forms of social insurance. Blind opposition, indignant repudiation, better denunciation of these laws is worse than useless. It leads nowhere and it leaves the profession in a position of helplessness as the rising tide of social development sweeps over it.

However, in 1920, the resolution to endorse compulsory health insurance was rescinded. Since then, the AMA has sought to preserve the independence and financial position as well as the technical competency and ethics of the physician. Like most of the population during the Depression, physicians had problems obtaining work, i.e., patients. Until recent years, the AMA, the professional agency of physicians, was a major factor in restricting the number of medical school students (Kessel, 1970). Throughout the thirties and forties it opposed Social Security legislation and voluntary health insurance since it did not want third-party intervention in medicine. In the late sixties when both had come into effect, the AMA, faced with an attempt to institute compulsory national health insurance, argued for increased voluntary health insurance instead of government involvement.

Over the years the power of the AMA has waned, as has its membership. In 1971, only 57.6 percent of all physicians were members, although the percentage of physicians in private practice who belong to the AMA is larger than that. Perhaps the main criticism of the organization among doctors is that it does not represent the physician's interests vigorously enough. There are left-wing groups in medicine such as the Medical Committee for Human Rights and the Physicians for Social Responsibility; however, their membership is small and is drawn generally from some of the Eastern cities, full-time employees of government agencies, and university medical schools. Much faster growing are the groups who attack the AMA from the right, such as the Association of American Physicians and Surgeons and the Congress of County Medical Societies. In the view of these and other physician groups who are unhappy with the "unprofessional" control over medicine, the answer is to unionize. Although AMA leadership remains opposed to true unionization, seeing it as a sellout of professional integrity, the physician's union movement is enjoying growing support. While less than 15,000 physicians are members of some type of union today, a national survey indicated that over 60 percent of America's doctors believe that physicians should unionize (Paxton, 1972). Another poll showed that more than half would strike as long as emergency services were not shut down (ibid.).

Specialty boards such as the American Board of Surgery and specialty associations such as the American College of Surgeons also have considerable influence on physicians and on the type of medical care received by consumers. The principal and almost exclusive objective of specialty boards and associations has been to upgrade the qualifications of specialists. Until recently, this has meant increasing the length of time needed for training and development of subspecialties, and sponsoring numerous continuing education programs and professional journals. Certification by a specialty board after rigorous examinations and proven abilities in practice is indeed a recognition of professional competency. Fellowship in a specialty college is also a meaningful peer recognition of competence.

Specialty groups have come under criticism for their inattention to national manpower requirements (Knowles, 1968). Recently, the surgical specialty groups have been addressing themselves to problems of overpopulation and considerations of overtraining.

Incomes of physicians are at an all-time high. The average take-home pay of office-based doctors before income taxes in 1972 was $42,700, and $62,500 for doctors incorporated in groups, according to a 1974 report prepared by the congressional research service of the Library of Congress. While these are averages, incomes exceeding $100,000 before taxes are not rare for some specialties such as pathology, surgical subspecialties, and even some general practitioners. Although these are earnings after the deduction of business expenses, many doctors complain that their practice expenses have been rising faster than their incomes. The 1975 crisis concerning soaring costs and difficulties of obtaining malpractice insurance is an example. Percent of expenses to billings vary widely from 15 to over 50 percent depending upon a physician's specialty and office services. The average doctor today spends as much time on each patient as he did in 1950—approximately 18 minutes. Although a physician collects over 91 cents of every dollar billed, the balance being bad debts or free care, the costs for high-profit office items such as injections, x-rays, and laboratory procedures have increased, and many more procedures are done in the hospital today, thus depriving the doctor of these large income-producing sources. Increasing burdens are also being placed on physicians' time and energies by peer review requirements of PSROs and the hospital utilization and quality review activities that are described in the next section of this chapter. Physicians could increase their productivity by delegating more tasks to other health personnel such as physicians' assistants or by working longer hours; the latter, however, places a strain on themselves and on their families.

Generally, a physician may earn more by working more, but not in the same ratio as the additional hours worked. These diminishing returns are being discovered by doctors, and many are changing their ways of practice. Because of a desire to delegate responsibilities such as finances, and to have more free time, doctors have been leaving solo practice and joining or forming more partnerships, expense-sharing group practices, and medical corporations. Foundations, HMOs, and other prepaid medical groups are becoming more common, as are salaried physicians who work limited hours.

In spite of all the criticism that is heaped on organized medicine today, it is clear from the high regard patients have for "their physicians" (confirmed from many surveys) that by and large doctors are totally dedicated to the welfare of their patients. At times expectations for the individual patient come into conflict with the organizational requirements of the large and complex hospital, hence conflict between physician and hospital. The increasing demands of society at large for cost and quality controls over medical care are naturally viewed as a threat to the traditionally sacred physician-patient relationship, hence conflict between organized medicine and the representatives of people—be they in government or from consumer groups.

HOSPITAL MEDICAL STAFF ORGANIZATION

The Joint Commission on Accreditation of Hospitals (JCAH)[1] states: "There shall be a single organized medical staff that has overall responsibility for the quality of all medical care provided to patients, and for the ethical conduct and professional practices of its members as well as accounting therefore to the governing board" (JCAH, 1970). While the governing board is recognized as having ultimate responsibility, the medical staff is considered to have responsibilities of "self-government" delegated to it by the governing board (AMA, 1964 and AHA, 1965).

The JCAH (1970) states:

Medical staff membership shall be limited to individuals who are fully licensed (by their state) to practice medicine and, in addition, to licensed dentists. These individuals, after having made formal application, may be granted membership on the staff in accordance with its bylaws, rules and regulations and within the bylaws of the hospital. Members of the medical staff must be professionally and ethnically qualified for positions to which they are appointed. Appointment to the medical staff is a privilege granted to the applicant by the governing body after considering recommendations made by the medical staff through established mechanisms. The medical staff must define in its bylaws the requirements for admission to staff membership and for the delineation and retention of clinical privileges.

Medical staff membership is usually categorized as:

Active medical staff: These are the individuals who deliver most of the care in the hospital and are the ones who are eligible to vote and hold office.
Associate medical staff: These are individuals who are being considered for active staff membership. Although they may not hold office, they may serve on committees and may be able to vote depending upon the hospital.

Other categories are courtesy, consulting, and honorary medical staff membership, which do not carry voting or officer privileges and have limited influence on the admission of patients.

Public or governmental hospitals as well as private hospitals may, and in general do, enforce rules controlling medical staff privileges so long as these rules bear reasonable, provable relationships to patient care and to the hospitals' professional

---

[1] About three fourths of the short-term hospital beds in the United States are in JCAH accredited hospitals. The JCAH is also discussed in Chapter 11 (Management of Quality).

standards. Indeed, during recent years, the trend of the law has been to enlarge the public hospitals' governing bodies' control of the institutions' medical standards (Southwick, 1967). On the other hand, nongovernmental hospitals are losing some of their freedom regarding medical staff privileges, particularly discriminatory practices unrelated to professional qualifications. For example, *Greisman v. Newcomb Hospital*[2] struck down a requirement in many hospitals that medical staff members must belong to the county medical society, and therefore the AMA, in order to be eligible for hospital privileges.

The JCAH requires medical staff bylaws, rules, and regulations to establish a framework for self-government and a means of accountability to the governing body (see "Guidelines" in the *Formulation of Medical Staff Bylaws, Rules and Regulations*, Chicago, JCAH, 1971). However, in a survey of a number of hospitals (Cadmus, 1967) some problems were found with bylaws including:

Unuse of and/or nonadherence to bylaws
Creation of bylaws by administrators without medical staff participation
Copying of model bylaws that are unrelated to the individual characteristics of the hospital

An example of the medical staff organization of a hospital that has both a chief of staff and a general medical staff president is portrayed in Figure 5-1.

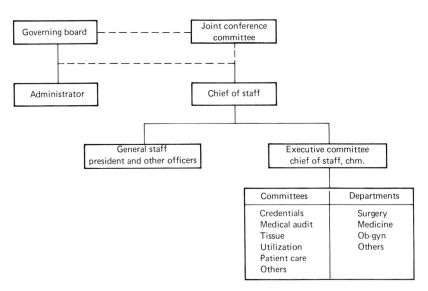

Figure 5-1 Example of a medical staff organization in a community general hospital. (Adapted from Kenneth J. Williams, "The Chief of Staff—The Hospital's Man or the Staff's Man," in C. Wesley Eisele (ed.), *The Medical Staff in the Modern Hospital*, McGraw-Hill, New York, 1967.)

[2]*Greisman v. Newcomb Hospital*, 40 N.J. 389, 192 Atlantic 2d. 817 (1963).

As noted in the previous chapter, the Joint Conference Committee is intended to serve as liaison between the governing board and the medical staff. It usually has no intrinsic authority but serves as a committee for formal communications between the board and medical staff. In an analysis of minutes from the Joint Conference Committees of three hospitals ranging in size from under 100 beds to over 300, Taylor (1967) found the following to be the most frequently discussed subjects over a three-year period: (1) equipment, (2) JCAH requirements, and (3) emergency room organization and procedures. Martin Stone (1971), Associate Director of the JCAH, suggested that the Joint Conference Committee has not been "overly impressive" as a liaison device. Harvey and Wallace (1972) concluded from their survey of 44 hospital administrators that Joint Conference Committees are ineffective devices for communication between trustees and medical staff.

The chief of staff has responsibility for "enforcing medical staff by-laws, rules and regulations" (JCAH, 1970). He is answerable to the board and not to the medical staff (Williams, 1967). Yet, in many, if not most, hospitals the chief is elected by the medical staff, and serves on a voluntary nonpaid basis for a term of up to about three years.

The chief of staff provides liaison between the governing board and the staff and between the hospital administration and the staff. He appoints all committees other than the executive committee whose members may be elected by the staff or appointed by the board or administrator or some combination of these. The chief of staff has leadership responsibility for quality control and for medical staff education, both of which are the major functions of medical staff organization.

The president of the staff in hospitals that have a chief of staff is more of a representative of the staff than of the hospital. He will frequently serve a one-year term or two consecutive one-year terms which are indicative of more of an honorary role. His primary task is to chair general medical staff meetings.

It is important to note that the terminology we have used is not consistent for all hospitals. This is especially true when the president and chief's roles are combined into one position in which case either term may be used. When there is only one position the JCAH refers to it as president (JCAH, 1970).

Another term for a head of a medical staff, and in this case, usually in larger teaching and governmental hospitals, is that of a medical director. He is usually a full-time hospital salaried and appointed chief of staff. In such institutions the organization chart might appear as shown in Figure 5-2.

In some hospitals, the medical director may report to the administrator, in others the medical director may report directly to the board, and, in a few, the administrator may report to the medical director. These roles and relationships are discussed in Chapters 9 and 16. The executive committee in hospitals with full-time medical directors frequently consist of full-time chiefs of medical departments such as surgery and medicine. There are other variations, for example, in university hospitals, but we will not add to the confusion with further elaboration.

The executive committee of the medical staff acts on behalf of the medical staff in addition to coordinating the activities and general policies of the various depart-

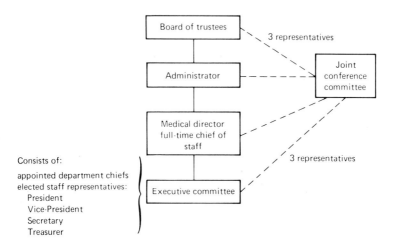

Figure 5-2 Example of a hospital organization with a full-time medical director. (*Source:* Kenneth J. Williams, "Why a Medical Director," in C. Wesley Eisele (ed.), *The Medical Staff in the Modern Hospital*, McGraw-Hill, New York, 1967.)

ments and services. It should meet at least monthly, with the administrator or his representative also in attendance, according to the JCAH. Its functions should include at least the following to meet JCAH standards:

Receive and act upon reports of staff committees

Consider and recommend action to the administrator on all matters of a medico-administrative nature

Implement approved policies of the medical staff

Make recommendations to the governing body

Take all reasonable steps to ensure professionally ethical conduct on the part of the staff members and to initiate such prescribed corrective measures as are indicated

Fulfill accountability to the governing body for the medical care rendered to patients in the hospital, and

Ensure that the medical staff is kept abreast of the accreditation program

Other committees are responsible for meeting other accreditation requirements and for maintaining high standards of care.

Medical Staff Selection

The Medical staff is required by the JCAH to establish a procedure to ensure a fair evaluation of qualifications and competence for appointment and annual reappointment to the staff. This is frequently done by a credentials committee in larger hospitals based on recommendations of the department to which the physician or dentist is applying for privileges. Procedures include a clear definition of privileges such as the types of surgical or medical procedures the individual is judged competent to perform. There must also be a mechanism for review of decisions and the right to be heard when requested by the practitioner. Final decisions are rendered by the governing board.

Medical Care Evaluation

According to the JCAH, each medical staff member must be held accountable for the appropriateness of care rendered to patients. Peer review procedures are performed by a number of committees as well as by departments in larger hospitals. These committees might include: a medical audit committee that reviews practices and outcomes against criteria or norms; a tissue committee that reviews tissues from surgery to provide surveillance over normal tissues removed, and analyzes necropsy reports; and a medical records committee that reviews the quality of medical records essential to effective evaluation as well as management of patient care. Utilization review is also required by third-party payers such as Medicare to ensure that beds and ancillary services are used appropriately and not unnecessarily. Departmental reviews are also required (or general medical staff reviews in smaller hospitals). These meetings must be held monthly to review the care and treatment of patients. This would include a review of selected deaths, unimproved patients, complications, and so forth. Additional meetings are recommended such as clinical pathological conferences (case studies) and necroposy reviews.

The medical staff is also required by the JCAH to participate in other patient care review activities such as pharmacy and therapeutic policies and other hospital departmental policies that affect patient care. This is frequently accomplished through a patient care review committee that includes members of the hospital administrative staff representing departments such as nursing and pharmacy.

For accreditation, the medical staff is required to provide a continuing program of professional education for medical staff members. This should include hospital-based activities and not just educational opportunities from outside the hospital.

Obviously, the medical staff organization and its activities are extremely significant in hospitals that meet standards of accreditation. In Chapter 9 (Management of Quality) we will consider accreditation, PSROs and other medical staff activities further.

We now move from the descriptive aspects of physicians and the medical staff to some of the major issues.

ISSUES

There are a number of major issues in hospital administration related to the medical staff. We will review salaried chiefs of service, remuneration of hospital-based specialists, and staff participation in management decision activities.

Full-Time Chiefs of Service

Having full-time salaried physicians in hospitals is not a new phenomenon; it has been part of the tradition in a number of European countries. It also occurs in the

United States in governmental institutions such as the Armed Forces, the Public Health Service, the Veterans Administration, and state and local hospitals. Many group practices have a salary-type method of distributing income, and some voluntary community hospitals have had salaried pathologists, radiologists, and other hospital-based specialists. University hospitals are frequently staffed predominantly with *strictly full-time*[3] salaried physicians. Increasingly, community hospitals with strong intern and residency programs have a full-time medical director and full-time salaried chiefs of services. Teaching and educational administrative requirements usually require full-time efforts in major teaching hospitals.

Arguments for and against salaried physicians have been discussed for years. Those opposed to salaried physicians contend that physicians paid on a fee-for-service basis will do more work and be more responsive to patients. There is evidence to support this, as noted in Chapter 2. On the other hand, there is evidence that the fee-for-service arrangement is more costly. There is no conclusive evidence, however, regarding quality under the two arrangements, since there is no universal definition of quality.

Organized medicine—i.e., AMA, state and county medical societies—has argued against salaried physicians in community hospitals and in the past against group practice in many communities calling it the "corporate practice of medicine." A number of states have laws against the corporate practice of medicine, most of which were passed in the 19th century. Many of the arguments related to corporate practice of medicine have concerned the methods of reimbursing pathologists and radiologists; these will be discussed in the next section. As recently as June 27, 1974 the AMA House of Delegates approved in principle that the AMA "study in greater detail the trend, prevalence, arrangements, and possible difficulties to hospital medical staffs as a result of control exercised by the governing boards appointments of salaried department heads and salaried chiefs of staffs . . ." (*Medical World News,* 1974).

During the 1960s increasing numbers of hospitals employed directors of medical education (DMEs). Many, however, found that it was difficult to separate education from quality care review and other medical staff administrative needs. Consequently, many DME positions evolved into full-time chief's positions. Continuing pressures for quality care and utilization review have placed further burdens on medical staffs, and more are employing full-time chiefs. Although the number of hospitals with full-time chiefs appears to be growing, most community general hospitals do not employ such persons since many physicians consider it a threat to the private practice of medicine.

Since the medical director and full-time department chiefs function as hospital rather than medical staff representatives, it is likely that the independence of the private practitioner is decreasing (Williams, 1967). Roemer and Friedman (1971), however, argue that in their survey they found a higher quality of care in addition to a better control of costs in hospitals with highly structured medical staff organizations employing full-time chiefs of staff and departments.

[3] A *strictly full-time* physician is one whose entire income from patients is channeled through the medical school or hospital and who is paid a salary. A *geographic full-time* physician is associated full-time with the medical school, but retains at least a major portion of his income from patient services.

The trend towards full-time chiefs raises questions about the changing role of the hospital administrator. The medical director or full-time chief may be an equal with the administrator, he may report directly to the administrator as chief executive officer to integrate the organizations, or he may be the chief executive officer with the administrator reporting to him. Currently, the prevailing mode in community hospitals appears to be that of medical directors reporting to a nonphysician chief executive officer, as suggested by Williams (1967). Ashley and Shmock (1972), however, suggest the medical director should be the chief executive officer since medical care is the major activity of the hospital. Trends and countertrends are evident with the VA moving away from physician chief executives while a few larger teaching hospitals have returned to physicians as chief executives.

We suggested in Chapter 2 that medical practice is becoming more institutionalized, centering around the community hospital. One can argue that full-time chiefs are either a cause or effect of this trend. Either way this has important implications for the organization and management of hospitals and for the roles of administrators. These implications are discussed in later chapters. Governing boards, medical staffs, and administrators must work out what is best to help achieve their own institutional goals and objectives.

Remuneration of Hospital-Based Specialists

Anesthesiologists, pathologists, physiatrists, and radiologists are physicians who manage hospital-based services of anesthesia, laboratories, physical or rehabilitation medicine, and x-ray, respectively.

In the 1930s and 1940s pathologists and radiologists were salaried at relatively low levels, since hospital income from their services were low. However, after World War II hospitals began increasing rates for laboratory and x-ray proportionately more than rates for hospital rooms because patients seldom complained as much about laboratory and x-ray charges as about room rates. Consequently, the large profits generated by these services were applied to losses from other hospital services.

Pathologists and radiologists, in addition to feeling exploited by hospitals, suffered an inferiority complex in relation to independent practitioners. They alleged that "being treated differently from other doctors, who normally bill directly and collect their own fees deprecates them in the eyes of the profession and public as 'hospital employees' rather than 'real doctors' " (Somers and Somers, 1967, p. 133). They also argued that "any hospital that employs doctors to render services for which it charges a fee is engaged in illegal 'corporate practice of medicine,' and the physicians so employed are engaged in 'unethical practice.' " Hospital administrators on the other hand argued that hospital-based specialists do not have the same doctor-patient relationships as independent practitioners; that they have a monopoly in the hospital wherein the patient has no choice; and that it is disconcerting and expensive for the patient to receive numerous separate bills. Consequently, hospital administrators and board members stated that they had ultimate responsibility, and therefore must have reasonable employer controls over these services.

The conflict came to a head with the development of Medicare in 1966: Should hospital-based physicians be reimbursed under the hospital portion (Part A) or the physicians' portion (Part B)? The result was that the physicians' portion of laboratory or x-ray services was placed under Part B and the hospitals' under Part A. The net result was an increase in separate billing by hospital-based physicians.

Currently arrangements with hospital-based specialists are usually on one of the following bases:

Salary from the hospital

Percentage of gross receipts, usually one-third of laboratory receipts in the case of pathologists or in a few cases a percentage of net laboratory profits, which places cost control as well as income incentives on the pathologist.

Lease arrangement whereby the hospital-based specialist leases space and maintenance services from the hospital and manages the service as an essentially independent operation.

There was a definite trend away from salary arrangements following the implementation of Medicare. Katz (1973) reported that over half the pathologists in the country were on a percentage arrangement and that a number of pathologists take home more than $100,000 annually before taxes. John Knowles, M.D., former director of Massachusetts General Hospital, now President of the Rockefeller Foundation, states: "It disturbs me when you get up into the $90,000 and $100,000 bracket at a time when cost of medical care is rising so fast and the radiologist is averaging a 40-hour week, you just can't justify that value placed on his services. It's just too much, when a pediatrician is working twice as hard and making $35,000 a year" (Katz, 1973).

Obviously, there is increasing concern about the remuneration of hospital-based specialists. Earnings differential among specialists is of concern to many physicians as well. One wonders whether, if medical staff members had participated in decisions regarding remuneration of hospital-based specialists and there had been a high degree of trust among the medical staff and trustees and administrators, such controversies and exploitations over the years might have been prevented.

Medical Staff Participation in Management Decisions

Medical staff membership on hospital governing boards was discussed in the preceding chapter. However, there is more to staff involvement in hospital decision activities than just membership on the governing board. Schulz (1972) found that in 20 percent of the hospitals in his two-state survey that had no medical staff members with voting privileges on the governing board, medical staff members reportedly participated actively in major decision activities by other means.

A number of authors and two major national study commissions have suggested that one of the primary factors contributing to the rising costs of hospital care and to problems in the management of hospitals is the lack of physician involvement in hospital management. Knowles (1966), for example, states that the medical profession controls over 88 cents of the hospital dollar, but is not held responsible nor accountable for costs. The Secretary's Advisory Committee on Hospital Effectiveness (U.S. Department of Health, Education and Welfare, 1968) was particularly emphatic about the importance of the physician's involvement in hospital management. The report related an interesting fable to underscore the point:

> The intelligent visitor from Mars was interrogating a hospital administrator on the purposes, functions, and administration of a hospital. The Martian was told that the doctors in the hospital order the procedures for patients and thus determine how the resources are used and what work members of the staff do—that the physicians decide which patients to admit and when to dismiss them.
>
> "And where do these important persons stand in your organization?" the man from Mars asked.
>
> "Actually, they stand outside the organization," the hospital administrator explained. "They are paid by our customers and they must observe certain rules, but by tradition the hospital must not interfere or try to influence their decisions."
>
> "But you must be joking!" the visitor exclaimed. "As anyone can plainly see, such an arrangement would be impossible to manage."
>
> The administrator acknowledged that it was not easy. The intelligent visitor was heard to mutter as he was leaving,
>
> "Impossible—or very, very expensive."

Other problems in hospital relationships may be the result of a lack of medical staff involvement. For example Harvey and Wallace (1972) in their survey of 44 hospital administrators reported that "With few exceptions, all [administrators] indicated a need for greater understanding among governing board members, the medical staff, and the administration." However, they did not draw the conclusion that greater medical staff participation in hospital governance and administration was the solution. Shortell (1974), in reviewing studies by Georgopoulos and Mann, Roemer and Friedman, and Neuhauser, suggests: "[these studies] imply that giving physicians increased participation in the affairs of the organization through salaried employment or other means may be an effective approach to issues of utilization-quality control and efficiency. . . ."

In a survey of hospital administrators in Illinois and Wisconsin, less than one-third of the hospitals reported that medical staff members participated actively in the review of income and expense statements, the selection of the director of nursing service, or the preparation of hospital objectives and program priorities (Schulz, 1972). In 40 percent, medical staff members reportedly participated actively in preparation of the hospital budget and in about 60 percent staff members reportedly participated actively in negotiations regarding remuneration of hospital-based specialists.

The lack of participation in major decision activities might be attributed to a number of factors:

Physicians are not interested in participating or may not feel competent to participate in such managerial activities.

Physicians feel it is a misuse of their training and time.

Administrators and trustees will not permit physicians to participate for fear of diminishing the authority and power of administrators and trustees. (Research in other settings, however, suggests participation may strengthen administrative power [Mulder, 1971].)

Questions also remain regarding how to provide for efficient yet effective physician participation and accountability. In addition to board and/or board committee membership, participation can be achieved through administrative committees and activities. Having full-time medical directors and department chiefs is another possibility. In Chapter 4, physician membership on governing boards was discussed. At this point we will consider physician participation in management decisions without trying to distinguish between governance and management decisions nor clinical and administrative decisions. Distinctions between governance and administrative and clinical decisions are becoming less clear since each impinges increasingly on the other; this is so even though all agree that medical decisions for specific patients are the prerogatives of the patient's physician within the constraints established by the medical staff, board, and administrative policies. For example, the privileges granted to a physician are usually defined by the medical staff, while the board and administration generally decide what types of illnesses will be served by the hospital.

We define physician participation in management decisions as having a number of physicians (or duly selected representatives of physicians who officially and effectively communicate with other physicians) discuss, deliberate, and help decide such issues as:

Definition of hospital goals and plans, and evaluation of institutional success in achieving goals through review of financial and other evaluative statements
Allocation of resources, e.g., money, personnel, and facilities
Obtaining resources, e.g., level of charges and facilities
Other management policies relating to how goals are to be achieved
Certain personnel decisions, e.g., selection of an administrator or other key administrative heads, defining qualifications, and deciding on levels of compensation

Another reason why organized medicine wants a greater voice in governance and administrative decisions (in addition to those cited in Chapter 4) is that it appears to be concerned about the growing power of hospital governing boards and administrators. In her warning about this, Anderson (1973), of the Office of General Council of the AMA, noted:

In some institutions, the situation has become so grave as to create a line of authority that goes from the attending staff to a salaried medical hierarchy which in turn is responsible to a hospital administrator often styled as President of the hospital and frequently, not only chief hospital executive, but the dominant voice on the hospital governing board. In the institutions where the hospital administrator occupies the role of hospital president and chairman of the hospital governing board, the only line of communication between the governing board and medical staff is through him. This is lay domination at its zenith and a trend that should be aborted as early as possible.

On the other hand, administrators and governing board members have been heard to complain that physicians don't really understand the problems of administering a large and complex institution operating under increasing internal and external constraints. It has been suggested that there is a conflict in goal priorities in hospitals with the physician concerned with providing service to the individual and the administration and board with maintaining the organization as a whole (Goss, 1963). At least, there are frequently suspicions of goal conflict since the administrator sometimes believes that physicians aren't really concerned with the welfare of the hospital and physicians sometimes believe the administration and board are really not concerned about the welfare of their patients. Participative management is recognized as a way to foster goal conformity and promote understanding (or cooptation). In other nonroutine industries participative management has been shown to increase satisfactions.

The primary expectation of national policy makers from physician participation in management decision activities is that it will help control hospital costs. Some ways in which it might help to do this are:

If physicians participated in decisions of management to reduce costs, they might be more supportive of efforts. For example, one hospital administrator was unable to reduce nurse staffing as recommended by industrial engineering consultants. Reportedly, this was because the nurses enlisted support from physicians to pressure the administrator not to implement the presumably more efficient staffing plan.

If physicians participated in decisions regarding allocation of funds and other resources, there might be a more effective evaluation of requests for more staff, equipment, or new services, and a greater willingness to say no to extravagant requests. Lay boards and administrators are frequently hard-pressed to refute claims from physicians, nurses, or other professionals who state that a new service, higher staffing levels, or more equipment will improve quality.

Physicians are oriented primarily toward the patients' needs and might therefore be more concerned about costs they incur. The board and administration may be more concerned about institutional growth and prestige, as well as quality, which tend to increase costs (Schulz and Rose, 1973).

If physicians participated in budget and other financial matters, they might be more knowledgeable and concerned about unnecessary utilization of beds and ancillary services. (This could foster higher costs, however, if participating physicians were, at least subconsciously, to help serve institutional goals of growth and maximizing income by increasing utilization.)

Closer communication between administration, board, and the medical staff through participative decision making might increase the knowledge and interest of the administrator and board in medical staff peer review activities and result in closer board surveillance of the effectiveness of such efforts. The governing board does have ultimate responsibility for the quality and costs of care delivery in the hospital.

On the other hand, one can see how increased medical staff participation might lead to problems even if it could be achieved at all.

It could diminish the influence of administrators, governing board members, and individual physicians. If physicians were given management information and a say in decision making, this, coupled with their status and technical expertise, might change their role and weaken professional-lay checks and balances. It might also place unusual power in the hands of a few physicians, thereby diminishing the independence of the individual physician further.

It could result in more goal conformity, thereby minimizing conflict, which promotes change. It could also result in management by consensus, which might well reduce institutional flexibility and delay the decision-making process.

It might foster even more rapid cost increases. For example, the following arguments might be made to show that it can help to increase costs:

Participation in management and governance activities would take away from the time a physician could spend on patient care, which would misutilize physicians.

A physician's training and orientation are antithetical to a management role and physicians are frequently believed to be poor managers.

Physician participation in budget matters, program plans, and so forth might use their influence to extract even more costly services and facilities. Physicians are oriented towards maximum service for their patients, not cost containment.

Physicians are already involved in the activity most related to their role in cost containment, that is, peer review to prevent overutilization of services.

A search of the literature found many opinions about physician participation, but little empirical evidence that would shed light on these questions. Schulz (1972a) found that, in the few cases where there appeared to be extensive participation, there was no statistical evidence of major differences in utilization of hospital services or hospital cost indicators.

While there appears to have been little experience with physician participation in the United States, Great Britain has recently reorganized its health service to allow physician participation in management decisions as national policy (Battistella and Chester, 1973). The nationalized organization for the delivery of health services in Great Britain is of course different from the system in the United States.

However, it appears that within the British National Health Service, using a management team approach, physicians are able to participate and be effective members of the team. Apparently, such participation gives physicians a greater voice and accountability for management decisions. It may improve satisfaction and it appears to develop physician support for decisions made. It does not reduce hospital costs, but apparently does result in savings that can be used for other purposes (see Schulz and Chester, 1975). It also calls for different roles within the hospital, which we discuss in Chapter 9. We discuss other conclusions and implications about physician participation in Chapter 16.

In conclusion, we suggest no group associated with the hospital is more important, frustrating, exciting, or unexpendable than the medical staff. While some physicians are reactionary, others are very progressive. It has been our experience that in a partnership with trust and understanding, physicians can be most supportive of goals, and will work hard to achieve them.

REFERENCES

AHA: *The Medical Staff and Your Hospital,* American Hospital Association, Chicago, 1965.

AMA: *Report on Physician-Hospital Relations, June, 1964,* Council on Medical Service Committee on Medical Facilities of the American Medical Association, Chicago, 1964.

Anderson, Betty Jane: "Hospital Governing Board and Medical Staff Relations," paper presented to the North Central Medical Conference Program in Bloomington, Minnesota, Oct. 20, 1973, reprinted in the *Milwaukee Medical Society Times,* 1973.

Ashley, John T. and Carlton L. Shmock: "The Medical Director in a University Teaching Hospital," *Journal of Medical Education,* vol. 47, no. 6, pp. 453-459, 1972.

Battistella, Roger and T.E. Chester: "Reorganization of the National Health Service," *New England Journal of Medicine,* vol. 289, pp. 610-615, 1973.

Bunker, John P.: "A Comparison of Operations and Surgeons in the United States, England and Wales," *New England Journal of Medicine,* vol. 282, no. 3, pp. 135-144, 1970.

Cadmus, Robert R.: "Medical Staff Bylaws, Rules and Regulations," in C. Wesley Eisele (ed.), *The Medical Staff in the Modern Hospital,* McGraw-Hill, New York, 1967, pp. 11-27.

Colombotos, John: "Social Origins and Ideology of Physicians: A Study of the Effects of Early Socialization," *Journal of Health and Social Behavior,* vol. 10, pp. 16-29, 1969.

Dennis, James L.: Speech delivered while Dean, University of Oklahoma School of Medicine. Currently, Dr. Dennis is Vice President for Health Sciences, University Of Arkansas Medical Center, Little Rock, Arkansas.

Freidson, Eliot: *Profession of Medicine,* Dodd, Mead, New York, 1972.

Goss, Mary E.W.: "Patterns of Bureaucracy Among Staff Physicians," in Eliot Freidson (ed.), *The Hospital in Modern Society,* Free Press, New York, 1963, p. 180.

Guest, Robert: "The Role of the Doctor in Institutional Management," in Basil Georgopoulos (ed.), *Organization Research on Health Institutions,* Institute for Social Research, University of Michigan, Ann Arbor, 1972.

Harvey, James D. and Samuel T. Wallace: "Are JCC's Effective Forums?" *Hospitals, J.A.H.A.,* vol. 46, pp. 49-52, 1972.

Janeway, Charles: "Family Medicine—Fad or for Real?" *New England Journal of Medicine,* vol. 291, pp. 337-343, Aug. 15, 1974.

JCAH: *Formulation of Medical Staff Bylaws, Rules and Regulations,* Joint Commission on Accreditation of Hospitals, Chicago, 1971.

JCAH: *Accreditation Manual 1970 Updated 1973,* Joint Commission on Accreditation of Hospitals, Chicago, 1973.

Katz, Delores: "Medicine's New Royalists," *Detroit Free Press,* Feb. 4, 1973.

Kessel, Ruben: "The AMA and the Supply of Physicians," *Law and Contemporary Problems,* vol. 35, no. 2, 1970.

Knowles, John: *The Teaching Hospital,* Harvard Univ. Press, Cambridge, Mass., 1966.

Knowles, John: Presentation at the AAMC annual meeting, Houston, Texas, Nov. 1968.

Knowles, John: "The Physician in the Decade Ahead," *Hospitals, J.A.H.A.*, vol. 44, pp. 57-62, 1970.

Levit, Edithe J., Melvin Sabshin, and Barber Mueller: "Trends in Graduate Medical Education and Specialty Certification," *New England Journal of Medicine,* vol. 290, pp. 545–549, Mar. 7, 1974.

Lewis, Charles E.: "Variations in Incidence of Surgery," *New England Journal of Medicine,* vol. 281, no. 16, pp. 880-884, 1969.

Medical Economics: "Art vs. Science," pp. 20ff., Oct. 29, 1973.

Medical World News: "Full-Time Physicians in Hospitals," pp. 41-47, October 4, 1974.

Mulder, M.: "Power Equalization through Participation," *Administrative Sciences Quarterly,* vol. 16, no. 31, 1971.

National Board of Medical Examiners: *Evaluation in the Continuum of Medical Education,* Philadelphia, 1973.

Paxton, Harry T.: "Unions Now?" *Medical Economics,* vol. 49, no. 9, pp. 31-43, 1972.

Pellegrino, Edmund: "The Changing Matrix of Clinical Decision Making in the Hospital," in Basil Georgopoulos (ed.), *Organization Research in Health Institutions,* Institute for Social Research, University of Michigan, Ann Arbor, 1972, pp. 301-328.

Rezler, Agnes C.: "Attitude Changes During Medical School: A Review of the Literature," *Journal of Medical Education,* vol. 49, pp. 1023-1030, Nov. 1974.

Roemer, Milton I. and Jay W. Friedman: *Doctors in Hospitals: Medical Staff Organization and Hospital Performance,* Johns Hopkins Press, Baltimore, Md., 1971.

Schulz, Rockwell: "Relationships Between Medical Staff Participation in Hospital Management and Costs of Hospital Care," Ph.D. dissertation, University Microfilms, University of Michigan, Ann Arbor, 1972a.

Schulz, Rockwell: "Physicians on Boards: Survey Examines Level, Extent of Participation," *Hospitals, J.A.H.A.*, vol. 46, pp. 51–54, 1972b.

Schulz, Rockwell and T.E. Chester: "Physician Participation in Hospital Management Decision: Expectations in the United States and Experiences in England" (forthcoming).

Schulz, Rockwell and Jerry Rose: "Can Hospitals Be Expected to Contain Costs?" *Inquiry,* vol. 10, pp. 3-8, 1973.

Shortell, Stephen: "Hospital Medical Staff Organization: Structure, Process and Outcome," *Hospital Administration,* pp. 96-107, Spring 1974.

Smith, Louis, C. Remund and Anne R. Crocker: "How Medical Students Finance Their Education," vol. 46, no. 7, pp. 567-574, 1971.

Somers, Herman M. and Anne R. Somers: *Medicare and the Hospitals: Issues and Prospects,* The Brookings Institution, Washington, D.C., 1967.

Southwick, Arthur F., Jr.: "Legal Aspects of Medical Staff Function," in C. Wesley Eisele (ed.), *The Medical Staff in the Modern Hospital,* McGraw-Hill, New York, 1967, pp. 65-85.

Stone, Martin: "J.C.A.H. Standards Emphasize Better Management, Physician Participation," *Modern Hospital,* Feb. 1971, pp. 108ff.

Taylor, Keith O.: "The Joint Conference Committee," in C. Wesley Eisele (ed.), *The Medical Staff in the Modern Hospital,* McGraw-Hill, New York, 1967.

U.S. Department of Commerce: *Statistical Abstract of the United States 94th Annual Edition,* Bureau of Census, Washington, D.C., 1973. Permission to quote received from Medical Economics Company.

U.S. Department of Health, Education and Welfare: *Report of the Secretary's Advisory Committee on Hospital Effectiveness,* 0-295-545, Washington, D.C., 1968.

Williams, Kenneth J.: "The Chief of Staff—the Hospital's Man or the Staff's Man?" in C. Wesley Eisele (ed.), *The Medical Staff in the Modern Hospital,* McGraw-Hill, New York, 1967, pp. 27-35.

Wolfe, Sidney: Presentation to Georgetown University Symposia on the Future of Science, reported in *Biomedical News,* p. 10, Jan. 1972.

Chapter 6

Hospital Programs: Nursing

"Nursing is a troubled profession." The trends and issues that underlie this commonly used phrase hold important implications for the administration of hospitals and other health care institutions and agencies. Most importantly, nursing service is a most, if not the most, critical component in fulfilling hospital objectives for patient care. Nurses constitute the largest single group of health professionals. In 1972, there were 778,000 employed RNs compared with 356,000 medical doctors.[1] About 65 percent of the RNs are employed by hospitals. The first section of this chapter will briefly explore nursing in transition as a background to current issues. The second section will consider issues in nursing, and the third will explore certain proposals, among them the role of nursing and the clinical nurse specialist.

[1]*Source:* American Nurses Association and American Medical Association as reported in *Source Book of Health Insurance 1972-1973,* Health Insurance Institute, New York City.

NURSING IN TRANSITION

The formal nurse training that was evolved in 1860 served as the basic model for nursing education until World War II. It was a matronly model that provided all bedside services in order to reduce the impact of environmental problems such as dirt. Later a model of tender loving care (TLC) was imposed on nursing. While TLC is still expected today, other expectations are changing dramatically. In years past, nursing service was essentially the entire hospital; other hospital employees were there to help the nurses, who in turn served the doctors. Nurses were clearly subservient to physicians; for example, they stood up when a physician entered the room, and they opened the door for him. Nevertheless, they had a close personal relationship with each physician and patient.

Before World War II, nurses served as administrators in a large number of hospitals. While that is still true in a relatively small number of hospitals today, in most the director of nursing is in a second- or third-level position reporting to the administrator, an assistant, or an associate hospital administrator. At that time, nursing education was primarily hospital in-service education with the student nurse providing a great deal of the patient service. It is interesting to note the emergence of conflict between medicine and nursing as early as 1905. Only 5 of the 160 medical schools at that time required any college work for admission to medical school. Attempts by nurses to establish the minimum requirement of a high school diploma as a qualification for nurse training were bitterly opposed by most of the medical profession as a threat to the profession (Alexander, 1972, p. 12).

Profound changes in nursing began during World War II and have been increasing at an accelerating rate since then. During World War II, with acute shortages of registered professional nurse personnel, the nursing field fostered the development of Licensed Practical Nursing (LPN) or, in some parts of the country, Licensed Vocational Nursing (LVN). The number of nurse aides also expanded rapidly since shortages in registered nurses continued until the mid-1970s. Registered nurse shortages were attributed to other employment opportunities for women, major hospital expansion, shortening of the work week, and reduction in services provided by student nurses. Whereas in 1950 51 percent of active nursing personnel in hospitals were registered nurses, by 1974 this dropped to only 33 percent. Meanwhile, many tasks formerly undertaken by nurses were being performed by others (see Table 6-1).

In the 1950s considerable unrest developed in nursing due to low wage levels, the long work week, rotating shifts, and the fact that other health professionals e.g., physical therapists, began doing tasks formerly performed by RNs. Collective bargaining developed in a few locations such as California and Minneapolis-St. Paul, but it was thwarted in many other areas because nurses and other hospital workers were excluded from national labor legislation until 1974. Other factors relating to collective bargaining are discussed in Chapter 13.

During the 1960s, major changes in nursing education occurred. Hospital diploma nursing education programs began closing due to a number of pressures, among

Table 6-1

Original RN functions and activities	Other health workers now providing the service
Diet therapy	Dietician and dietetic aid
Social service—related to disability, hardship, etc.	Medical social worker
Central supply service-cleaning, wrapping supplies, sterilizing packs, etc.	Central supply technician and worker
Medical records—maintenance of charts, records, discharges, abstracts, etc.	Registered medical record librarian
Recreation therapy—activities, games, amusements, reading materials, etc.	Recreation therapist and volunteers, candy stripers, etc.
Rehabilitation therapy	Physical therapist, occupational therapist
Operating room, delivery room—scrub nurse, circulating nurse, etc.	Operating room technician
Bedside nursing	Licensed practical nurse, aide, orderly, volunteer
Nursing specialties—recovery room, postoperative nursing care, monitoring devices, hypothermia techniques, uses of pacemakers, oxygen tents, cannulae, etc.	Inhalation therapist, biomedical engineering technician
Employment interviews (for nursing service)	Personnel director
Administrative tasks	Ward or unit manager and ward secretary

Adapted from Robert E. Kinsinger, "Training Health Service Workers: The Critical Challenge," *Proceedings* of the Department of Labor, HEW Conference on Job Development and Training for Workers in Health Services, Washington, D.C., Feb. 14-17, 1966, p. 27.

them the high cost of nursing education to hospitals, the pressures of the American Nurses' Association for baccalaureate and associate degree education, and the expectations of high school graduates for a college degree. Hospital nursing diploma education programs declined from over 900 in 1960 to less than 650 in 1970, while students in hospital diploma programs declined from nearly 95,000 to 71,000 during the same period (ANA, 1970-71). In addition to the increase in four-year baccalaureate programs, two-year associate degree programs emerged along with the two-year community college development in the United States.

Table 6-2 describes the various levels and initial educational programs in nursing. The term *nurse* covers all of these, yet there is a wide range in training and in roles. There are separate licensing examinations for registered professional nurses (associate degree, diploma, and baccalaureate) and for licensed practical or vocational nurses.

In spite of education differences, Alutto et al. (1971) found that regardless of any initial personality similarities or differences, graduating nurses from associate, diploma, and baccalaureate programs did not differ in terms of cognitive commitments to professional nursing, employing organizations, and clinical specialties. However, other research suggests that education may affect behavior (Highriter 1969; Davis 1974).

In the 1960s and early 1970s trends toward (1) clinical nurse specialists, (2) nurse clinicians, and (3) nurse practitioners developed.

1 Clinical nurse specialists have a master's degree with education in such specialties as pediatrics, obstetrics, or psychiatry. There is also a trend toward certification of specialists. Objectives are to return the nurse to direct patient care and to provide for greater comprehensiveness, continuity, and coordination of patient services, with the clinical specialist functioning as a partner with the physician rather than in a subservient role (Brown, 1971). This development is discussed in more detail in a later section of this chapter.

2 The nurse clinician is a middle-level position of nursing practice that is attained by demonstrating advanced clinical competence in providing leadership for the nursing team. The nurse clinician functions more as a generalist. She may be prepared at any level, i.e., diploma, bachlor's, or master's level.

3 The nurse practitioner, a term frequently used to express the expanded nursing role, usually, but not always, functions in an ambulatory patient care setting. This nurse may be a graduate of any level nursing program from the associate degree to the master's. She needs four months to one year of apprenticeship or formal training to become a pediatric nurse practitioner, obstetrical nurse practitioner (midwife), family nurse practitioner, etc. In most cases she works closely with a physician (Murray, 1973). However, a few have "hung out their own shingle." Nurse practitioners tend to function in areas that overlap with traditional doctor functions, e.g., taking of medical histories, physical assessment, screening of patients, management of long-term care. The problem is that these areas are the ones in which the role of the physician's assistant is developing, and conflict arises between the male-dominated ex-military medical corpsmen and the female-dominated extended nursing practitioners (Reverby, 1972). Physicians' assistants and conflict are discussed in the next chapter.

Table 6-2 Levels and Educational Programs in Nursing

Profession	Total length of professional training beyond H.S.	Indicator of academic structure	Indicator of academic achievement	Certifying bodies	Geographical location of training	Basic skills
Registered nurse—master's degree	5-6 academic years	1-2 years academic interspersed with clinical training in a specialty, e.g., pediatrics or psychiatry. Or, nursing administration or education.	M.S., nursing	University standards and NLN	University hospital & community health agencies	More independent responsibility for quality of patient care. Responsibility for staff and patient education.
Registered nurse—baccalaureate degree	4 years, and summer sessions	Four years academic interspersed with clinical experience, usually in the last two years.	B.S., nursing	State Board of Nursing, University Standards and NLN	University hospital and community health agencies	Psychosocially biologically oriented—concern for total patient and family well-being.
Registered nurse—diploma	27-36 months	1 year academic 2 years clinical courses and experience	Diploma granted by hospital	State Board of Nursing and NLN	Hospital	More task-oriented e.g., catheterization, paracentesis, thoracentesis.
Registered nurse—associate degree	Two years	2 years academic interspersed with clinical experience	Associate degree, nursing	State Board of Nursing and NLN; State & Local educational rules and regulations	Junior colleges; Hospital	More task-oriented e.g., catheterization, paracentesis, thoracentesis
Licensed practical nurse (LPN)	One year	One year academic and clinical experience	Diploma & licensure	State Board of Nursing; State and local rules and regulations	Vocational technical school; Hospital and nursing home	Technical task-oriented "bedside care"

Adapted from Avedis Donabedian et al., *Medical Care Chart Book*, Bureau of Public Health Economics, University of Michigan, Ann Arbor, 1968.

While the distinctions between general duty nurse, head nurse, nursing supervisor, nurse clinician, clinical nurse specialist, and nurse practitioner have apparently been accepted and understood within nursing, this does not appear to be the case with physicians, hospital administrators, and others. We will discuss some of these distinctions, particularly the clinical specialist, in a later section of this chapter since it appears that these roles are gaining wider acceptance.

While clinical nursing and specialization are currently being emphasized at the master's degree level, nursing administration is being deemphasized in university nursing schools. Some nursing schools have either eliminated the master's degree program in nursing service administration, or are offering minimal elective courses in administration to be taken in conjunction with the clinical nursing major. Miller (1972) suggests that nursing administrators in teaching hospitals should have advanced clinical nursing knowledge as acquired in master's clinical nurse specialization programs in addition to training in administration. Others suggest that administration is the key factor and that individuals trained in hospital and health services administration are qualified to fill positions such as director of nursing service in a hospital.

The American Nurses' Association (ANA) and American Hospital Association (AHA) (1971) state that nursing registration (RN) is a prerequisite for a director of nursing service. It is assumed that an individual with an RN would have a greater understanding of requirements of nursing care and advantages in communicating with other RNs, and would be able to direct the development of the nursing care program. However, it is also true that administration is problem- not discipline-centered. In the administration of nursing services, the organization and management component is not significantly different from that of other professional groups.

Nursing in ambulatory settings is also experiencing many changes, particularly in relation to nurse practitioners and extended roles. Nurses in community mental and neighborhood health centers, and in family and pediatric office practices, are providing services in ambulatory and home care and performing tasks that were formerly the sole prerogative of physicians, such as taking patient histories and giving a complete physical examination (Brown, 1971).

We now turn to further exploration of these trends and other issues drawing particularly on a National Commission for the Study of Nursing and Nursing Education (Lysaught, 1970).

ISSUES IN NURSING

The National Commission for the Study of Nursing and Nursing Education (Lysaught, 1970) calls nursing a "troubled occupation." Problems in nursing stem from many of the same sources that create problems in the delivery of health care, and are related to the rapid rate of change in our society.

Growth of Population and Increasing Consumer Demands

The population explosion has placed increasing strains on our health system; nursing, representing the largest health professional group, has experienced some of the greatest pressures. While the productivity of physicians has increased substantially largely due to the delegation of tasks and responsibilities to nursing, that of the nursing profession, which is not able to automate, has not. The delegation of medical tasks to LPNs and nursing assistants has increased administrative work, the growth of allied health professionals has clouded roles, and expanding technologies have created demands for greater specialization within nursing. Although the number of nurses to 100,000 population increased from 268 in 1960 to 380 in 1972 nationally, demand exceeded supply of nurses through the 1960s (U.S.DHEW, 1974). Moreover, ratios vary widely ranging from 176 nurses per 100,000 population in East South Central United States to 509 in New England (ANA, 1971). Part of the shortage was due to a large number of RNs being employed part-time (29 percent in 1970). Moreover, the working life of an RN is about 20 years, or less than half that of the general labor force. It is also interesting to note that nurses spend less than half their time in direct patient care activities. For example, staff nurses spend on the average 41 percent of their time in direct patient care activities with 25 to 30 percent of the balance in planning and coordinating care and in communication related to patient charts. Head nurses spent 15 percent, and nurse supervisors only 7 percent in direct patient care, (Lysaught, 1972). Recently, shortages of nurses have disappeared in many locations with a number of hospital administrators now reporting waiting lists of applicants.

Increasing consumer expectations of quality health care as a right have affected nursing by increasing the need for nurses in ambulatory and outreach care programs. Consumers are also dissatisfied with an apparent diminishing of TLC as technical and administrative demands on nurses increase.

Knowledge Explosion

The knowledge explosion has affected nursing as it has other disciplines. Patients undergoing cardiovascular surgery or renal dialysis, or those in coronary care units and other specialized services require specialized nursing care. The knowledge explosion has also affected nursing education, resulting in increasing numbers of master's and doctoral programs. In 1960, 1,197 master's and 6 doctoral students graduated, but in 1971-1972 over 2,000 master's and 27 doctoral students graduated (U.S.DHEW, 1974).

Women's and Professional Rights and Opportunities

Since approximately 99 percent of registered nurses are women, the profession is not unaffected by the women's rights movement. However, nursing has been faced with professional chauvinism as well as male chauvinism. Nurses are not only no longer willing to subsidize patient care through low wages, they are also no longer willing to serve as handmaidens to physicians—they want to be treated as colleagues.

Career mobility is also a problem in nursing. For example, there is very limited vertical mobility. An RN cannot build on her training and experience if she wishes to become a physician; she or he must start over. The same is true for a nursing attendant (nurse aide) who wishes to become an LPN or an RN. However, within nursing education, steps are being taken to provide for proficiency examinations which would take into account knowledge and skills in order to accelerate baccalaureate or other training.

The status of nurses appears to be lower than that of women in other fields such as business, government, medicine, and teaching (Corwin and Taves, 1963). In a survey of student nurses and personnel in three major hospitals they found that compared to student nurses who had a relatively high image of nursing on the average, the image that the general duty nurses held seemed to be especially low. However, head nurses had a somewhat better image of nursing than general duty nurses. They also found that other nursing personnel had an even lower image of nursing.

Recognition in nursing is usually attained through supervisory positions, with higher pay for the nursing administrator rather than for the clinical nurse. Argyris (1965) suggests that nurses believe an administrator is a second-class citizen. He also suggests that a nurse is free to "blow her top" only in reference to the administrator and this is another factor which gives nursing administration a low-status image. On the other hand, Taves et al. (1963) found that nursing personnel who have higher ranking official positions in the organization are more satisfied with their jobs than lower ranking personnel.

Cost and Quality Control

Increasingly, all health professionals, including nurses, as well as health institutions, will come under more stringent cost and quality controls. There is growing evidence that a great deal could be done to control costs of nursing service more effectively. For example, the Illinois Commission on Nursing (1971) found in its study of 31 community hospitals in that state that:

> Variations in nursing hours per patient day (NHPD) from hospital to hospital were substantial (3.78 to 5.50). They cannot be explained by an apparent need of patients. . . . The study showed no significant relationship between nursing input (NHPD) and output (patient care requirements and the feeling that these requirements are met).
>
> The study furnished substantial evidence of poor scheduling techniques . . . it was apparent that most hospitals in the study determined their staffing needs on the basis of number of beds rather than on the basis of patient census.
>
> Generally, more nursing hours were expended where there was poor use of nursing skills.
>
> The use of labor-saving devices as measured in this study did not produce a decrease in NHPD.
>
> Ironically, measures of relative sophistication in nursing service administration, developed in the study, established a direct correlation between sophistication and NHPD—that is, the higher the sophistication, the greater the number of hours . . . also there was no relationship in the amount of supervision provided and total hours per patient day.

Connor (1961) reports from his research that when available nursing hours increased, there was no increase in direct patient care, but instead an increase in personal time.

In a study of 19 Massachusetts hospitals, Harris (1970) reports low productivity of nurses and overstaffing.

Medical and surgical nursing service represents 20 to 25 percent of total hospital costs; consequently, nursing is more vulnerable to charges of waste than other departments. Studies mentioned previously also note the lack of use of explicit measures of nursing effectiveness as well as efficiency although considerable effort is now going into developing effectiveness measures. In reviewing the literature Foster (1973) reports on nursing's role and opportunities in budgeting and cost controls. It is likely that cost containment efforts will put additional pressures on a "troubled profession."

Other Pressures and Problems

The recent National Commission on Nursing carefully considered issues in nursing and we will quote liberally from this widely respected report (Lysaught, 1970). The Commission, for example, examined nursing in the light of a number of common characteristics of professional groups, as listed below:

> *Level of Commitment.* By such a standard, nursing is certainly placed in an ambivalent position. Setting aside the fact that approximately one-third of those students in preparatory programs drop out before completion of the course, it has been shown that nurses leave their profession at a much higher rate than physicians, engineers, lawyers or teachers. . . .
>
> Many agree that the very function of nursing adversely affects the commitment to a professional career. Davis et al. (1966) state, ". . . one of the more persistent themes to emerge from our field work is that of progressive disenchantment of students with hospital nursing. . . . This would seem to be the thrust of the Willard report (1967) when it characterized nursing as a "fragmented task oriented service."
>
> *Long and Disciplined Education Process.* The second characteristic common to the professions is that of education—a lengthy and vigorous process that incorporates both theoretical and applied content. Throughout the history of American nursing, individuals have striven to change and improve the content, and the process of nursing education. Only the uninitiated observer, however, could feel the results have been satisfactory and the major problems solved.
>
> If some nursing leaders thought that nursing education within the college environment would solve the professional problems, they were headed for disappointment. Bridgeman (1953) found severe shortcomings of nursing educational standards. Strauss (1966) feels that collegiate nursing is still hampered by a number of problems: a variety of educational institutions and degrees, the low academic prestige of nursing within the college or university, a heritage of affiliation with professional schools of education and the induced strain between practitioners who came from diploma schools and educators who are intent on eliminating any but collegiate schools of nursing. . . .
>
> Within the collegiate schools, there is no common agreement on what constitutes the content of the "long and disciplined educational process." Even as a few schools are beginning major curricular overhauling, some critics are suggesting

that collegiate schools are preparing "well rounded nurse generalists" when they should be producing "highly skilled specialists" (Davis et al., 1966). Similarly there are criticisms of the separation of collegiate nursing education from nursing practice and direct patient care—the feeling that the collegiate educators have overplayed their hand in divorcing nursing education from the hospital or from other care facilities.

Perhaps the most ubiquitous criticism of the present state of nursing education as a professional discipline is the lack of research in that discipline and the institutional system providing it. . . .

In short, then, there are difficulties in nursing education that stem from the location, content and the development of content. Furthermore, these problems stack up against nursing in its efforts to satisfy the professional characteristics of a "long and disciplined educational process." Clearly the trend is toward a greater utilization of institutions of higher education; the trend is less clear when we examine the need for reapproachment between education and service that will strengthen meaningful research into the form and content of nursing education.

Unique Body of Knowledge and Skill. One of the most persistent problems faced by nursing is that of defining what nursing is, and what is distinctive about it. This of course stems from the close historical relationship between medicine and nursing, both of them involved in the clinical care of the patient. This dilemma has been heightened by the frequent attempts to define nursing in terms of procedures or techniques that emphasize skill at the expense of knowledge and understanding.

Nursing care is related to medical care and the demarcation between the two professions might be likened to a Venn diagram in which there are both intersections and mutual subsets: a patient might be receiving care during a specified period of time from a physician, a nurse, a therapist and a fellow family member.

Glaser (1966, p. 26) suggests, "It has been easy to define the areas of special nursing competence. . . . But every professor depends on the knowledge accumulated through research and writing, and in this respect, the basis of American professional nursing has been stunted. . . ."

Discretionary Authority and Judgement. Nursing has traditionally been "embedded within a hierarchy of authority" in which its autonomy has been largely circumscribed (Strauss, 1966, p. 62). Most of the medical and nurse practice acts now written place sharp limitation on the authority and judgmental exercise of the nurse. In day-to-day situations, however, Hughes (1958) has recorded that doctors frequently fail to fully exercise their authority and judgement and that the nurse has to exercise more than is legally reserved to her.

Active and Cohesive Professional Organization. It would seem that the American Nurses' Association (ANA) should meet these criteria (of self-governance, source of professional self-discipline, standards, ethics, and cohesiveness). Here again, we find nursing struggling toward, but not yet attaining a completely successful professional association that is characteristic of other disciplines. . . .

In 1967 only 25 percent or just over 200,000 of the registered nurses in the nation belonged to the ANA. In addition, nursing encompasses large numbers of auxiliaries and para-professionals who may or may not share nursing's professional concerns, but who are ineligible for membership in the ANA. Beginning with the first course in practical nursing in 1890, there has been an unending struggle over the roles, the education and control of various aides to nursing.

Nursing, further, has a unique situation to consider: the existence of another national organization that appears to serve many of the same functions as the ANA. The National League for Nursing (NLN) is an organization that . . . includes representatives from nursing, practical nursing, aides, orderlies, allied health professions and lay bodies—accreditation, one of the prime functions of most professional bodies, has resided traditionally with the League rather than the ANA.

Most professional organizations also have a major role in achieving prestige for their members and in determining to some extent the distribution of rewards within the profession. In recent years the ANA has become much more militant in matters of salary and benefits, and has used a number of tactics to apply pressure on hospitals and administrators who fail to meet salary demands. In some cases, the points of argument covered nursing service and the conditions of patient care as well as basic money concerns. This forceful approach to pay and working conditions has not always found favor with those inside and outside nursing—some find it closer to the work of a labor union than a professional group—but this tactic has succeeded in improving salary levels, and most likely accounts for some of the increased membership in recent years.

Whether or not nursing does, or should, enjoy professional status is not the only issue. It is obviously faced with serious problems that affects the major functions of the hospital. Argyris (1965) suggests that there are basic problems such as frustration of the dominant predispositions of nurses. He reports that nurses in the hospital he studied were not able to effectively fulfill such predispositions, e.g., being self-controlled, indispensable, compatible, and expert. Corwin and Taves (1963) suggest that the "drive to gain professional status and achieve a unique place of importance within the hospital's division of labor, inevitably brings the group into conflict with lay administration and physicians who are jealous of their prima donna status within the hospital scheme." Scott (1966) states that "the nurses' drive for professionalism may be based on carving out a special niche for themselves in which they can operate relatively independently from control by other groups and which allows them to claim superior status" (p. 52). Christman (1972) suggests nurses are more a captive of the administrator than of the physician. A number of the problems we have discussed in this section are not unique to nursing. We will therefore explore some of them further in the next chapter after discussing the roles of other health professionals. We also suggest a few possible solutions to some of the problems as they manifest themselves in the institutional setting. Two major issues, the role of nursing and the development of clinical nurse specialists, are discussed below.

PROPOSALS FOR NURSING

Role of Nursing

The U.S. Department of HEW Secretary's Committee to Study Extended Roles for Nurses (1971) concluded that "In this period of rapid transition, the identical procedure performed on a patient may be the practice of medicine when carried out by a physician or the practice of nursing when carried out by a nurse" (p. 12). In trying to define the nurse's role in relation to the physician's role some have suggested nursing is concerned with care while medicine is concerned with cure. Many physicians and nurses will dispute such a separation, noting current overlaps in both areas. Others, including physicians, administrators, and nurses see nursing as "discreet tasks" designed to help and comfort patients in a dependent role carrying out the orders of the physician. While some specific treatments may be done by either a physician or a nurse on occasion, there is relatively little overlap in roles. In this model, the nurse is not seen to require much background knowledge in order to carry out her functions (Hale, 1966). The National Commission (Lysaught, 1970, pp. 61-62) argues against this as being an unrealistic hierarchical arrangement.

Another model suggested by nursing groups emphasizes a decision-making role for nurses. While it designates a separate domain of expertise and practice this approach views nursing as a team effort interacting with the physician and other health workers. It sees nursing as separated into professional (decision-making and leadership) and technical (cure and care services) activities. This approach stems from increased emphasis on the behavioral sciences. It also represents a determined effort by the profession to develop a science of nursing that will permit accurate prediction and control of the outcomes of nursing intervention (Lysaught, 1970, p. 62-63).

The National Commission for the Study of Nursing (Lysaught, 1970, p. 64-76) recommends an interactive model that provides for nursing assessment, intervention, and instruction for patients that varies by patient condition and environmental setting. More specifically it suggests a dynamic model for nurse-physician interaction within this setting, based on patient needs. An example of the reciprocal roles of the physician and nurse in an ambulatory setting is depicted in Figure 6-1 (Lewis, 1969).

Needless to say the role of the nurse is not clear and is in a state of transition, or in the words of Mauksch (1972), "churning." Almost all proposals suggest an expanded role for nurses. We believe that the dynamic interactive model suggested by the National Commission is the most appropriate since it relates to the needs of a given situation. As Lambertsen (1973) suggests, nurses must be prepared to function within unstructured or ambiguous patterns. Physicians and nurses need flexibility in their relationships. As suggested earlier in this chapter, numerous environmental factors will affect the nurse's role. Certain planned activities currently under way such as educational changes, development of physician's assistants, federal studies and demonstration programs, and institutional licensure will also have an important influence. These are discussed further in the next chapter and in the final chapter where we consider the future.

Clinical Nurse Specialist

In 1943 Frances Reiter, a nursing educator, coined the term "nurse clinician" to describe a "superior kind of nurse, distinguished by the depth of her clinical knowledge and by her ability to form collegial relationships with physicians and representatives of other health disciplines" (*Hospitals*, 1973, p. 135). Now, more than 30 years later,

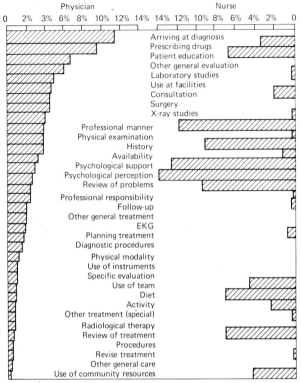

Figure 6-1 Nurse and physician relationships in reference to activities in an ambulatory care setting. (*Source*: Charles E. Lewis et al., 1969.)

there is considerable interest in such roles as clinical specialists, nurse clinicians, and nurse practitioners.

Clinical specialization is assumed to parallel the major medical services such as medicine and surgery. It is the role that is receiving most attention in the larger hospitals. The definition of a clinical nurse specialist does not appear to be very clear even from a review of 181 articles on the subject (Hummel, 1972). However, the literature search showed a considerable degree of consensus about the clinical specialist's roles in the health care delivery system. There was substantial agreement that it involved direct patient care activities (90 percent specified this), interdisciplinary activities (87 percent), developing innovative and experimental approaches to patient care (86 percent), consultation (82 percent), and staff development (66 percent). Patient care was given priority over these activities by 44 percent of the authors. Brown (1970) defines the position as one in which the nurse is "generally outside the organizational line on the chart in order to move where and when she thinks she is most needed. She is a consultant who acts as a practitioner, teacher and supervisor; her primary role in cooperation with the physician may be viewed as that of representative of the patient's interests within the concept of comprehensive coordinated and continuing care" (p. 69).

Whatever it is, the concept is enjoying increasing interest and application among nursing groups. At this state of development it is more important to examine what clinical specialization is attempting to accomplish. It appears from a review of the literature and discussions with those closest to its development that the clinical nurse specialist is expected to:

Help cope with advancing knowledge and technologies. New patient care services such as cardiovascular surgery, renal dialysis, and neonatalogy require advanced nursing knowledge and skills.

Help return the nurse to the patient so she can focus on patient rather than just system needs. This means more accountability and responsibility to the patient and more independence from physicians and nonnursing duties. Accountability also means concerns for costs in relation to benefits.

Broaden as well as expand roles of nurses, particularly in ambulatory care settings, nursing homes, and other places currently all but ignored by health professionals. Presumably the *health* of the consumer will be the focus of attention rather than just intermittent crisis care.

Function more in a collegial team setting as opposed to the current hierarchical relationships. Implied is the training of the clinical specialist in a team setting rather than the current isolation from medicine and other health professions.

Develop more of a professional status for nursing within the previously mentioned criteria for a profession.

A number of studies on the functioning of the clinical nurse specialist in hospitals report improvements in patient care and satisfactions of nurses, physicians, and patients. Simms (1965) reported favorable reactions from patients who were to undergo open heart surgery to improvements resulting from the specialized skills and humanistic approach of clinical nurse specialists. Little (1967) reported improved care for tuberculosis and alcoholism patients through the use of clinical nurse specialists, although some operational problems arose due to the fact that the approaches of the specialists were sometimes in conflict with hospital policies. Georgopoulos and Christman (1970) concluded that clinical specialists brought about impressive gains in patient care and in the performance of other staff workers within an experimental medical and surgical area at University of Michigan hospitals. Barrett (1972) reported that physicians on a surgical unit with nurse specialists reacted favorably in terms of patient care and relationships between doctors and nurses. Ayers (1973) found the initial response of hospital staff members to the clinical nurse specialists to be curiosity, some mistrust, and hostility, much of which subsided as the specialists proved themselves to be competent bedside nurses. The greatest difficulty was with medical social workers, who perceived conflict over professional territory. "The factor that most affected the specialists in developing their roles was the perceived ambiguity of their tasks, duties and functions" (Ayers, p. 141). While most evaluations report many benefits from the use of nurse specialists, to date we have not seen a cost-benefit analysis of the concept. There is considerable research activity to develop outcome measures for nursing care, and with such measures cost-benefit studies should be more feasible.

The changing and expanding role of nurses is evident in a 1973 law enacted in the state of Washington, which permits RNs the right to perform such functions as observation, assessment, diagnosis, care of counsel, and specifies that nurses are directly responsible to the consumer for the quality of nursing care rendered. Both the Washington State Medical and Hospital Associations had opposed the bill; however, the hospital association withdrew its opposition after the legislation was amended to include the phrase "provided, however, that nothing herein shall affect the authority of any hospital . . . concerning its administration and supervision" (*Hospital Week*, 1973).

Other changes directly related to nursing service are being proposed and tried. For example, both the Duke University and University of Florida Hospitals removed nursing services from the direct line authority of the hospital administrator and placed them under the nursing school dean. In both cases, they went back to placing nursing under the hospital administrator. Vanderbilt University Medical Center collapsed all aide categories—dietary aide, nurses' aides, etc. -into that of a general health worker who supports the patient, nurse, and physician, and developed a team of physician, nurse, and general health worker who work together with the same patients (Christman, 1972). This innovation develops team and patient-team rapport and continuity. Other innovations such as service unit management are discussed in the next chapter.

It is apparent that most of the steps being recommended and followed to solve the problems of a "troubled profession" are directed toward improving the knowledge and skills of nurses through more education, specialization, and professional independence. One cannot argue, without any data to the contrary, that such steps will not improve the quality of nursing care and enhance professional stature. Issues related to quality, professionalism, conflict, and cost in nursing and other hospital professions are discussed further in later chapters.

Administration of Nursing Services

The administration of nursing services has been downgraded as an issue because the emphasis has been on enlarging the patient care role of nursing. We, however, believe that there are issues in nursing administration that are at least as troublesome, and that may contribute to problems in patient care. The finding of the Illinois Commission on Nursing (1971) that nurse staffing doesn't relate to patient needs, and other similar findings, implies mismanagement. Turnover rates in nursing service of over 60 percent per year may be beyond management's control, but they at least underscore problems in the management of nursing service. Strikes by nurses such as the 1974 strike in San Francisco where a major issue was nursing influence in management also reflect managerial problems. Sister M. Francesca Lumpp (1974) in describing the "disappearing leader" in nursing service administration found some major dissatisfactions among 268 directors of nursing service in Catholic health facilities. Highest priority dissatisfactions were: (1) nurses' resistance to change; (2) lack of communication, understanding, and cooperation among hospital departments; (3) lack of prepared personnel; (4) difficulty in motivating personnel; and (5) physicians' lack of understanding of the nurses' role. Lower priority dissatisfactions were: (1) lack of policy decisions emanating from the hospital administrator; (2) lack of nursing department budget; (3) lack of continuity of care between hospital and outside agencies; and (4) poor working relations between the director of nursing and the hospital administrator. By way of comparison satisfactions were listed as work to: (1) effect improvements in patient care; (2) promote professional growth among the nursing staff; (3) build strong working relationships between medical and nursing staff; (4) interpret nursing for other persons on the health team; (5) be a change agent in delivery of health care; and (6) grow professionally and personally in a challenging position.

We suggest that nursing has been essentially isolated from the administration and governance of many hospitals. In a major discussion on the role of the director of nursing service at the 1973 annual meeting of the American Society for Hospital Nursing Service Administrators (*Hospitals,* 1974) there emerged substantial reported evidence that directors of nursing are not recognized as functioning at the top administrative level. In the Society's survey of 483 heads of nursing it was found that only 35 percent of the women had the title of "assistant hospital administrators," or the equivalent; others had department head titles such as "director of nursing service." It was also reported that a large number (including some with assistant administrator titles) do not even attend medical staff executive committee meetings along with the administrator. We suspect that few hospitals include nursing directors in board meetings even though nursing is the largest and most important single service in the hospital. We have heard administrators say they do not share overall hospital financial reports with *their* "director of nursing." On the other hand, the Illinois Commission reports, and other evidence indicates, that administrators and governing boards do little managing of nursing service as long as physicians and patients are not complaining about nursing.

As pressures for cost containment and cost effectiveness measures grow, management of nursing services must be strengthened. This doesn't necessarily mean a hierarchically oriented supervisory scheme. On the contrary, we suggest a participative management scheme, which would also utilize such techniques as management by objectives. Moreover, we suggest that a management team concept would be appropriate for most hospitals. In this arrangement the director of nursing services would essentially function as a partner with the hospital administrator and physician members of the team. These alternatives are discussed in Chapter 9.

REFERENCES

AHA: "Position of the Administrator of the Department of Nursing Service in Hospitals," *Hospitals, J.A.H.A.*, vol. 45, pp. 130–131, 1971.

Alexander, Edythe L.: *Nursing Administration in the Hospital Health Care System,* C.B. Mosby, St. Louis, 1972.

Alutto, Joseph A., Lawrence Hrebiniak, and Ramon Alonso: "A Study of Differential Socialization for Members of One Professional Occupation," *Journal of Health and Social Behavior,* vol. 12, pp. 140-147, 1971.

ANA: *Facts about Nursing,* American Nurses' Association, New York, 1970-71 edition.

Anderson, Odin W.: *Toward an Unambiguous Profession? A Review of Nursing,* Center for Health Administration, Series A6, Chicago, 1968.

Argyris, Chris: *Diagnosing Human Relations in Organizations: A Case Study of a Hospital,* Yale University Labor and Management Center, New Haven, Conn., 1965.

Ayers, Rachel: *The Clinical Nurse Specialist,* City of Hope National Medical Center, Duarte, Calif., as reported in *Hospitals, J.A.H.A.,* "The Clinical Nurse Specialist," p. 141, Feb. 1, 1973.

Barrett, Jean: "The Nurse Specialist Practitioner: A Study," *Nursing Outlook,* vol. 20, no. 8, pp. 524-527, 1972.

Bridgeman, M.: *Collegiate Education for Nursing,* Russell Sage Foundation, New York, 1953.

Brown, Esther Lucile: *Nursing Reconsidered: A Study of Change,* parts 1 and 2, J.B. Lippincott Company, Philadelphia, 1971.

Christman, Luther: "Observations by L. Christman and Discussion," in Basil Georgopoulos (ed.), *Organization Research on Health Institutions,* Institute for Social Research, University of Michigan, Ann Arbor, 1972.

Connor, Robert J.: "A Work Sampling Study of Variations in Nursing Work Load," *Hospitals, J.A.H.A.,* vol. 35, p. 404, 1961.

Corwin, R.G. and Marvin J. Taves: "Nursing and Other Health Professions," in H.E. Freeman, S. Levine, and L.G. Reeder (eds.), *Handbook of Medical Sociology,* Prentice-Hall, Englewood Cliffs, N.J., 1963, pp. 187-212.

Davis, F., V.L. Olesen and E.W. Whittaker: "Problems and Issues in Collegiate Nursing Education," in F. Davis (ed.), *The Nursing Profession,* John Wiley, New York, 1966.

Davis, B.G.: "The Effect of Leads of Nursing Education on Patient Care: A Replication," *Nursing Research,* vol. 23, pp. 150-155, Mar.-Apr. 1974.

Donabedian, Avedis, S. J. Axelrod, C. Swearingen, and J. Jameson: *Medical Care Chart Book,* Bureau of Public Health Economics, University of Michigan, Ann Arbor, 1968.

Foster, Katherin Davis: "Annual Administrative Review: Nursing," *Hospitals, J.A.H.A.,* vol. 47, pp. 143-150, 1973.

Georgopoulos, Basil and Luther Christman: "The Clinical Nurse Specialist: A Role Model," *American Journal of Nursing,* vol. 70, no. 1030, May 1970.

Glaser, W.A.: "Nursing Leadership and Policy: Some Cross-National Comparisons," in F. Davis (ed.), *The Nursing Profession,* John Wiley, New York, 1966.

Hale, T.: "Problems of Supply and Demand in the Education of Nurses," *New Eng. Jr. of Med.,* vol. 275, no. 19, p. 1048, 1966.

Harris, David H.: "Nursing Staffing Requirements," *Hospitals, J.A.H.A.,* vol. 44, pp. 64ff., 1970.

Highriter, M.E.: "Nurse Characteristics and Patient Progress," *Nursing Research,* vol. 18, pp. 484-500, Dec. 1969.

Hughes, Everett et al.: *Twenty Thousand Nurses Tell Their Story,* Lippincott, Philadelphia, 1958.

Hummel, Patricia: "Identification of Different Approaches to Clinical Specialization in Graduate Education in Nursing," USPHS Division of Nursing Project, Grant Number 1-D10-NU-09535-01, 1972 (unpublished).

Hospitals: "The Clinical Nurse Specialist," *Hospitals, J.A.H.A.*, vol. 47, pp. 135-141, 1973.

Hospitals: "A Profile of the Nursing Service Administrator," *Hospitals, J.A.H.A.*, vol. 48, pp. 65ff., 1974.

Hospital Week, published by the American Hospital Association, Chicago, Mar. 23, 1973.

Illinois Commission on Nursing: *Nurse Utilization: Illinois, A Study in Thirty-One Hospitals 1966-1970*, vol. 3, Illinois Study Commission on Nursing sponsored by the Illinois League for Nursing and the Illinois Nurses Association, 1971.

Lambertsen, Eleanor: "Let's Get the Nurse's Role into Focus," *Prism*, September 1973, pp. 19ff.

Lewis, Charles E., Barbara Resnik, Glenda Schmidt, and David Waxman: "Activities Events and Outcomes in Ambulatory Patient Care," *New England Journal of Medicine*, vol. 280, pp. 645-649, 1969.

Little, D.: "The Nurse Specialist," *American Journal of Nursing*, vol. 67, p. 552, 1967.

Lumpp, Sr. M. Francesca: "The Disappearing Leader Syndrome in Nursing Service Administration," *Hospital Progress*, pp. 6-8, Jan. 1974.

Lysaught, Jerome: *An Abstract for Action*, National Commission for the Study of Nursing and Nursing Education, Jerome Lysaught, Director, McGraw-Hill, New York, 1970.

Lysaught, Jerome P.: "The House Reunited: It Must Not Fall," *American Journal of Public Health,* vol. 62, no. 7, pp. 957-962, 1972.

Mauksch, Hans O.: Nursing: Churning for Change," in Howard Freeman, Sol Levine, and Leo. G. Reeder (eds.), *Handbook of Medical Sociology*, 2d ed., Prentice-Hall, Englewood Cliffs, N.J., 1972, pp. 206-230.

Miller, Doris I.: "How Should We Prepare Our Nurse Administrators?" *Hospitals, J.A.H.A.*, vol. 46, pp. 120-126, 1972.

Murray, Raymond H. and Shirley A. Ross: "Training the Nurse Practitioner," *Hospitals, J.A.H.A.*, vol. 47, pp. 93ff., 1973.

Reverby, Susan: "Health: Women's Work," *Health Pac*, pp. 15-20, Apr. 1972.

Scott, W. Richard: "Some Implications of Organization Theory for Research on Health Services," *Milbank Memorial Fund Quarterly*, vol. 44, no. 4, part 2, 1966.

Simms, L.L.: "The Clinical Nursing Specialist: An Experiment," *Nursing Outlook*, vol. 13, no. 26, 1965.

Strauss, Anslem: "The Structure and Ideology of American Nursing: An Interpretation," in F. Davis (ed.), *The Nursing Profession*, John Wiley, New York, 1966.

Taves, Marvin, Ronald G. Cronin, and J. Eugene Haas: *Role Conception and Vocational Success Stratification*, Ohio State University Press, Columbus, 1963.

U.S. Department of Health, Education and Welfare: *Extending the Scope of Nursing Practice*, a report of the Secretary's Committee to Study Extended Roles for Nurses, Washington, D.C., 1971.

U.S. Department of Health, Education, and Welfare: *Health Resources Statistics, Health Manpower and Health Facilities, 1974*, DHEW Publication No. (HRA) 75-1509, p. 202.

Willard, W. R. (Chairman): *Nurse Training Act of 1964 Program Review Report*, U.S. DHEW, PHS Publication 1740 (commonly known as the Willard Report), 1967.

Chapter 7

Other Health Professionals and Hospital Programs

The proliferation of health professions in recent decades has been one of the primary factors contributing to the increasing complexity of health services and health services administration. As in nursing, this has created role changes, ambiguities, and conflicts.

In this chapter we consider health professionals other than nurses, including pharmacists, who are also attempting to expand their role, and physicians' assistants, a relatively new health vocation that affects the delivery of health services and the roles of others. Opportunities for programs of outreach that can help hospitals meet some of the broader health needs described in Chapter 1 are also suggested. Finally issues of coordination of programs and licensure of professionals are considered at the end of this chapter.

The U.S. Department of Labor (1970) lists 225 different health vocations. Approximately 125 of these are considered as allied health professionals. Moreover, there are 250 secondary or specialist designations within the 225 vocations. Table 7-1 lists 12 of the 125 health professions and gives their educational characteristics and skills.

As the reader already knows, terminology, definitions, and classifications in health systems are confusing. Nevertheless, to use one source, Greenfield (1969) divides health manpower into four separate classifications: (1) the autonomous professionals, which include physicians, osteopaths, dentists, podiatrists, and optometrists; (2) the allied health professionals, which include nurses, psychologists, cytotechnologists, medical technologists, occupational and physical therapists, pharmacists, medical social workers, and many others; (3) the allied health technicians, which include x-ray technicians, nurses with an associate or diploma degree, medical technicians, and medical and dental assistants; and (4) the allied health assistants, which include licensed practical nurses, nurses' aides, and other categories of aide personnel.

As categories of health vocations have expanded, so have numbers within most of them. While in 1950 there were 3.3 other health professionals for each physician, by 1967 there were more than 10.3 (*Medical Care Chart Book*, 1972). In 1960, the health industry employed 2.6 million persons or 4 percent of the civilian labor force. By 1974 the number rose to 4.5 million, with over 2.5 million employed by hospitals. Within the nongovernmental not-for-profit short-term hospital, the increase from 2.44 employees per patient day in 1963 to 3.14 employees per patient day in 1973 is partially explained by the proliferation and expansion of programs and professions.

Increased numbers of allied health professions have led to the formation of a Commission for the *Study of Accreditation of Selected Health Educational Programs* (SHASEP) to address the following points:

> Professional education in these fields . . . which have become an increasingly vital component of the nation's health services . . . is being seriously encumbered by the costly maze of accreditation requirements and procedures imposed by the multiplicity of professional associations that characterize this important health manpower sector.
>
> The public interest requires that a means be found to promote collaboration between professional associations in allied health and educational institutions in these fields in an effort to create a new system of accreditation that will make possible a coherent, flexible, rational approach to manpower development.

PHARMACISTS AND PHYSICIANS' ASSISTANTS

We have chosen to review pharmacists because pharmacy represents one of the major treatment and expense categories in the hospital and there appear to be more issues associated with it than with some other categories. Physicians' assistants are presented because this is a relatively new field that could have a major influence on the organization and delivery of health services; however, they do function primarily outside of the hospital. Other health fields are not omitted because they are unimportant, but because this book is an overview and it was therefore necessary to limit its scope.

Pharmacists

Many will attribute the real advances in medical treatment since the 1930s to spectacular progress in drug therapy. It is estimated, for example, that 95 percent of the

TABLE 7-1 Selected Characteristics of Representative Members of Health Care Team

Profession	Total length of professional training beyond H.S.	Basic curriculum structure	Indicator of academic achievement	Certifying bodies	Geographical location of training	Basic skills
Dietitian	5 yr	4 yr academic training 1 yr dietetic internship	B.S.—Foods and nutrition certificate for internship completion	American Dietetic Assn. (ADA)—registry exam (trend toward state licensure)	University setting Hospital, nursing homes, etc.	1 Determination of appropriate diet content for treatment of specific diseases 2 Source of information and advice to physicians
Inhalation therapy or respiratory therapy	Usually 2 yr, one summer	1st yr: 70-80% didactic training; 20-30% clinical training 2nd yr: 70-80% clinical training; 20-30% didactic training	Associate degree, inhalation therapy	American Assn., of Inhalation Therapists (AAIT)—registry board AMA-AAIT—review and *approval of schools*, state and local educational rules and regulations	Vocational technical school Hospital	1 Performs selected tests used in diagnosis of pulmonary diseases 2 Performs selected treatments for patients having pulmonary diseases
Laboratory assistant	12 mo	20% didactic training 80% clinical Experience in affiliated lab.	Diploma and certification	Amer. Society of Clinical Pathologists (ASCP) Amer. Medical Tech. Assoc. State and local educational rules and regulations	Vocational technical school Hospital	1 ECG techniques 2 Hematology 3 Urinalysis 4 Bacteriology 5 Serology 6 Chemistry

Table 7-1 (continued)

Profession	Total length of professional training beyond H.S.	Basic curriculum structure	Indicator of academic achievement	Certifying bodies	Geographical location of training	Basic skills
Medical technologist	4 yr	3 yr (90 credits) (basic sciences, liberal arts, etc.) 1 yr: 60% didactic training, 40% clinical experience in lab. (includes 3 mo. internship)	B.S. in med. technology Certificate upon completion of internship	AMA ASCP University approval	University setting Hospital affiliated lab.	Laboratory practice and theory: Chemistry Immunology Bacteriology Hematology
Occupational therapy	4 yr 10 mo	4 yr academic (liberal arts and professional subjects)—some "preclinical" experience, 10 mo. clinical experience	B.S. occupational therapy Certificate for completion of clinical experience (trend toward master's degree in O.T.)	Americ. Occ. Therapy Assn. AMA–university approval	University setting Hospital	Manual arts and crafts, practice in functional prevocational and home-making skills and activities of daily living. Sensorimotor, educational, recreational and social activities for patients
Pharmacy technician	1 mo	On-the-job training under supervision of trained technician and pharmacist	None	None	Hospital	1 Drug dispensation 2 Preparation of selected drugs 3 Maintainance of records
Pharmacist-B.S.	5 yr plus usually 1 yr internship	1st 2 yr: liberal arts; 3rd thru 5th yr: professional courses & basic sciences	B.S. pharmacy	University standards & state licensure	University setting	1 Knowledge of drug action & human physiology 2 Responsibility for drug dispensing

Table 7-1 (continued)

Profession	Total length of professional training beyond H.S.	Basic curriculum structure	Indicator of academic achievement	Certifying bodies	Geographical location of training	Basic skills
						3 Source of information to physician, nurse, patient Same as B.S. but more depth
Doctor of Pharmacy (Referred to as Pharm D.)	6 yr plus 1 yr internship	3rd thru 6th yr: professional courses	Doctor of Pharmacy	University standards and state licensure	University setting	
Pharmacist-M.S. hospital pharmacy or Pharm. D.	2-3 yr beyond B.S.	1 yr academic 1 yr residency or combination of the above in 2-3 yrs.	M.S. hospital pharmacy or Doctor of Pharmacy	University standards and state licensure	University setting Hospital	1 More highly developed understanding of clinical implication of drug use or 2 Improved development of management skills in hospital pharmacy
Physical therapist	4-6 yr; 4 mo. internship	4 yr academic 4 mo clinical experience	B.S., physical therapy	University standards Amer. Registry of Physical Therapists (certification) AMA	University setting Certificate for completion of clinical experience	Therapy programs for patients involving physical means, e.g., exercise, heat, massage
Radiological (x-ray) technician	24 concurrent months 1 New trends: 4 yr programs leading to B.S. in radiological technology 2 2 yr training programs in vocational technical schools	Combinations of didactic training (physics, electronics, etc.) and clinical experience; 1/8 didactic training; 7/8 clinical experience	Certificate from hospital	Amer. Registry of Radiological Technologists (ARRT) AMA Amer. College of Radiologists	Hospital	Performance of radiographic examination

Table 7-1 (continued)

Profession	Total length of professional training beyond H.S.	Basic curriculum structure	Indicator of academic achievement	Certifying bodies	Geographical location of training	Basic skills
Social worker, B.S.	4 yr	4 yr didactic training—small amount of "field" experience	B.S., social work	University standards	University Selected agencies	1 Knowledge of human behavior (small groups and organizational life) 2 Structure and function of community agencies 3 Understanding of development of social policy 4 Planning and evaluation of treatment using above knowledge (casework, group work, and community organizations)
Social worker, M.S.	1 to 2 yr beyond B.S.	Didactic training—50% clinical experience—50%	M.S., social work	University standards	University hospital or health agency	1 More depth knowledge practitioners 2 Supervisor of social work practitioners

Source: Adapted from *Medical Care Chart Book*, 5th ed., Department of Medical Care Organization, School of Public Health, University of Michigan, Ann Arbor 1972.

drugs in use today were unheard of in 1950. On the other hand, medication errors such as inappropriate prescribing or dispensing of drugs contribute to health hazards. On the financial side, expenditures for drugs in fiscal year 1972-1973 was nearly $8.8 billion or nearly 10 percent of total health care expenditures.

While drug therapy has become increasingly important, the pharmacist in the community and in the hospital is experiencing a role crisis. In years past, the neighborhood pharmacist compounded drugs and was a primary source of health service, advising customers on therapy for minor ailments or telling them where or how to seek proper medical service. This role has changed dramatically, since most drug stores are now retailing centers owned by large chains that employ pharmacists to "count pills, insert them in bottles and type labels" (Derzon, 1971). At the same time, the training of pharmacists has been extended to at least five years.

Pharmacy services in hospitals have grown and a specialty of "hospital pharmacist" has developed, with a number of universities offering a Master's or a Doctor of Pharmacy Degree in hospital pharmacy. However, we still find pharmacists in many hospitals just counting pills and labeling bottles. On the other hand, in some hospitals there is centralization and accountability of drug use control by the hospital pharmacy department, which results in a more meaningful role for the pharmacist (Brodie, 1966). In these and some other hospitals the pharmacist truly serves as a consultant to physicians providing advice about the 1,200 drugs generally available, plus more than 6,000 drug combinations that can be issued in a variety of dosage forms and under numerous trade names. It has been frequently reported that "detail men" (salesmen representing drug companies) are still a primary source of "education" for practicing physicians (Greene, 1972). The clinical pharmacist on the other hand is trained to provide more objective and presumably more effective advice to physicians.

Pharmacists in some hospitals have managerial functions as well, such as responsibility for central supply and hospital purchasing in addition to pharmacy. Pharmacists in such roles have titles such as "assistant administrator for materials management."

An expanded role for the pharmacist has been proposed, called a "clinical pharmacist." A task force on the pharmacist's clinical role has proposed that he or she could perform the following functions (*Journal of the American Pharmaceutical Association*, 1971):

Prescribing drugs
Dispensing and administering drugs
Documenting professional activities
Direct patient involvement
Review drug utilization
Education
Consultation

Presumably most pharmacists support this expanded role as do a number of physicians (Hynniman and Lamy, 1971). However, the *Journal of the Indiana State Medical Association* scoffed at the idea of bestowing the designation of "clinical" pharmacist and the practice of letting pharmacists make hospital rounds with a physician to give on-the-spot advice on drugs. The article went on to call the clinical pharmacist "an interloper without portfolio as a therapist" (Greene, 1971, p. 35). A hospital administrator on the other hand suggests "the [pharmacy] profession is changing because it wants to preserve and expand its professionalism" (Derzon, 1971, p. 12).

In a few hospitals, such as those of the University of California at San Francisco and the University of Wisconsin at Madison, the role of the pharmacist has expanded to the point where he or she responds to cardiac arrest calls, takes drug use histories from patients, dispenses drugs and advises patients at the bedside, consults actively with physicians, and monitors drug therapy (Varnum, 1973).

There is general agreement that pharmacists today are overtrained and/or under-utilized. While the expanded role appears to yield a number of benefits such as more informed patients, nurses, and physicians, and reduced medication errors, it is not at all clear to us that added benefits compensate for added costs. We suggest that the development of hospital clinical pharmacy will be thwarted unless rigorous research shows that benefits in terms of health outcome measures are widely judged to be worth the costs.

Physicians' Assistants

We want to briefly consider the relatively new field of physician's assistant (PA). This field has important implications for physicians and other health professionals including its overlap with nursing, and its effect on the delivery of health services. Figure 7-1, developed by Barbara Bates, M.D., who had been a nurse, figuratively represents the relationships between nursing, medicine, and physicians' assistants. It shows some overlap among these three groups in meeting psychological needs and tasks instrumental to diagnosis and treatment. The physicians' assistant usually functions within the sphere of medicine overlapping to some extent with nursing with regard to tasks instrumental to diagnosis and treatment and to a more limited extent in meeting psychological needs.

The physician's assistant program has developed with strong support from physicians and out of a concern that much of a physician's time is spent on functions that do not effectively utilize his or her training and skills. It has been estimated, for example, that pediatricians spend at least half their time in tasks that do not properly utilize their advanced training. Other reasons for developing physician's assistants, in addition to increasing productivity of physicians, were to utilize the skills and training of medical corpsmen returning from Vietnam, to help alleviate nursing shortages, and to attract more males into health services. Moreover, there has been a reluctance in nursing to assume more tasks under physician supervision.

The first formal training program was developed at Duke University in 1965. By 1972, there were more than 112 training programs across the country. Titles and type of training vary considerably. Most PAs are in primary care. Table 7-2 lists selected examples. The Board of Medicine, the predecessor organization of the National Academy of Sciences' Institute of Medicine, has attempted to clarify the differences by

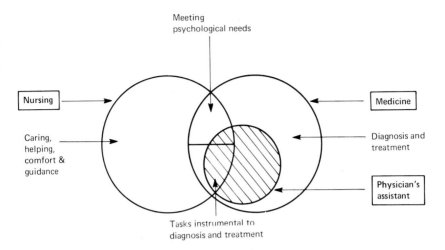

Figure 7-1 Role of physician's assistant who has military service corps background in relation to nursing and medicine. (*Source:* Barbara Bates as presented by Andrus, Len Hughes, and John P. Gayman in H. F. Conn, R. E. Rakel, and T. W. Johnson (eds.), *Family Practice*, W. B. Saunders, Philadelphia, 1973, Chapter 10.)

setting up categories of Type A, B, and C that parallel both the nursing hierarchy (professional, technical, and practical respectively), and the American Academy of Pediatrics definitions (associates, assistants, and aides). At the insistence of organized medicine, physicians' assistants function under the direct supervision of, and in almost all cases are employed by, physicians. Such relationships have been written into statutes in a number of states. In certain rural areas, for example, in Alaska and Wyoming, physicians' assistants may work over 100 miles away from their doctors maintaining communication via telephone or other communication devices.

Smith et al. (1972) found that a PA can increase the productivity of a physician's general office practice by 40 to 75 percent. Another study found that the use of one PA (in a private office practice with two pediatricians) increased total office income by $17,000 with no additional overhead, thus more than covering the PA's $7,600 salary (Smith, 1973, p. 18). Another study in Colorado found that physicians charged patients for PA services from 75 to 100 percent of what they would charge if they had performed the service themselves. One may conclude from these studies that PAs will indeed increase the productivity (and income) of physicians, and thereby the availability of health services, but, other things being equal, will probably do little to reduce the cost of health care.

Other studies have shown that PAs are well-accepted by middle-class consumers. However, they have not been uniformly well-received by either low-income individuals, who might profit most from increased availability of medical services, or by high-income individuals (Pondy, 1970).

PAs have not been particularly well-received by some nurses who feel they could fulfill the role themselves if given a chance and some additional training. In 1972

Table 7-2   Examples of Physicians' Assistants and Practitioner Training Programs

Title of PA	Example of educational institution	Length of program	Credential awarded	Minimum requirements
Physician associate	Brooklyn-Cumberland Hospital and Long Island University	2 years	A.A.	High School Diploma
Physician assistant in family practice	University of Oregon Medical School	1 year, 3 months	Certificate	RN
Medex	University of Washington Medical School	1 year, 3 months	Certificate	Prefer former independent duty corpsmen
Pathology assistant	University of Alabama at Birmingham	2 years	B.S.	Junior college or hospital corpsmen experience
Family nurse practitioner (Primex)	Cornell University New York Hospital School of Nursing	18 weeks, 7½ months in practice	Certificate	RN currently employed and sponsored by ambulatory services agency

Source: Training Programs for Physician Support Personnel, U.S. Department of Health, Education and Welfare Publication No. (NIH) 72-183, May 1972, as reported by Reverby (1972).

there were at least 40 nurse practitioners or nurse clinician training programs that could prepare a nurse to perform many of the PAs' tasks. On the other hand, most hospital nurses state they are unconcerned about PAs because the roles are quite distinct. Conflict however occurs when PAs as physicians' representatives give orders to nurses that appear to be independent of physicians' supervision. Eleanor Lambertson, Dean of Cornell's Nursing School stated, "It is not who does what, but who prescribes and who delegates to whom . . ." (Reverby, 1972). The President of the American Nurses Association stated, "Nurses should not take orders from such assistants because a profession does not take orders from an assistant" (Reverby, 1972).

Because this is a relatively new field, it is difficult to properly assess its influence on the management of health institutions and the delivery of health care. Potentially PAs could have a greater impact on hospitals if, for example, they were employed to fulfill some tasks formerly or currently done by interns or residents or if hospitals utilize PAs for outreach services. Clearly, however, if PAs continue to grow in number this is likely to have a major impact on the need for more physicians, opportunities for expansion of services to promote health and prevent disease, roles of nurses, and so forth.

OTHER HOSPITAL PROGRAMS

Throughout this book, we have attempted to stress the role of the hospital in the larger health system. In this section, we want to briefly discuss outreach services to which a hospital, group practice, or other health institution might look for opportunities to help meet some of the broader health needs of a community. We will examine outreach services in relation to environmental health, promotion of health, prevention of illness, treatment, and rehabilitation.

Environmental Health

We suggested in Chapter 1 that many components of the environment have a majo. bearing on health. Seldom is the hospital considered to have a role in environmental health and there is little evidence that it currently does. We suggest several ways in which it might.

Neighborhood health centers have demonstrated ways in which to deal with environmental factors, e.g., by fostering educational improvements and training the undereducated for health careers, or by exposing and helping to correct housing and sanitation problems. Other ways include supporting economic improvements as well as legislative changes designed to reduce illness and accidents due to alcoholism, drug abuse, pollution, and highway and leisure-time hazards.

American hospitals might follow the lead of Great Britain, where a community health physician is being developed whose task is to identify health needs in the community and then help to bring together the environmental, social, and health services needed to meet them. Few hospitals, group practices, or other health institutions and agencies take a proactive role in improving health in its broadest sense. Almost all are reactive trying to repair the damage that has been done. Obviously, it takes time and money to improve health, as neighborhood health centers have found. However, at the time of this writing research and demonstration funds have been available, and the health institutions interested in innovation and leadership would probably find funds for such efforts because they would be a unique approach for the traditional treatment centers. If the projects and achievements of community physicians in Britain are rigorously evaluated, we suspect that demonstrated benefits would result in making public funds available for further projects.

Occupational Health

Occupational health services offered by a community hospital is the kind of an outreach program that would probably be able to support itself in addition to having a measurable impact on improving health. The majority of industries in the United States employ fewer than five hundred people. Many small factories are marginal in relation to the heatlh standards and requirements of the Occupational Safety and Health Act (OSHA). A number of small manufacturing companies have been put out of business because of workmen's compensation. Such companies are afraid to call in state agencies for fear they might be cited for failure to meet standards. Moreover, they don't know where to turn for help, even if they are aware they have problems. Community hospitals could provide services to such firms, charging a fee to support their efforts. They could serve as intermediaries between industries needing help and state services, providing education and support rather than police services. Rural hospitals might meet a particular need by aiding farmers who work in a most hazardous industry, although funding for such an ongoing service might be difficult to obtain. The need for occupational health services is evident; hospitals and/or physician organizations such as group practices and HMOs have human and technical resources to help meet these needs and improve health in their community.

Health Promotion

Belloc (Haggerty, 1972) reports he and his colleagues found that five factors in the way people live—the amount of sleep, diet, alcohol consumption, regular exercise, and tobacco use—were significantly associated with health. Moreover, the relationship was cumulative—the more positive factors present, the better the health. He reports that people of 55 to 64 who had good health habits had the same health (as determined by their functioning) as 25- to 34-year-olds who had bad habits.

As we suggested in Chapter 1, the evidence is overwhelming that individuals can do much to promote their own health. It is well known that people learn best when they have problems that need answers. Hospitals could do much to educate their patients to good health practices. Hospitals and other health institutions could be centers for consumer health education teaching both patients and the community at large (Somers, 1975). They could also seek to develop activated health consumers—that is, those who know how and when to seek service, how to judge quality, and what their rights are. As recently as 1970 Somers and Somers (1973) identified only 50 hospitals in the entire United States with a planned health education program. A number of studies have shown the effectiveness of patient education activities:

Egbert (1964) at Massachusetts General Hospital randomly assigned 97 patients who had come to the hospital for elective abdominal surgery and divided them into two groups. The 51 patients in the control group were treated in the routine manner. They were told nothing about postoperative pain and were given very little information about what was going to happen to them. The 46 patients in the experimental group were told about the postoperative pain they would feel—where they would feel it, how severe it would be, how long it would last. They were told that the pain was caused by spasms in the muscles under the incision, and taught breathing exercises to relax those muscles and relieve most of the pain. They were also told that if the exercises didn't work, they should ask for medication. Following surgery, the patients in the experimental group requested 50 percent fewer narcotics for pain relief than the 51 patients in the control group. Moreover, patients in the experimental group were able to go home an average of 2.7 days earlier than those who received no health education.

A study was done by Avery et al. (1972) of two groups of asthmatics who used the emergency room of a Baltimore hospital. Twenty-nine patients were placed in small-group classes that discussed the causes of asthma and what the patients could do to alleviate the symptoms. They talked about smoking, diet, general health measures, pollen and dust control, and use of drugs. The other 29 patients received no instruction, but were treated in the usual manner when they had asthma attacks and came to the emergency room for help. At the end of four months, the patients in the experimental group had made 55 fewer visits to the emergency room. The hospital calculated that it has saved $6 in emergency room costs for every dollar it had spent on health education.

Rosenberg (1971) reports on a study of 100 patients with congestive heart failure. Fifty patients and their families received information and counseling about the causes of congestive heart disease, and the role of diet and medication in controlling the disease. The other 50 patients received no special education. At the end of a year, the 50 patients in the education group had spent only one-third as many days in the hospital as the other 50 patients.

Levine (1973) reports a study of 45 hemophiliacs at New England Medical Center in Boston. The patients were taught how to give themselves injections at home to control bleeding. In the year before they received the instructions, each patient spent an average of $5,780 on medical care. The year after the study began, the average yearly expense had dropped to $3,209.

Roccella (1974), who reviewed the above studies, comments, "Although additional more carefully controlled studies of the effect of education of patients and the public would be helpful, there is significant evidence that education of patients could reduce the cost of health care." Here is another opportunity for hospitals to take a leadership role in improving the health and economy of the community.

An individual's place of employment is probably the most convenient and controlled place to provide health education. Certainly, employers have a big investment in the health of their employees. Yet, Kerr (1973) suggests there is virtually no preventive medicine program in industries employing under 500 workers, which represent three-fourths of all workers in U.S. industries. Hospitals and/or other health institutions could be of major assistance in improving the health of employees, particularly in smaller companies. Some of the more progressive companies have programs for their top executives in which the company physician assesses the health potential of the individual and outlines a promotion program to achieve his or her potential for an optimal state of physical and mental healthfulness. Surely, group practices, hospitals, and others can be of assistance in extending such programs.

Prevention and Diagnosis

We suggested a number of ways health institutions can help to control environmental factors in order to prevent accidents and disease. Health screening of high-risk populations is a capability within reach of most health institutions and such services are expanding. Outreach services to prevent alcoholism and treat and rehabilitate alcoholics should be considered as more hospitals establish detoxification, treatment, and rehabilitation units.

Information services can provide worried individuals with information on diseases, symptoms, and sources for help. Some hospitals and agencies have telephone dial access tapes that people can phone to get information.

Home Care Services

Currently hospitals provide outstanding treatment and rehabilitation inpatient services. Numerous studies found evidence of unnecessary admissions and length of stays in hospitals (Zimmer, 1972; Gertman and Bucher, 1971). Home care services by hospitals or effective referral programs to community health agencies and visiting nurses associations can help to alleviate such problems. Studies have also shown over-utilization of nursing home services with estimates of 16 to 23 percent of persons in nursing homes who could be in their own, or in low-rent, homes if home care nursing, dietary, and housekeeping services were available (Markgren, 1972).

Home care outreach services can provide many health and social benefits to the infirm as well as possible financial benefits to patients and those who finance health services. In their study of home care and extended care in the Kaiser Foundation Health Plan in Portland, Oregon, Hurtada et al. (1972) found that such services, when *integrated* with a hospital, clearly contribute to the rehabilitation of a significant number of patients, reduce hospital utilization, and thereby offset costs of the added service.

We have suggested just a few of the opportunities for outreach services. If hospitals and other health institutions and agencies are truly concerned about the health of their community and clients, they must begin to explore opportunities for meeting these broader needs.

ISSUES

We have discussed a number of issues related to the selected professions we have reviewed in this chapter. Four major issues associated with health programs and health professionals are: coordination, control of quality, cost, and conflict. Organizational arrangements to improve coordination of the patient care team are discussed in this section, and licensure, certification, and accreditation are presented as factors in quality control, which are covered in Chapter 11. Costs are considered in Chapter 12 and conflict in Chapter 13.

Coordination of Programs

Coordination of hospital programs must be considered both from the perspective of the overall hospital organization (macrosystem) with all its departments and services, and from that of patient care or the nursing unit (microsystem) with all the bedside and ancillary services required for each patient. Both systems are complex. Goals of the macrosystem are geared more toward institutional effectiveness and efficiency while goals of the micro- or bedside system are oriented more toward effective and efficient treatment for the individual patient. Goals at the macro- and microsystem levels are not always compatible even though patient care is the primary mission of the hospital.

Coordination can be both vertical (hierarchical) and horizontal (lateral). Neuhauser (1972) suggests techniques for maintaining coordination in Table 7-3, showing both hierarchical and lateral coordination, as well as the characteristics and relationships that affect them. In the hospital a nurse or other professional will function as part of a task force in lateral coordination in cooperation with other health professionals in order to serve individual patients. At the same time, the nurse will have hierarchical responsibility to the individual physicians for delegated functions and to nursing and hospital administration for overall effectiveness and efficiency. Simultaneous hierarchical and lateral coordination is usually referred to as a matrix-type organization.

Croog (1963) suggests that the hospital administrative organization emphasizes maintenance of operation or organization. Some hospital administrators strive for strong central hierarchical organization along classical lines of management to provide for more effective and efficient functioning. Heydebrand (1973) suggests that the greater the degree of task complexity (as found in a teaching hospital in contrast to a psychiatric hospital, which has more routine tasks and a homogenous work force), the greater the likelihood that different modes of coordination will be present (i.e., more internalized professional work norms and lateral, interdepartmental coordination). Therefore, bureaucratic-hierarchical modes of coordination will be less significant in complex task situations such as exist in intensive care general hospitals, and coordination is best shifted to the subunit level.

Starkweather (1970, p. 27) also suggests a more decentralized organization to promote coordination at lower levels. He states, "Organizational performance, defined here as the ability of the hospital to properly articulate and coordinate components necessary for the delivery of effective hospital care to patients, is significantly lower in large hospitals." He found in his survey of "six selected hospitals which were alike virtually in all respects except for size . . ." that the larger hospitals were poorer performers in admission time lag, bed turnaround time, and accuracy of dietary services. To cope with this problem Starkweather recommends a decentralized management with considerably greater delegation of authority than is prevalent in larger hospitals today. He calls for a management troika of specialists in administration, nursing, and medicine for each 100-bed unit as the basic decision-making unit (see Figure 7-2).

The service unit management concept (SUM) attempts to provide for greater coordination at the nursing unit for delivering service to the patient as in Starkweather's model; however, SUM does not necessarily call for decentralizing top management or a management troika. Several versions of SUM are in use, and vary in at least two ways: (1) the place of SUM in the hospital organization, e.g., the unit manager reporting to a hospital administrator or nursing administrator in the hospital

Table 7-3 Techniques for Maintaining Coordination

Technique	Examples
I. *Hierarchical Coordination*	
(a) Traditional scalar hierarchy	The classical organization chart, hierarchically imposed rules and regulations.

When the organization's tasks become too complex and too rapidly changing the traditional hierarchy is inadequate and other coordination mechanisms are brought into play.

(b) Staff personnel and departments	"Assistants-to" who back up the hierarchy, staff, planning, clerical personnel.
(c) Automation	Information processing and decision making by computers.
II. *Lateral Coordination*	
(a) Management committees, task forces	Used to coordinate activities between hierarchically separate departments and people.
(b) Direct contact by individuals from different departments to solve problems.	Individual contacts, face to face, telephone, or in writing.
(c) Work teams made up of members from different departments at the production level	The patient care team using the patient's medical record as a coordinating device.
(d) Integrators, integrating departments	Unit managers, scheduling departments, expeditors.
III. *Structural characteristics effecting need for coordination*	
(a) Self containment	Decentralization through independent autonomous subunits (product departmentalization) needing less interunit coordination.
(b) Less specialization	Specialists require coordination while generalists perform a larger range or tasks.
(c) Duplication	Duplication of service departments to coordinate with decentralized production departments; for example, having inpatient and outpatient pharmacy, x-ray, etc.
(d) Decentralization and professionalization (appropriate for complexity not coordination)	Push decisions down to lower levels and increase worker goal congruence. Professional education may lead to ability to coordinate one's work without close supervision.
IV. *Environmental relationships*	
(a) Buffer departments	Admissions office, discharge planning, purchasing, personnel, public relations.
V. *Resource characteristics related to coordination*	
(a) Input inventories	"Floor stocks" provide surplus production inputs and lessen the need for close interdepartmental coordination, but at the price of higher inventory costs.
(b) Queues	As a way of minimizing coordination or as a result of lack of coordination, e.g. waiting lines at cafeteria or x-ray.
(c) Delays	If more coordination is required then the task can be carried out over a longer period of time.
(d) Stabilizing the production	Advanced scheduling and booking avoids the problems associated with peak loads.

Source: Duncan Neuhauser, "The Hospital as a Matrix Organization," *Hospital Administration*, Fall 1972 as modified from Jay R. Galbraith, "Organization Design: An Information Processing View," M.I.T. Sloan School of Management, Cambridge, Mass., Oct. 1969 (mimeographed). Reprinted with permission from the quarterly journal of the American College of Hospital Administrators, *Hospital Administration*.

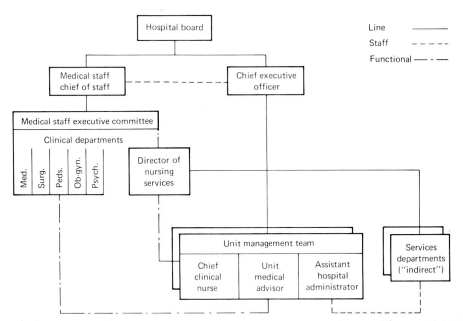

Figure 7-2 Proposed large hospital organization authority and relationships. (*Source:* David B. Starkweather, "Rationale for Decentralization in Large Hospitals," *Hospital Administration*, p. 39, Spring 1970. Reprinted with permission from the quarterly journal of the American College of Hospital Administrators, *Hospital Administration*.)

organization; and (2) the responsibility of the unit manager for numbers of beds, types of tasks, and activities (Jelinek, 1971). Objectives of SUM are:

1 Reduction in cost
2 Improvement in quality care
3 Saving nurse time—and permitting her or him to spend more time at the patient's bedside
4 Increasing personnel satisfaction, and
5 Setting the stage for further improvements

Jelinek found in his study that SUM did not reduce personnel cost (rather, there was some increase in cost). It improved quality, according to his index of judgment of professional nurses and perception of nurses on the unit. It did relieve the professional nurse from some nonprofessional activities but it also increased personal, unoccupied, and standby time. SUM units were found to have higher personnel satisfaction than non-SUM units. And reportedly it did help to set the stage for further improvements. Munson (1972, p. 136) reports that "[SUM] Programs which take over the scut work and leave nurses free to nurse are easy to start because they please nurses initially, but are hard to maintain. Programs which seek to manage a setting in which professionals can practice patient care are more threatening initially because they start with the assumptions that nurses should change, but have more intrinsic vitality if they survive."

There appears to be an increasing interest in unit management organizational arrangements; however, evidence to show that it is the only or even a right answer to the problem of improving effectiveness and efficiency of patient care is far from conclusive. It may improve coordination at the patient care level; however, one administrator who adopted the program reported to us that it handicapped overall hospital coordination and it was expensive. He suggested it was likely to be one of the first activities eliminated if the hospital had to curtail costs sharply.

Further research applying organization theory, e.g. technology, tasks, and structure to the hospital should be helpful in evaluating and developing various modes of coordination.

Licensure, Certification, and Accreditation of Health Professionals

Control of quality, role definition, and mobility of health professionals are functions that have been primarily in the province of state licensure or certification or registration by the various professional groups. These activities were initially established to set standards to improve the quality of service and protect consumers. However, there is increasing concern that they do not set appropriate standards or properly protect consumers; rather, they tend to protect the professions, create inflexibility, fragment services, prevent career mobility, limit progress, and foster inefficiencies in the delivery of health services (Cohen 1973, Hershey 1973).

Licensure is the process by which an agency of government grants permission to persons to engage in a given profession or occupation by certifying that those licensed have met some minimal criteria, usually by passing a standard test and/or attending an accredited program. States license anywhere from 14 to 30 health professions, and criteria for licensure can vary widely between states. Many states also have practice acts that legally define the scope of practice of medicine, nursing, and other professions. Licensing boards are usually dominated by professionals in the field. In most states, once a person is licensed there is no further evaluation of his or her competency, and seldom are licenses removed even when there are gross abuses of consumers.

Recently there have been proposals for a number of changes such as reorganization of licensure boards with public representation and institutional rather than state licensure. Institutional licensure would place responsibility or institutions for appropriate use of personnel, and institutions would be evaluated and licensed if they effectively defined and controlled qualifications of personnel. Proponents of institutional licensure suggest that it would lead to far more effective quality control, offer flexibility in providing more efficient and effective health services, promote upward and lateral mobility, and correct other shortcomings of state licensure (Hershey and Wheeler, 1973), (U.S. DHEW, 1971). There is, however, strong opposition to institutional licensure particularly by the American Nurses Association, on the grounds that it would handicap mobility and diminish professional control.

Another proposal for correcting some of the problems of state licensure is to set up a national certification program that would standardize criteria across the nation (U.S. DHEW, 1971). National certification would recognize that all citizens have a right to high-quality professional services and would help to promote national mobility of health professionals among other stated benefits. Other proposals include reform of present personnel licensure to include more flexible definitions of professional practice, reform of educational prerequisites for licensure, and through enactment of general delegatory provisions such as amendments to the laws to permit the supervised practice of new paramedical professions, e.g., physicians' assistants.

Certification or registration is the process by which an agency or association grants recognition to an individual who has met certain predetermined qualifications. Certification is usually done by a private group or professional association. It has been attacked on the grounds that it fosters some of the problems associated with guilds e.g., preventing upward mobility among health professions. It is difficult, for example, for licensed practical nurses to obtain credit for their previous experience if they want to become registered nurses. Equivalency examinations, however, are used in some professional schools to equate nonformal learning with learning achieved in academic courses or training programs. Proficiency examinations can also be used to promote upward mobility as well as to monitor periodically the qualifications of health professionals.

Accreditation is the process by which the AMA and/or the appropriate professional associations set their standards and then evaluate and recognize an institution or program of study if it meets these standards. As of January 1973, the AMA accredited some 22 different allied health occupations and 2,665 programs. A number of health professionals are reportedly unhappy with AMA dominance over their profession (Reverby, 1972). Brown (1973) suggests that organized medicine has controlled these occupations to its own benefit.

In another recent development, the federal government is spending over $5 million for grants to analyze tasks of health professionals. Preliminary results indicate substantial discrepancies in the understanding and roles of health professionals and many opportunities for improving their utilization and qualifications. As a result of research findings, many changes could develop in controlling quality, role definition, and mobility of health professionals. These changes will have a major impact on the management of health institutions.

REFERENCES

Avery, Charles H., Lawrence W. Green, and Sidney Kreider: "Reducing Emergency Visits of Asthmatics: An Experiment in Health Education," Testimony, President's Committee on Health Education, Pittsburgh, Pa., Jan. 11, 1972.

Brodie, Donald C.: *The Challenge to Pharmacy in Times of Change,* American Pharmaceutical Association and American Society of Hospital Pharmacists, Washington, D.C., 1966.

Brown, Carol A.: "The Division of Laborers: Allied Health Professions," *International Journal of Health Services,* vol. 3, no. 3, pp. 435-444, 1973.

Buchanan, Paul C.: "Laboratory Training and Organization Development," *Administrative Science Quarterly,* pp. 466-477, Sept. 1969.

Cohen, Harris: "Professional Licensure, Organizational Behavior and Public Interest," *Health and Society, Milbank Memorial Fund Quarterly*, vol. 51, no. 1, pp. 73-95, Winter 1973.

Coleman, James S.: *Community Conflict*, Free Press, Glencoe, Ill., 1957.

Croog, S. H.: "Interpersonal Relations in Medical Settings," H.G. Freeman, S. Levine and L. G. Reeder (eds.), *Handbook of Medical Sociology*, Prentice-Hall, Englewood Cliffs, N.J., 1973.

Derzon, Robert: "Should the Role of the Pharmacist be Redefined?" Joe B. Graber and Donald Brodie (eds.), *Challenge to Pharmacy in the '70's*, USPHEW, reproduced by National Technical Information Service, Springfield, Va., 1971.

Egbert, Lawrence D. et al.: "Reduction of Postoperative Pain by Encouragement in Instruction of Patients," *New England Journal of Medicine*, no. 270, pp. 825-827, Apr. 16, 1964.

Georgopoulos, Basil and Lloyd Mann: *The Community General Hospital*, Macmillan, New York, 1962.

Gertman, Paul M. and Bruce M. Bucher: "Inappropriate Hospital Bed Days and Their Relationship to Length of Stay Parameters," presented at APHA Annual Meeting, Minneapolis, Minn., Oct. 11, 1971.

Greene, Clyde C., Jr. "Mutual Concerns of the Physicians and the Pharmacist in Patient Care," in Joe B. Graber et al. (eds.), *Challenge to Pharmacy in the '70's*, reproduced by National Technical Service Information Service, USPHEW, PB 203 019, pp. 32-38.

Greenfield, Harry: *Allied Health Manpower*, Columbia University Press, New York, 1969, pp. 24-28. Other writers have developed different categories based upon certain characteristics associated with each position.

Haggerty, Robert J.: "The Boundaries of Health Care," *Pharos*, pp. 106-111, July 1972.

Hershey, Nathan and Walter S. Wheeler: *Health Personnel Regulation in the Public Interest*, California Hospital Association, Sacramento, 1973.

Heydebrand, Wolf U.: *Hospital Bureaucracy*, Dunellen Publishing Co., New York, 1973.

Hurtado, Arnold V., Merwyn Greenlick, and Ernest Saward: *Home Care and Extended Care in a Comprehensive Prepayment Plan*, Hospital Research and Educational Trust, Chicago, Ill., 1972.

Hynniman, Clifford E. and Peter P. Lamy: "Physicians View the Pharmacist," *Journal of American Pharmaceutical Assoc.*, NS 11, pp. 158-163, April 1971.

Jelinek, Richard: SUM (Service Unit Management): *An Organizational Approach to Improved Patient Care*, W. K. Kellogg Foundation, Battle Creek, Mich., 1971.

Journal of American Pharmaceutical Association: "Report of Task Force on the Pharmacists' Clinical Role," vol. NS 11, no. 9, pp. 482-485, Sept. 1971.

Kerr, Lorin: "Occupational Health—A Discipline in Search of a Mission," *American Journal of Public Health*, vol. 63, no. 5, pp. 381-385, 1973.

Levine, Peter and Anthony F. Britten: "Supervised Patient Management of Hemophilia," *Annals of Internal Medicine*, vol. 78, pp. 195-201, 1973.

Markgren, Paul: "The Impact of Low Rent Housing for the Elderly on Institutional Care," University of Wisconsin, Department of Urban and Regional Planning, Jan. 1972 (mimeographed).

Medical Care Chart Book, 5th edition, Department of Medical Care Organization, School of Public Health, University of Michigan, Ann Arbor, 1972.

Munson, Fred C.: *Crisis Points in Service Unit Management Programs*, Sept. 1972 (unpublished). Available from author at Program and Bureau of Hospital Administration, School of Public Health, University of Michigan, Ann Arbor.

Neuhauser, Duncan: "The Hospital as a Matrix Organization," *Hospital Administration*, Fall 1972.

Pondy, Louis R.: "A Study of Patient Acceptance of the Physician's Assistant," unpublished paper, Duke University, Feb. 1970.

Reverby, Susan: "The Sorcerer's Apprentice," *Health Pac Bulletin*, no. 46, pp. 10-16, Nov. 1972.

Roscella, Edward J.: *Public and Patient Education Consideration in Reducint Health Care Costs*, Presentation at Michigan Public Health Association Manual Meeting, April, 1974.

Rosenberg, Stanley G.: "Patient Education Leads to Better Care for Heart Patients," *HSMHA Health Reports*, vol. 86, pp. 793-802, Sept. 1971.

Smith, Kenneth R.: *Health Practitioners: Efficient Utilization and the Cost of Health Care*, Monograph, Economics Research Center, University of Wisconsin, Madison, Jan. 1973, 30 pp.

Smith, Kenneth R., Marianne Miller, and Frederick L. Golladay: "An Analysis of the Optimal Use of Inputs in the Production of Medical Service," *Journal of Human Resources*, no. 7, pp. 208-225, Spring 1972.

Somers, Anne and Herman Somers: Research Quarterly Cassette on Patient Education, American College of Hospital Administrators, Chicago, Ill., 1973.

Somers, Anne: "Consumer Health Education: An Idea Whose Time Has Come?" *Hospital Progress*, pp. 10-11, Feb. 1975.

Starkweather, David B.: "Rationale for Decentralization in Large Hospitals," *Hospital Administration*, pp. 27-45, Spring 1970.

Tannenbaum, A. S.: "Control in Organizations: Individual Adjustment and Organizational Performance," *Administrative Science Quarterly*, p. 236, Sept. 1962.

U.S. Department of Health Education and Welfare: *Report on Licensure and Related Personnel Credentialing*, Washington, D.C., 1971.

U.S. Department of Labor: *Job Descriptions and Organizational Analysis for Hospitals*, rev. ed., Washington, D.C., 1970.

Varnum, James W.: "Administrators View of Unit Dose Drug Distribution System," *Canadian Journal of Hospital Pharmacy*, pp. 13-16, Jan.-Feb. 1973.

Zimmer, James G.: "Length of Stay and Hospital Bed Misutilization," presented at APHA Annual Meeting, Atlantic, N.J., Nov. 13, 1972 (mimeographed).

Chapter 8

Tasks and Functions
of the Administrator

If the spouse of an administrator asked, "What did you do today?" nine times out of ten he or she is likely to respond, "I've been in conferences and on the phone all day." Chances are the question won't be asked again although the response was truthful. If the question were, "What did you accomplish today?," on most days the administrator would be hard-pressed to think of anything. While the outcomes of administrators' efforts are elusive in the short range, their impact on the hospital in improving access to care, quality, and cost containment over the longer range is very strong, and they constitute the single most important influence.

In this chapter we will attempt to describe what an administrator does in terms of his or her time, responsibilities, tasks, and functions. In the next chapter the changing role of the administrator is considered.

HOSPITAL ADMINISTRATORS

It is important to note that hospital administration involves considerably more than the positions of hospital administrators and assistant administrators. As we have suggested previously much of the administration of hospitals and other health services is provided by physicians, nurses, and other health professionals in addition to managerial functional specialists, who will be discussed in the next chapter. The Commission on the Education for Health Administration (Austin, 1974) has defined health administration as ". . . planning, organizing, directing, controlling, and coordinating the resources and procedures by which needs and demands for health and medical care and a healthful environment are fulfilled by provision of specific services to individual clients, organizations and communities."

Westphal (1969) has estimated that as many as 30,000 administrative positions exist in the health service industry. He projected a need for 2,000 graduates of health care administration programs annually by 1979. In 1973, 970 students graduated from the 38 master's programs in health services administration in the United States and Canada. Increasing numbers of students are also being prepared for health administration through baccalaureate programs and on-the-job work-study programs. However, many if not most of the 30,000 administrative positions are filled by health professionals and others without formal administrative training. The Commission on Education for Health Administration (1975) estimated that fewer than 25 percent of executive-level positions in the medical care system are filled by individuals who have had formal entry level education in health administrative. It is, however, the chief executive officer, hospital administrator, president, executive vice president, or whatever his title, and his top assistants who concern us in this chapter.

In a 1965[1] Cornell survey with about 4,000 respondents, Dolson (1966) characterized hospital administrators as follows: Two-thirds were between 35 and 55 years old, 79 percent were men, 72 percent college graduates, 43 percent had advanced degrees, 50 percent were in their jobs for less than 6 years, with average tenure about 7 years. Women were found to account for just over 20 percent of the hospital administrators. Since then we would suspect that this percentage has declined since fewer Catholic hospitals are now headed by nuns. The percent with advanced degrees has probably increased. About 12 percent of hospital administrators were physicians. We would suspect that the percent of administrators who are physicians has not increased—more probably there has been a further decrease.

Murray et al. (1968) surveyed how administrators of Catholic and non-Catholic hospitals spent their time and found no significant differences between the two. In a similar study in a large teaching hospital Connors and Hutts (1967) identified six functions performed by hospital administrators: extramural tasks, controlling, planning, personnel tasks, organizing, directing, and coordinating. Extramural tasks refers to self-development, teaching and lecturing inside and outside the hospital, and relationships with agencies, individuals, and groups external to the hospital. The chief executive officer spent nearly 37 percent of his time in these activities. An American College of Hospital Administrators Task Force (1973) suggests that hospital chief executives spend 25 to 75 percent of their time on extramural affairs depending on the type of hospital

[1] The most recent broad-based study available; however a number of studies are underway in 1975-1976 under research contracts from the Bureau of Health Resources Development in HEW.

and its environment as well as on individual preferences. Table 8-1 summarizes the results of the Connors and Hutts and Murray studies. Some differences in time can be explained by differences in hospital sizes, with administrators in larger hospitals spending more time in planning and extramural activities. Differences in methodologies preclude interpretation of variations in the Connors and Hutts and Murray studies.

Connors and Hutts (1967) also examined the specific tasks performed by administrators (Table 8-2). Note the time devoted by the chief executive officer to health industry activities, group administrative meetings, and policy formulation and implementation. The assistant administrators, on the other hand, were more concerned with departmental operations, and physical facilities and equipment. There were also differences among the assistant administrators. For example, Administrator B spent much more time on departmental operations, Administrator D on health industry activities and public and community relations, and Administrator D and E were involved in financial and business management. Also, much of the junior administrator's time (Administrator E) was concerned with education, probably special projects in the education task.

This study not only shows the general dimension of the tasks and functions performed by administrators, but it also points out the variations in specific individual assignments within a hospital.

Davis and Henshaw (1974) surveyed hospital administrators who were graduates of Columbia University Graduate Program in Health Services Administration (73 percent were chief administrative officers and the rest second-level administrators; two-thirds worked in large urban settings, over half within large black and Spanish-speaking communities). They found the results shown in Table 8-3 on administrators' perception of importance to the institution, time spent, and their level of responsibility with regard to various decision areas.

Table 8-1 Percent of Administrator's Time Spent on Various Activities

Activity	Connors and Hutts (1967) Teaching hospital	Murray et al. (1968) non-Catholic hospitals All in study	400 beds or more	1-99 beds
Planning	25.8	25.5	31.2	23.3
Directing and coordinating	4.5	24.6	20.7	23.6
Extramural	36.9	20.9	22.7	16.2
Personal	3.4	11.8	13.5	13.9
Controlling	16.5	11.4	8.6	10.9
Organizing	12.9	3.9	3.1	4.1
Operating	—	1.9	0.3	8.0

Source: Anthony R. Kooner, "The Hospital Administrator and Organizational Effectiveness," *Organization Research in Health Institutions,* Basil Georgopoulos (ed.), The Institute for Social Research, University of Michigan, Ann Arbor, 1972, p. 361.

Table 8-2 The Nature of Administrative Activities

Activity	Percent of time spent by administrators in a teaching hospital					
	A (Chief exec.)	B	C	D	E	Average
		(Assistant administrators)				
Departmental opera-tion (nonspecific)	10.8	22.2	31.6	10.1	7.7	16.5
Health industry activities	29.9	11.9	8.4	20.4	10.7	16.3
Administrative education	10.5	15.6	9.1	1.5	28.4	13.0
Public and com-munity relations	2.8	4.9	2.2	31.5	5.6	9.4
Systems	1.9	7.6	14.0	2.1	18.9	8.9
Financial and business management	6.3	8.6	0.7	13.9	11.9	8.2
Physical facilities and equipment	4.5	14.7	13.2	2.9	2.1	7.5
Group administrative meeting	8.2	7.0	3.8	7.4	11.2	7.5
Policy formulation and implementation	9.5	0.8	4.1	2.9	–	3.5
Personnel management	1.0	1.8	5.5	1.4	1.5	2.2
Legal and governmental	1.6	0.2	2.5	5.5	0.7	2.1
Clinical service operation	4.1	2.3	1.4	–	0.2	1.6
Administrative research	4.5	0.6	2.2	–	0.2	1.5
Other	2.1	1.8	1.3	0.4	0.9	1.3
Medical center oper-ation (nonspecific)	2.3	–	–	–	–	0.5
TOTAL	100.0	100.0	100.0	100.0	100.0	100.0

Source: Edward J. Connors and Joseph C. Hutts, "How Administrators Spend Their Day," *Hospitals, J.A.H.A.,* vol. 41, p. 48, Feb. 16, 1967. Reprinted, with permission, from *Hospitals, Journal of the American Hospital Association.*

There are a number of interesting findings in Table 8-3. For example, there is a high correlation between importance to the hospital and the amount of time spent, but low correlation between these two and level of responsibility. Quality and evaluation ranks in the bottom half, cost control (financing expenditures) ranks number 1 in importance and time and number 3 in level of responsibility, yet financing (income) ranks 7 and 8 in importance and time spent, but 1 in responsibility.

TABLE 8-3   Results of a Survey of 161 Columbia University Hospital Administration Graduates' Perception of Importance to Hospital, Time Spent, and Level or Responsibility for Various Decision Areas

Decision Area	Importance to hospital	Time spent	Level of responsibility
Financing (expenditures)	1	1	3
Medical staff relations	2	2	5
Physical plant, equipment, construction	3½	5	4
Health care delivery	3½	4	7½
Administration of professional departments	5	3	2
Financing (income)	7	8	1
Community relations	8	7	10
Outside agencies; governmental and voluntary	9	9	6
Quality control and evaluation	10	10	7½
Governing body	11	11	14
Legal aspects and litigation	12	13	13
Education programs	13	12	11
Shared services	14	14	12
Research programs	15	15	15

Source: Samuel Davis and Stanley Henshaw, *Decision Analysis in Hospital Administration: A Tool for Curriculum Revision* (monograph), Association of University Programs in Health Administration, One DuPont Circle, Washington, D.C., Apr. 1974, pp. 5 and 7.

We now move into a description of tasks and functions of administration drawing upon general management literature.

TASKS AND FUNCTIONS OF ADMINISTRATION

Among the tasks and functions of administration are (1) establishing or helping to establish institutional goals and objectives, (2) planning, strategies, policies, and tactics to achieve goals, (3) establishing a managerial climate for carrying them out, (4) establishing and controlling systems and subsystems, and (5) integrating systems.

Hospital Goals and Objectives

Since we discuss goals and objectives in Chapter 4 and elsewhere in this book, we will not go into them again here. It is important to note, however, that goals and objectives should be the basis for evaluating the administrator and his effectiveness. We refer the reader to the literature on management by objectives and to ACHA (1973) Task Force V report for descriptions of evaluations of administrators based on objectives.

Planning, Strategies, Policies, and Tactics

Planning   Planning has also received considerable emphasis in both management and hospital literature and is discussed in Chapter 10. Strategies, policies, and tactics are just beginning to receive emphasis in the management literature and we will briefly review some of the basic definitions here.

Strategies　Cannon (1968) thinks of strategies as *directional action decisions.* We believe this is a significant definition. In the first place, it identifies the need for *direction.* For example, should the hospital build a new facility for extended care patients? This is not something the administrator will decide upon his own, but he will have much input into the governing board on the subject, with participation from others, even though the idea may have originated with him in the first place.

Many other directional-type decisions can be identified. For example, overall questions concerning outreach services, laboratory facilities to expand diagnostic services, special equipment (radium therapy), specialized activities such as open-heart surgery, and countless related issues all require directional decisions. They are directional because they identify areas of emphasis as well as monetary expenditure. All the services can be useful to some patients; the basic question always is, Will there be sufficient demand or is it better to enter into some type of shared-service arrangement?

A second major component of the definition relates to the word *action.* The concern here is that something actually should happen. None of us has trouble recalling a situation where we sat around a conference table for a long period of time and decided to move in a certain direction. Then, nothing happened; there was no action; the decision was not implemented. There is nothing easier than making decisions without action. What is needed is to include the action or implementation phase in the original strategic decision.

This brings us to the third word in the definition of strategy, the word *decision.* Administrators must engage in the making of decisions. This is no different for the hospital administrator than for any other kind of manager. An important factor is to know when to make a "rapid decision," and when the decision can be delayed, or perhaps not made at all. Many decision-making models have been proposed. Indeed, an entire new science of decision theory has developed. When one deals with strategy, there is usually time to get the necessary data, so that decisions can be made on the basis of something more than wild hunches. Throughout this book, references are made both directly and indirectly to strategy and decision making.

Policy　Policy is usually defined as a guide to action. The administrator must be responsible for seeing to it that necessary policies are developed. Generally, errors consist either in having no policies at all with everything done by word-of-mouth, or in having such a tremendous number that the organization is inundated with them.

There are really no precise guidelines that administrators can employ. They do realize that if the same type of questions keep coming up or changes are not forthcoming, either there is no policy or one that is not clearly understood. The problem is generally to effectuate a change before it is too late. Also, administrators must keep in touch with their organizations. Perhaps this is why participatory management has become more popular; it provides a means for the administrator, as well as middle-management people, to receive feedback.

Newman and Logan (1971) emphasize the significance of policy as follows:

> Strategy concentrates on basic directions, major thrusts and overriding priorities. The full implication of the strategy, however, is clarified by thinking through the more detailed policy that guides execution of the strategy. Central management must actively participate in shaping policy (a) partly because working through the policy implications is an excellent way to check the practicality of a basic concept and (b) especially to make sure that the intent of strategy is correctly interpreted into the work of the various departments of the company.[2]

It should be noted that policies can be useful in avoiding conflict insofar as they guide positive behavior. However, too many detailed policies can also stifle the initiative of subordinates who spend all their time referring to policy.

Tactics   It is somewhat difficult to distinguish between strategy and tactics and some may decide that there is no need to do so. Generally strategy has to do with the entire effort whereas tactics relates to the various parts or subunits of the whole. Thus, the concept of establishing an extended-care nursing home can be viewed as strategy. Once the initial decision has been made, the actual construction and operation become tactical in nature. The point of significance is that the actual operations may preclude the realization of the original strategic decision, for example, because of unexpectedly high operating costs or changes in reimbursement expenses from federal and state sources. Thus, there have been many strategic decisions which have gone awry because of the failure of the tactics used to achieve the anticipated goals.

Whatever the terminology used, administration must engage in the establishment of overall strategy. In some instances this may involve initiating or facilitating major goal setting regarding the type and extensiveness of patient care. It is a wise administrator who recognizes the significance of this activity in the strategic formulation stages and, even more importantly, in the implementation stages of policy and tactics. In fact, it is quite likely that administrators will fail to fulfill their job responsibilities by inattention to policy and tactics. Some may view administration as involving only these functions, but we believe they should also be involved in strategic decisions.

ESTABLISHING THE MANAGERIAL CLIMATE

Hospitals have personalities in the same way as people do. Their personality is not something tangible; it is made up of the sensations and impressions of those who come in contact with the hospital. Such impressions are generated by the values held by those who govern the hospital and the physicians who use it. Quite naturally administrators and other staff play a major role in the development of these values since the organization tends to reflect those who govern and use it. Hage and Dewar (1973) in their study of health institutions found that the values of the elite in the organization had a

---

[2] William H. Newman and James P. Logan, *Strategy, Policy and Central Management*, South-Western Publishing Co., Cincinnati, Ohio, 1971, p. 9.

greater influence on the institution than organizational characteristics. Moreover, one cannot discount the factor of tradition or past history because usually administrative people must be compatible with each other and the organization. Despite this situation, the administration manages change, and where a change in managerial climate is called for in order for the hospital to present a different image, it must recognize the need and be capable of meeting it.

The philosophy of administration and hence of administrators has been changing quite perceptibly in recent decades. Yoder (1970) comments that:

> . . . in current discussion of administration, the trend clearly favors less authoritarian, more permissive strategies. Historic policy and style is viewed as overly autocratic; its critics describe it as "hard." Modern strategies are designed to encourage more negotiation and wider participation. Critics of this style have labled it "soft" (p. 157).

Neuhauser (1972) makes a similar kind of analysis when he describes the situation in organization theory.

> It does not take much reading in organization theory to discover a major divergence of opinion among those writers who praise the efficiency of large formal organizations and the centralized hierarchical authority structure associated with it. (Max Weber, Henri Fayol, and Georgopoulous and Mann for hospitals come to mind.) In contrast, the human relations writers have focused on the human problems apparently inherent in such organizations, including Likert, Katz and Kahn, and Argyris for hospitals and have recommended more participation in decision making by workers. They are in fundamental disagreement as to the degree to which procedures should be specified hierarchically and imposed on organization members. Both schools of thought believe they have found the best way to run an organization (p. 8).

Another group of writers argue that the type of management style depends upon circumstances, e.g., the degree of specialization in the hospital. This has been referred to or labeled as the *situational or contingency theory of management*. As Neuhauser points out, this may really call for another approach, namely matrix organization. He defines matrix organization thus: "The existence of both hierarchical (vertical) coordination through departmentation and the formal chain of command and departments (the patient care team) is called a matrix."

In searching to explain why changes occur in managerial philosophy and style, one must turn to change in society itself. Tannenbaum and Davis (1969) state that values are in a state of transition. They set forth a number of propositions to describe the direction of change in society.

> **1** Away from a view of man as essentially bad toward a view of him as basically good
> **2** Away from avoidance or negative evaluation of individuals toward confirming them as human beings

3 Away from a view of individuals as fixed towards seeing themselves as being in process

4 Away from resisting and fearing individual differences toward accepting and utilizing them

5 Away from utilizing an individual primarily with reference to his job description toward viewing him as a whole person

6 Away from walking-off with expression of feelings toward making possible both appropriate expression and effective use

7 Away from taskmanship and game-playing toward authentic behavior

8 Away from the use of status for maintaining power and personal prestige toward use of status for organizationally relevant purposes

9 Away from distrusting people toward trusting them

10 Away from avoiding facing others with relevant data toward making appropriate confrontation.

11 Away from a view of process work as being unproductive effort toward seeing it as essential

12 Away from a primary emphasis on competition toward a much greater emphasis on collaboration

A second explanation for changes in managerial style is based on changing concepts of power. Zalesnik (1970) states that "organizations operate by distributing authority and setting a stage for the exercise of power" (p. 48).

In a related article, Ways (1970) says,

the . . . general trend of twentieth-century society, particularly in the United States, is toward a wider distribution of power, a broadening of participation by individuals in controlling their own lives and work.

This situation in the United States stems from two developments.

. . . the first, widely discussed in the sixties, is a sharp and insistent demand of the desire for material goods: food, house, cars, clothing. The second revolution concerns the psyche. It pertains to the dignity, status, personality, significance, and power of individuals. Many of the aims of the second revolution can be summed up in a word: Participation.

This change in society is reflected in the attitudes of employees themselves. Rush (1969) in a National Industrial Conference Board study comments that

. . . [there] is a growing realization that the employee is, indeed a new breed. He appears to have different values, different needs, different motivation than his predecessor. He is better educated, he is a product of the knowledge explosion, he is more aware politically, socially, and economically, he is more demanding, he is less easily managed by traditional controls, and he is generally more sophisticated. . . . There is evidence that management is trying hard to understand the new work force's motivation and business.

The report continues by suggesting that industrial managers are turning to the behavioral scientists to aid them in their understanding of social changes. In our opinion, this approach is equally productive for health service administrators.

What have the behavioral scientists learned from their research? Cross (1970) says that

> . . . the behavioral scientists have summarized a half century of their research under a few major headings that may be considered as operational principles. They are: (1) human behavior depends both on a person and his environment; (2) human behavior always makes sense to the individual; (3) human behavior is influenced by the individual's needs which vary from person to person and from time to time; and (4) human behavior is influenced by emotion and feeling more than by logic.

There are many forces at work which shape the administrator's values and hence the values of the organization he leads. Kralewski (1971), in a report adapted from a paper presented to the California Hospital Association's annual meeting, identifies a number of characteristics of leadership for the hospital administrator.

> First of all, leadership must be based on a health systems approach and an orientation toward comprehensive health services available to all members of our society. . . .
> Leadership must be based on a continual willingness to test the market and innovate. . . .
> The administrator in this setting (large-scale organizations responsible for a variety of services) must develop leadership styles that maximize the potential of these technical specialties at all levels of the organization. . . .
> The administrator will have to develop a leadership style that is at least somewhat detached from the personal internalized administrative role of the past that was typified by the small family organization (pp. 8-13).

The leadership characteristics point to a trend for the future as well as to changes in administrative style. Hence it is only through leadership, i.e., initiation, integration, facilitation, and support of others, that the administrator can implement both social and institutional changes to improve access to health care, quality of care, and containment of health care costs.

ESTABLISHING AND REVIEWING SYSTEMS AND SUBSYSTEMS

Austin (1974), in a report to the Commission on Education for Health Administration, suggests a systems approach for administrators. He points out that "administrative functions can be classified as having two sets of counter-tensions, internal and external to the conversion process itself" (the transformation of inputs into outputs). Austin explains these two sets of countertensions as follows:

> Internal management functions relate to the administrator's interaction with elements in his organization. Formal decision processes at the executive level

include: (1) organization of resources; (2) budgeting and financial control of the conversion process; and (3) management and evaluation of organizational performance. An effective administrator will carry out these functions while recognizing the importance of the informal aspects of organizational life in the development of a management philosophy.

The second category of administrative functions are those external to the conversion process, related to the interaction of the administrative unit with its environment. Executive decision processes include: (1) program planning and policy decisions; (2) coordination of organizational activities with other elements of the community, other community organizations, etc.; and (3) evaluation of the outcomes of the conversion process.

Administrators participate in the formation of the total system (the hospital) and its various subsystems—nursing services, dietary services, etc. The administrator may have many staff experts such as systems engineers as well as department supervisors themselves. It is likely that administrators and their staff will be more concerned with redesigning or reappraising an existing system and giving approval for changes than with formulating a new system. In determinating changes as well as evaluating results, the chief executive officer and his or her staff may well consider systems analysis. Systems analysis is an aspect of general systems theory. We cannot explore the concept in depth here, but merely touch on some general ideas that are provocative. Churchman (1968) suggests that there are five basic considerations to be kept in mind in thinking about systems. These are:

... (1) the total system objectives and more specifically, the performance measures of the whole system; (2) the system's environment: the fixed constraints; (3) the resources of the system; (4) the components of the system, their activities, goals and measures of performance; and (5) the management of the system (pp. 29-30).

Administrators are involved in implementing the systems concept. In fact, they are key persons, for without their support the system just will not operate effectively. Because the very nature of this book is based on the systems concept, our purpose in this chapter is only to point out the role of the administrator in system planning and implementation.

INTEGRATIVE SKILLS

From Adam Smith's early pin-making example to the present, we observe an increasing emphasis upon specialization. Specialization is about the only way of handling exploding knowledge. We plan for specialization, organize for it, and control for it. However, with specialization comes the need for its twin function, integration.

Integration is particularly significant from a systems point of view. Much has been written about the nature of conflict in hospitals (Schulz and Johnson, 1971). In fact, whenever two systems meet in any form or fashion, there is potential for conflict. A similar situation often exists with regard to specialists. Administrators must be prepared to meet these contingencies; they need skills for resolving conflicts as well as for integration and control. In addition, these types of skills must be performed in the atmosphere of the hospital.

The primary role of the administrator is to provide leadership to facilitate action toward appropriate goals. He or she must help motivate the staff, as well as advise superiors and colleagues about the environment and design of his or her unit and of the total organization. Certain competencies are required by the role in order to deal with internal and external affairs. A careful review of information, including both theory and practice, suggests the following competencies to be appropriate: (1) coordination; (2) communication; (3) fact-finding, investigation, or research; (4) evaluation or appraisal (of people and programs); (5) management development and education; and (6) negotiation.

One can argue that these competencies are nothing more than a redefining of the functions of administration. While conceding this point we also suggest that these particular competencies relate to *implementation* as opposed to *determination* of policies and procedures. Implementation is a subject that has been neglected in administrative literature. In addition, most of these concepts permit the use of findings from the behavioral sciences as well as traditional managerial or administrative theories and practices.

Coordination

There exists the need for competency in coordinating diverse work concentration roles, in order to unify these efforts to achieve total goals or objectives.

Another aspect of coordination concerns the implementation of what can be called group solidarity. Each individual in the organization should understand and appreciate his or her significance and relationship to others. Sometimes this is considered a part of morale or attitudes toward others as well as to the total organization. Naturally, it is impossible to order one person to relate well to another. It is possible, however, to explain the importance of good relationships. The behavioral scientists can assist through their work on personality and attitude formation. For example, attitude surveys conducted annually will alert administration to changes in employee attitudes toward unions or changing states of morale. Information is available concerning not only the nature of attitudes and their development, but also the modification of attitudes. Armed with this kind of information, the administrator can be much more effective in achieving coordination both internally and externally with other agencies and resources important to the hospital's role in meeting community health needs.

Communication

Someone once said that if we could solve the problems inherent in communications, we would indeed solve most of the problems not only of an organization but also of the world. But it is somewhat disconcerting to note that as we improve communication facilities, we seem to achieve less understanding.

A key problem in communication is the assumption that others hear and understand what we say and write. Usually, we make no effort to ascertain whether or not our message is received. Too, if we discover that our message is not understood, we usually conclude that it is not our fault but that the problem rests with the receiver for not listening or for being too obtuse to understand.

If the administrator discovers that he is not "getting across" to his staff, he often resorts to memoranda or policy statements. Before long, these become the way of life and very little attention is given to face-to-face communication. For many people the written word is more difficult to understand than the spoken one. This is true because, in most cases, if the reader encounters an obscure passage, he does not have the opportunity to question the writer. A high level of profundity is not achieved by using unintelligible language.

Most people can think about five times as rapidly as they can speak. This suggests that there is all kinds of room for static, ranging from "turning off one's hearing aid" to rewriting or restating the speaker's message. Thus, we sometimes rely on visual aids to help keep the listener's attention. But oftentimes the listeners give so much attention to the visuals that they do not hear the message!

A final thought related to the competency of communication involves the art of listening. Communication is a two-way street and administrators must listen to what staff members tell them both directly and indirectly. Much of what has been said about the receiver applies to the transmitter of information because it concerns the feedback of understanding in words and behavior.

Fact Finding, Investigation, or Research

Every administrator must make a number of decisions each day. Some are made after much fact-finding and analysis; others must be made immediately and are based upon knowledge and experience. To assist them in this, administrators often have staffs or perhaps departments of advisors who are specialists in certain areas or who provide them with advice and assistance when continual research and evaluation are necessary. These units, e.g., budgets and finance and personnel, are usually referred to as staff departments. Administrators have, in fact, delegated a degree of authority in order to obtain the necessary facts and to be assured that certain services are provided for their staff and for the organization. In addition, administrators are constantly acquiring facts through their own observations, in reading, or in studying the situation in their departments or divisions.

An important aspect of fact-finding is its innovative potential. Too little attention has been given to innovation because so much time and effort is spent on problem solving. The idea seems to be that if all your problems are solved, you have a viable department. In most situations, this is an unattainable goal. Perhaps a better approach would be to give more attention to innovation. All the problems might not disappear, but the attitude would be positive rather than negative. There is a need for effective innovation both in managing workers and organizing work; despite the progress being made in this area, it may still be the most neglected and have the most potential for increasing productivity.

Managerial style in fact-finding and investigation is an important element. Situations where consensus is important would call for attention to group decision-making processes, whereas situations calling for immediate decisions that cannot be delayed necessitate individual fact-finding usually based upon administrative experiences in similar situations.

Fact-finding, investigation, and research are the most important ways of identifying community needs and expectations. A great deal of information is available from other sources in the community such as planning and public health agencies; however more attention must be given to this important responsibility of administration.

Evaluation or Appraisal

Another competency needed by administrators is the ability to evaluate people, programs, and the overall effectiveness of the hospital in meeting community needs and expectations. Evaluation of people is necessary not only with regard to prospective employees but also in terms of clientele relationships and interpersonal behavior. In addition, administrators are constantly required to evaluate progress in terms of expected achievement, merit, and continuation.

Certainly, administrators must constantly make judgments about others. Often this is done with great reluctance, but this reluctance does not remove the responsibility. Invariably, administrators and managers ask how the evaluation or appraisal process can be improved. Sometimes it is suggested that the system or technique should be improved, whereas a study of the perceptual process itself is required. The following quotation by Costello and Zalkind (1963) illustrates this point:

> We conclude our discussion of perception with a few straight-forward suggestions for raising the probability of more effective administrative action. One suggestion is that the administrator become aware of the intricacies of the perceptual process and thus be warned to avoid arbitrary and categorical judgments and to seek reliable evidence before judgments are made. A second suggestion grows out of the first—increased accuracy in one's self-perception can make possible the flexibility to go slowly, to seek evidence, and to shift positions as time provides additional evidence about others.
>
> However, not every effort that is designed to improve perceptual accuracy will do so. The dangers of too complete reliance on formal training for perceptive accuracy are suggested. . . . The danger is that a little learning encourages the perceiver to respond with increased sensitivity to individual differences, without making it possible to gauge the real meaning of the differences he has seen (pp. 53-54).

The authors conclude with a summary made by Taft (1955) after he reviewed 81 studies in this field: There seem to be three main elements in our ability to judge others—having suitable judgmental norms, judging ability, and motivation. If our background is similar to that of the subject, we can easily use appropriate *norms* to make our judgment. *Judging ability* seems to combine both general and social intelligence, with perhaps another specific factor of nonanalytic judgment or "intuition." *Motivation* is probably the most important area—if we are motivated to judge our subject accurately and if we feel free to be objective, we are likely to achieve our aim, provided we have the necessary ability and can use appropriate judgmental norms.

In making evaluations, the administrator must first establish the general organizational structure and the jobs to be performed. Then individual employees must know what is expected from them on their jobs. This management-by-objectives approach provides a sound basis for evaluation. Measurable institutional objectives based on community needs are essential to evaluation of institutional effectiveness.

Management Development and Education

One of an administrator's objectives is to develop management throughout the hospital and bring about behavior change in his staff members so that institutional goals can be changed. This usually requires an educational effort on his part. There is no dearth of theories of education, which range from extreme progressivism to traditionalism.

The need for better management in a complex system such as a hospital, which has few trained managers particularly in professional areas, is evident. The administrator cannot manage the institution by him- or herself. Another significant aspect relates to retraining. Most people will agree that change is occurring at an increasing rate. This tends to create technological obsolescence in all positions, including that of the administrator. Thus, a part of the educational activity must be directed to training and retraining administrative personnel as well as staff members in related areas. Unless this situation is recognized, we may very well see increasing numbers of men and women who are too young to retire and too old to learn. Management development and education must be a continuous activity that includes planned programs for keeping current with changing styles of administration.

Community education is another major facet of education that has been described elsewhere in the book.

Negotiation and Creative Problem Solving

A bargaining transaction, Commons (1951) says, has three steps: (1) negotiations, which end when the parties agree on intentions, (2) the contract or "commitment," which imposes upon the parties obligations for future performance and payment; and (3) administration or performance of agreed-upon obligations, which completes the transaction when carried out by both parties.

There is little doubt that the administrator spends considerable time negotiating both with agencies outside the hospital and with staff members within, especially regarding their working arrangements and conflict resolution. It is somewhat unfortunate that the term *negotiation* has become associated to such a great extent with the collective bargaining process. The term actually implies reaching a mutual agreement between the two parties involved.

There are many examples of negotiation in administration. Increasingly administrators must negotiate with third-party payers, regulatory agencies, planning groups, and so forth. Internally, for example, there are elements of negotiation in the hiring functions. Often certain adjustments are made in the duties assigned, depending upon the interests and abilities of the person to be hired and the needs of the health service organization. If no agreement is reached, it is either because the person is not acceptable or the organization or the position is not acceptable to the person. A similar negotiation activity often exists in salary determination.

Now, what can be said in connection with developing the competency of negotiation? First, one should recognize the part that emotions play in a negotiation session. Ideally, this activity is or should be rational. Unfortunately, tempers are likely to be short and sometimes critical attitudes are present that are not conducive to objectivity.

A second thought relates to the kind of authority exercised. If the negotiation conference is one-sided in favor of the administrator, a unilateral decision will be reached. In fact, we can say this is an arbitrary decision and the administrator is in the role of an arbitrator. On the other hand, the decision may be tossed to the other party whose answer will be accepted by the administrator. True negotiation should be somewhere between these extremes.

Ideally, the administrator will strive for creative problem solving (Maier, 1964). This implies moving away from a win-lose (I win-you lose, or vice versa) situation to a win-win (I win-you win) end result. In this case the administrator will turn from a "choice" to a "creative problem-solving" situation with both parties focusing on mutually agreed-upon goals.

SUMMARY

Administrators perform a variety of tasks and functions that quite naturally vary by position and job assignment. Administrative personnel must establish a managerial climate consistent with the needs of the hospital. As part of their assignment, administrators participate in establishing objectives and strategies to meet community and institutional needs as well as becoming involved in policy and procedural implementation. They help design the hospital systems and encourage the formation of various subsystems. They are responsible for seeing to it that these systems function properly. In this connection they require a number of integrative skills. Their primary aim is to develop an effective hospital system in which all components function as a team to meet community needs first, institutional needs second, and individual employee, physician, and administrators needs third.

In the next chapter we explore different roles of administrators.

REFERENCES

ACHA (American College of Hospital Administrators) Task Force V (1972): *Principals of Appointment and Tenure of Executive Officers,* Jerome Bieter, Chairman, Chicago, Ill., Aug. 1973.

Austin, Charles: "What Is Health Administration?" *Hospital Administration*, pp. 14-29, Summer 1974.

Cannon, J. Thomas: *Business Strategy and Policy*, Harcourt, Brace and World, New York, 1969.

Churchman, C. West: *The Systems Approach*, Dell Publishing Company, New York, 1968.

Commission on *Education for Health Administration*, Health Administration Press, Ann Arbor, Mich., 1975.

Commons, John R.: *The Economics of Collective Action*, Macmillan, New York, 1951.

Connors, Edward J. and Joseph C. Hutts: "How Administrators Spend Their Day," *Hospitals, J.A.H.A.*, vol. 41, Feb. 16, 1967.

Costello, Timothy W. and Sheldon S. Zalkind: *Psychology in Administration: A Research Orientation*, Prentice-Hall, Englewood Cliffs, N.J., 1963.

Cross, Joseph L.: "Open Letter to a New Manager," *Personnel Journal*, February 1970.

Davis, Samuel and Stanley Henshaw: *Decision Analysis in Hospital Administration*, (monograph), Association of University Programs in Health Administration, Washington, D.C., Apr. 1974.

Dolson, Miriam T.: "How Administrators Rate Different Tasks of Importance," *The Modern Hospital*, June 1965.

Dolson, Miriam T., Rodney White, and Paul Van Ripper: "Study Reveals What Administrators Earn," *Modern Hospital*, Apr. 1966, pp. 103-106.

Hage, Jerald and Robert Dewar: "Elite Values Versus Organizational Structure in Predicting Innovation," *Administrative Sciences Quarterly*, pp. 279-290, Sept. 1973.

Kovner, Anthony R.: "The Hospital Administrator and Organizational Effectiveness," in Basil Georgopoulos (ed.), *Organization Research on Health Institutions*, Institute for Social Research, Ann Arbor, Mich., 1972.

Kralewski, John Edward: "Leadership in the Evolving Health System," *Hospital Administration*, Spring 1971.

Maier, Norman F.: "Maximizing Personal Creativity Through Better Problem Solving," *Personal Administration*, vol. 27, 1964.

Murray, R. T. et al.: "How Administrators Spend Their Time: Research Report," *Hospital Progress*, vol. 49, pp. 49-58 as reported in Kovner, op. cit.

Neuhauser, Duncan: "The Hospital as a Matrix Organization," *Hospital Administration*, Fall 1972.

Newman, William H. and James P. Logan: *Strategy, Policy and Central Management*, South-Western Publishing Co., Cincinnati, Ohio, 1971.

Rush, Harold M. F.: *Behavioral Concepts and Management Application* (Personnel Policy Study no. 216), National Industrial Conference Board, Inc., New York, 1964.

Schulz, Rockwell and Alton C. Johnson: "Conflict in Administration," *Hospital Administration*, vol. 16, Summer 1971.

Taft, R.: "The Ability to Judge People," *Psychological Bulletin*, vol. 52, pp. 1-21, 1955.

Tannenbaum, Robert and Sheldon A. Davis: "Values, Man and Organizations," *Industrial Management Review*, Winter 1969.

Ways, Max: "More Power to Everybody," *Fortune*, May 1970.

Westphal, Robert: "Educating for the Future," *Hospital Administration,* vol. 6, pp. 81-94, 1969.

Yoder, Dale: *Personnel Management and Industrial Relations,* Prentice-Hall, Englewood Cliffs, N.J., 1970.

Zalensnik, Abraham: "Power and Politics in Organizational Life," *Harvard Business Review,* May/June 1970.

Chapter 9

Changing Roles of Hospital Administrators

If you were to ask a hospital administrator, "What is your role in the hospital?" he or she is likely to respond with a statement such as "to see to it that the hospital meets community needs efficiently and effectively." Or, as one administrator responded, "to manage 'my' institution and serve community needs 'better' than anyone else." There are different role models that an administrator can have to fulfill these objectives. We suggest that there is no one best role for all hospitals; it will vary according to a number of internal and environmental factors. Roles are determined by others and by many institutional and environmental characteristics such as size and control of hospital, or whether it is teaching or nonteaching. The personal characteristics and styles of the administrator also affect roles. Moreover, administrators have multiple roles to fill, such as task roles and social roles.

In spite of the difficulty in defining roles, it is important to attempt to classify them. A definition and classification of roles should help administrators and board members to understand and improve relationships and responsibilities; it may also help in reducing conflict due to role ambiguity, selecting appropriate models for individuals to pursue, and selecting and training administrators. Moreover, we suggest that roles change as the hospital environment changes and a classification of roles should help to evaluate the effects of such changes.

In this chapter we outline four general models that may be used both to describe roles from an historical point of view and to make projections for the future. In the first section (Role Models—an Overview) we examine roles in light of the limited published research at this time. In the second we suggest four models to describe changing roles of administrators in the context of external and organizational factors. The third section contains some general conclusions.

We base this chapter on the limited available literature, on preliminary research findings from a number of current projects of the authors, and on subjective inferences from exposure to a number of hospitals over the years. Our projections for the future are speculative, but we hope they will provide a frame of reference within which the readers can draw their own conclusions.

ROLE MODELS—AN OVERVIEW

Connors and Hutts (1967), Murray et al. (1968), Dolson (1965), and others have examined administrative roles from a task viewpoint. The American College of Hospital Administrators has been developing profiles of administrators for the past several years, and various programs in hospital and health administration have conducted surveys on their graduates' positions, collecting data on such factors as tenure, salary, and age. The Brunell Institute in England (Rowbottom et al., 1973) has studied the roles of hospital administrators in England using a social analysis methodology. Currently a number of studies on the roles of administrators are under way, or just beginning. Roles have also been studied in other settings. For example, Parsons (1960) and Petit (1967) classified managerial roles as technical, organizational, and environmental.

Katz and Kahn (1966) suggest a role model from which we have adapted Figure 9-1. Starting from the inside of the model, i.e., line 1 (from role sender to role receiver), Katz and Kahn describe a role episode. It includes four concepts:

> *Role expectations* which are evaluative standards applied to the behavior of any person who occupies a given organizational office or position; *sent role*, which consists of communications stemming from role expectations and sent by members of the role set as attempts to influence the focal person; *received role* which is the focal person's perception of the role-sendings addressed to him, including those he "sends" to himself; and *role behavior* which is the response of the focal person to the complex of information and influence he has received (p. 182).

Arrow 2 is a feedback loop. The degree to which a person's behavior conforms to the expectations held for him or her at one point in time will affect the state of those expectations at the next point. For example if the focal person's response to the

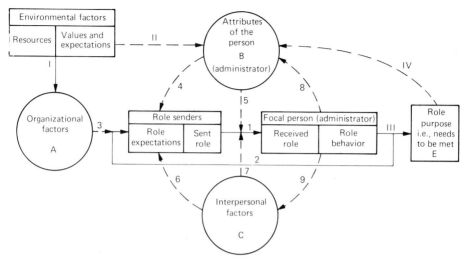

Figure 9-1 Theoretical role model (Adapted from Daniel Katz and Robert L. Kahn, *The Social Psychology of Organizations*, Wiley, New York, p. 187, 1966.)

role sender is hostile, the role sender is likely to expect of and behave toward the focal person far differently than if the focal person's response was submissive. An example of a role episode between a physician and administrator might be as follows. The physician in requesting a new service for the hospital might "expect" the administrator to be resistant because he perceives the administrator to be most concerned about costs. The physician may then send an intimidating role of "You better get this service or I'll take my patients elsewhere." The administrator as focal person perceives the physician will expect him to be more concerned about costs and perceives that the physician will indeed take his patients elsewhere. Consequently, to avoid risk and conflict the administrator's behavior could be one of submission. Feedback of this to the role sender might change the physician's expectations and/or reinforce an intimidating behavior on the part of the physician.

We know, however, that there are other factors in roles, such as *organizational factors* (A), which in this case might be a very strong governing board organization in a competitive hospital community situation, combined with open staffs, a surplus of beds, and low occupancy. This situation allows the physician to make a threat with some likelihood of carrying it out and having an impact on the administrator. *Attributes of the person* (B) e.g., personality characteristics of the administrator, will affect the role sender's expectations and sent role (line 4); it will also affect the role episode and *interpersonal factors* (C) (line 5) such as, Is there trust between the two (line 6)? Interpersonal factors will affect the role episode and over time the attributes of the administrator (line 7). Role behavior of the administrator will ultimately affect his attributes (line 8) e.g., if the administrator continually reacts defensively to threats his personality will change over time and it will also affect interpersonal factors (line 9). We suggest that this model can be helpful to readers in diagnosing problems in role relationships and behavior. In Chapter 13 role conflict and ambiguity are discussed and are related to the internal role factor.

In the balance of this chapter we are more concerned with external role factors that we have added to Katz and Kahn's model. *Environmental factors* (D) consist of resources, values, and expectations that affect organizational factors (line I). For example, Is this a wealthy suburban area that has expectations and resources for a prestigious medical center? If so, it might have a strong and prestigious governing board, and thus affect organizational factors. Environmental values and expectations will also influence the values and attributes of the administrator (line II). He or she will probably hold or adopt many of these environmental values and expectations.

To us *the role purpose* (E) is the output for the role behavior of the administrator (line III). The purpose of the role of the administrator is to help move the organization to meet needs of society i.e., improve health, improve access to health services, improve quality of service, contain costs, and achieve institutional objectives in relation to these output objectives. What administrators perceive as needs will also affect their attributes (line IV). Are the values of the administrator and the environment, e.g., circle of friends and community power groups, to improve health or to build the prestige of the hospital and the administrator? While these are not mutually exclusive there is substantial evidence of conflict between values and objectives of and for the hospital and administrator. For example, an administrator might argue that a second open heart surgery unit in the community, i.e., at his or her hospital is important, for comprehensive services to patients. However, the underlying value may be the prestige for the hospital and administrator that open heart surgery brings, and that an outreach home care service may not bring, even though it might improve health of the community more effectively. We, of course, suggest that while administrators will reflect the values, expectations, and resources of the environment, their purpose is to identify needs of the community, and help to influence values, expectations, and resources of the environment to meet community needs.

In this chapter we suggest different role models for the administrator in reference to changing environments and purposes, and relationships to organizational factors of governing boards, medical staff, and other members of the administrative team. We use the term *hospital administrator* in a generic functional sense that could include titles that vary from hospital superintendent, to director, administrator, vice president, president, and so on. We have, however, avoided the use of such titles because they may or may not relate to meaningful role models (Wren, 1974). Current empirical research on the roles of administrators can be expected to develop better models than those presented here, but we believe our role models, which relate primarily to organizational factors, environmental factors, and role purpose, are adequate to draw some conclusions about the changing needs of hospital administration.

Table 9-1 summarizes our description of roles of administrators in relation to the periods of time when the roles were most prevalent, organizational characteristics,

Table 9-1 Roles of Administrators in Relation to Time Periods & Characteristics of the Organization, Board, Medical Staff & Administrative Team

Role of Administrator	Time period	Organizational characteristics	Board characteristics*	Medical staff characteristics	Administrative team** characteristics
Type A: *Business manager* Responsible for procuring supplies and personnel for physicians and con-serving limited resources	1920s to 1950s Free enter-prise but limited funds	Informal	Board holds hopsital in trust for donors to hospital Weatlhy trustees may be important funding sources Board may be primarily influenced by individual physicians who bring in paying patients	MDs with most patients have dominant in-fluence MDs function individually with board, administra-tion, nursing, etc., rather than collectively through a staff organization	Few functional spe-cialists Nursing dominates employee staff and they relate directly with individual MDs
Type B: *Coordinator* Boundry spanner Develops external role and becomes more influ-ential as he negotiates for resources	1950s to 1970s Growth & prosperity Rise of third party payers	More formal lines of communication Administrator begins to serve as major source of communi-cation	Board serves more as a repre-sentative link to the com-munity	MDs begin to function col-lectively through medical staff organization rather than individually	Functional specialists begin to develop Other department heads relate more to administrator than to individual MDs
Type C: *Corporate chief* Relies on formal author-ity for influence & functions more like a private corporation president Controls management information	1970s— Developing scarcity of resources & increasing external regulatior	Hierarchical-classical organization	Board is *used* to obtain com-munity support as well as communicate community expectations to hospital	Medical staff organization bargains collectively with administrator and board	Stronger functional specialists who pro-vide information to and help to support the administrator

151

Table 9-1 (continued)

Role of Administrator	Time period	Organizational characteristics	Board characteristics*	Medical staff characteristics	Administrative team** characteristics
Alternative for the future Type D: *Management team leader* Functions as a partner with board members, medical staff, director of nursing and other administrative team members. Relies more on knowledge, attitudes, skills, and sharing information than on formal authority and control of information to move the hospital toward desired goals	1970s, 1980s— Developing scarcity of resources and increasing external regulation	Matrix—open systems organization	Board is increasingly concerned about internal matters to cope with optimal regulation and scarcity. Board has more internal members Board sets objectives & evaluates total operations with information systems	Medical staff is actively involved and shares accountability for management decisions	Strong administrative team which relates directly and in partnership with administrator, board members, medical staff, and other employees

*These are characteristics that relate to administrator's roles. We do not suggest they affect ultimate legal responsibilities of boards that have been increasing in recent years.

**Administrative team is defined as functional specialists (e.g., controller, personnel director, director of systems engineering), director of nursing service, pharmacy, etc.

and characteristics of the board, medical staff, and administrative team. We suggest four role classifications:

A. Business manager
B. Coordinator
C. Corporate chief
D. Management team leader

It is important to note that not all administrators or hospital organizations fit neatly into one of these roles; many administrators are in a transitional stage moving from one category to another, and in varying situations they will assume different roles. Although time periods are given in which each role was most prevalent, examples can be found of hospitals and other health services that would fit into each one of these models today.

Type A: Business Manager

The business manager's role is one that was typical of the 1920s, 1930s, and 1940s with regard to managerial tasks and relationships with the board and medical staff. A common title for the administrator was that of hospital superintendent. He or she was clearly under the direction of the board of "trustees" who had responsibility for external affairs, raised and controlled funds, and set policy for the hospital. In the past trustees were also more involved in internal matters such as personnel relations and building plans. Perrow (1961) has effectively described such an historical role of trustee domination over organizational factors initially. With the rise of specialization Perrow noted that individual physicians then dominated organizational factors. In an environment of treating the sick and injured it was the purpose of the business manager's role to supervise the task of obtaining supplies and personnel resources needed by individual physicians and to manage scarce funds and facilities within policies set forth by the board of trustees.

Such a role is still prevalent today in some institutions. For example, a number of medical group practice administrators function in this way, although others function in a Type D role. Administrators in some large public hospitals function as business managers in cases where the board has more of a supervisory role (Pfeffer 1973). In some university hospitals, where the medical school administration and faculty also function as the board, the role of the administrator could be that of business manager. We know of an administrator who developed a Type D role, but later returned to a Type A because the medical school administration and some faculty believed his position had become too strong.

The organization in this setting is informal with the individual physicians dealing directly with influential trustees. Historically, nursing dominated the administrative team, as there were few other employed health professionals. Since the administrator is less influential than in other models it is unusual to find strong functional specialists in this model. Trustees and individual physicians tend to deal directly with administrative team members rather than through committees or a hierarchical administrative structure under this model.

Type B: Coordinator

Environmental and organizational factors changed in the 1950s and 1960s. Hospital services and community relations became more complex, and the individual physician's autonomy declined due to increased specialization and stricter requirements for accreditation. With the decline of dependency on fund raising and increasing external influences such as the Joint Commission on Accreditation, came a decline in the board's control. Employee relations also became more critical because of increasing employee specialization, scarcity of skilled personnel, and the threat or development of collective bargaining. The administrator was the logical and needed coordinator for employee, medical staff, board, and external agencies as well as manager for the employee organization. A Type B administrator often finds himself in a boundary position serving as a catalyst or referee. He also gains in influence as information systems improve, particularly if he keeps information to himself, and he serves as communicator or negotiator with external forces such as JCAH and third-party payers.

This is a role that is still prevalent today in nongovernmental, not-for-profit, short-term hospitals. Many, however, appear to be in a transition toward the Type C role. Below is a description of the job duties of an administrator from the U.S. Department of Labor[1] that seems to fit the Type B role.

ADMINISTRATOR

Executive Director/Executive Vice President

Hospital Administrator

JOB DUTIES

Administers, directs, and coordinates all activities of the hospital to carry out its objectives in the provision of health care, furtherance of education and research, and participation in community health programs.

Is responsible for the operation of the hospital, for the application and implementation of established policies, and for liaison among the governing authority, the medical staff, and the departments of the hospital.

Organizes the functions of the hospital through appropriate departmentalization and the delegation of duties. Establishes formal means of accountability from those to whom he has assigned duties. Regularly schedules interdepartmental and departmental meetings, where appropriate, to maintain liaison between the medical staff and other departments. Names appropriate departmental representatives to the multidisciplinary committee of the hospital.

Prepares reports for, and attends meetings with, the governing body regarding the total activities of the institution as well as governmental developments which affect health care. Provides for personnel policies and practices that adequately support sound patient care and maintain accurate and complete personnel records.

Reviews and acts upon the reports of authorized inspecting agencies. Implements the control and effective utilization of the physical and financial resources

---

[1] U.S. Department of Labor, *Job Description and Organizational Analysis for Hospitals and Related Services*, Manpower Division, 1971.

of the hospital. Employs a system of responsible accounting, including budget and internal controls.

Participates, or is represented, in community, state, and national hospital associations and professional activities which define the delivery of health care services and aid in short-and long-range planning of health services and facilities. Provides an acceptable public relations program.

Pursues a continuing program of formal and informal education in health care, administrative, and management areas to maintain, strengthen, and broaden his concepts, philosophy, and ability as a health care administrator.

Delegates administrative responsibilities to associate administrators and to department heads.

The American College of Hospital Administrators Task Force V suggested in 1973 that this description applies to a historical rather than a current role.

In the Type B model the organization becomes more formalized with the administrator serving as a link between medical staff, board, and administration committees. Functional specialists such as controllers and systems engineers begin to develop, usually coming to the hospital directly from industry and needing the administrator as a communications intermediary with the professional groups.

Type C: Corporate Chief

Trends described in the coordinator's role continued into the late sixties and seventies and fostered a chief executive's role for hospital administrators more akin to the role of president of a private corporation. Indeed, increasing numbers of administrators are receiving the title of president and are being elected to board membership.

The American College of Hospital Administrators (ACHA) has supported a more dominant or authoritative role for the hospital administrator as chief executive. The ACHA Task Force V has recommended and its Board of Governors has endorsed the following role for the chief executive officer:

The hospital chief executive officer is the person basically responsible for skillfully leading the hospital towards securing and maintaining health for the people it has chosen or been mandated to serve.

The chief executive officer's responsibilities are comparable to those of the president of a business or industrial service corporation which is labor intensive with a high degree of professional input and which requires extensive capital investment. In many communities, the hospital is the largest employer in the area.

The chief executive officer, in effect, could be called a "social change agent." As a professional, he or she should view the hospital as a social instrument for change. The chief executive officer is responsible for planning policy and program development subject to approval by the governing body, so that the organization, in cooperation with other organizations, contributes its share of the total response required by community needs. The chief executive officer may also manage the hospital so as to execute approved plans, or may delegate authority for this responsibility to another hospital administrator in the organization.

The chief executive officer's responsibilities are analogous, in the world of music to a combination of those of the composer and the orchestra conductor, and in the world of drama, to a combination of the playwright, the producer, and the director.

Reference is made in the above section to the "corporate role." This is the corporate organization of business and industry in which the chief executive officer (president) is a dominant figure on the board of directors, which is usually headed by a chairman. When "corporate role" or "corporate organization" is applied to the hospital field, the implication is that the hospital chief executive officer should have broad responsibilities and accountability paralleling those of the corporate chief executive officer (pp. 32-33).

By way of comparison a study conducted by the National Industrial Conference Board (1969), involving 300 chief executive officers in the United States and Canada, cited the following core responsibilities of the chief executive officer:

1 Determining objectives and plans
2 Establishing priorities and allocating resources in accord with plans and priorities
3 Formulating policies that establish the value system of the company
4 Determining basic organization structure
5 Developing a successor
6 Maintaining key external relationships principally with government
7 Maintaining relationships with the board of directors
8 Control—establishing standards and maintaining surveillance of performance

These eight responsibilities appear to generally coincide with the task force description and our Type C role.

The Type C role appears to be more authoritarian and closer to the classical theories of bureaucratic hierarchical management espoused by Max Weber (1921), Henri Fayol (1930), R. C. Davis (1951), and others. The ACHA Task Force calls for "administrative skill in participative management," which to us suggests a manipulative use of participation.

The ACHA role definition and task force report make little reference to chief executive-medical staff relationships except to state that "a strong, viable joint conference committee is probably the best single organizational tool for . . . relating the medical staff organization *to* the chief executive officer and board of trustees" (emphasis ours). The implication of the ACHA and our Type C role is that the medical staff plays a bargaining rather than a participatory role. However, a number of authors suggest that a medical director be employed by the hospital and report to the chief executive officer to help integrate the medical staff. That would probably also be consistent with both the Task Force's conception of the chief executive officer and our Type C role.

If the hospital administrator indeed serves as a corporate president with commensurate authority, it is likely that the medical staff will become further isolated from active participation in hospital management decision activities. Organized medicine appears to be concerned about this possibility. Anderson (1974), of the Office of General Council of the AMA, recently spoke of such concern stating:

> In some institutions, the situation has become so grave as to create a line of authority that goes from the attending staff to a salaried medical hierarchy which in turn is responsible to a hospital administrator, often styled as president of the hospital and frequently not only chief hospital executive, but the dominant voice on the hospital governing board. In the institutions where the hospital administrator occupies the role of hospital president and chairman of the hospital governing board, the only line of communication between the governing board and medical staff is through him. This is lay domination at its zenith and is a trend that should be aborted as early as possible.

Such mistrust and concerns are promoting the development of physician unions and collective bargaining, which further separates medical staff and hospital administrative organizations. An ultimate result of this hierarchical arrangement may be the establishment of a physician as chief executive officer, in an effort to integrate the medical staff and hospital administrative organizations. In other hierarchically organized systems such as hospitals in other countries, a physician frequently serves as chief executive officer.

The governing board in a Type C situation has a diminished influence in the hospital. With increasing external control and regulations such as price controls, rate review, labor negotiations, certificate of need, and areawide plans, the influence of the governing board has decreased in recent years. Pfeffer (1973) suggests that the role of the board is to provide a link with its environment. He found in a survey of 23 private nonprofit nonreligious hospitals that obtaining support and resources from the hospitals' environment was the primary function of the boards in settings other than hospitals. This may result in boards being used to manage the organization's environment as if they were instruments of corporation executives as has been found in for-profit industries (Pfeffer, 1973 and 1972; Vance, 1964; Zald, 1969; and others).

Under the Type C hospital administration role, the administrative team becomes stronger, but in a classical line or staff relationship to the administrator. The increasing complexities of the organization and their negotiation function require administrators to have better management information systems. Control of information is recognized as an important source of power (Filley and House, 1969). Strong functional specialties providing information to the administrator help to support the administrator's power and the hierarchical arrangement.

Davis and Henshaw (1974) surveyed Columbia University Health Services Administration graduates regarding their influence over hospital decision making. Respondents were asked what gave them, as hospital administrators, more influence over the important decisions in their institutions—formal decision-making authority, or control over the organizational process. About 76 percent of the 161 respondents used stated control over the organization process (20 percent stated formal authority and 4 percent said they were equal). They were further asked which specific methods of control over management processes were most effective; 84 percent said "influencing what is perceived to be a problem," 80 percent said "deciding who should be involved in a particular decision," 69 percent said "influencing the flow of information to particular individuals or groups," and 56 percent said "information gathering." This suggests that these administrators may use information as an important means of developing power consistent with a Type C role.

Type D: Management Team Leader

As a management team integrator and leader the administrator functions in a participative management role more as a partner with the board, medical staff, nursing staff, etc. Type D is a proactive leadership role rather than a reactive coordinative role like Type B. It assumes that in order to develop a more effective team approach at the patient care level, a team should be developed at the top management level. Administrators bring the management team to consensus and coordinate decision making. The Type D administrator promotes responsible management at all levels of the organization by sharing information openly, working with the management team to define objectives and problems, and letting the team either make decisions or determine who should be involved in making them; he uses management by objectives and other behavioral principles rather than authoritarian techniques (Likert, 1961; Bennis, 1965). The goal would be to integrate the medical staff into major governance and management decisions through participatory practices rather than to rely on the line authority through a medical director.

The role calls for team decisions, but does not relieve the administrator of the responsibility to see that decisions are implemented. Behavior of the administrator outside of the management team would be more "situational" (Fiedler, 1967; Vroom and Yetton, 1973). A Type D role is based on strong group process and interactive skills. It assumes a confident administrator who relies on management for results based on agreed-upon goals. The difference between Type C and D lies more in the approach than in the objectives of the role. Type D plays down the chief executive's legitimate authority and accentuates team accountability and responsibility in achieving goals. Participative management in other settings has been found to increase the influence of the administrator to achieve proper institutional goals (Mulder, 1971). And if participative management is utilized properly (not manipulatively) it may help remove some of the adversary roles and resolve excessive conflict in hospitals (Schulz and Johnson, 1971). It emphasizes administration in the broadest sense to include nurses, physicians, and others in the hospital who in fact manage services as a part of administration.

In the Type D model, the board takes a more active role in establishing objectives and evaluating operating results against explicit objectives. It would be logical in this model for the board to include the administrator, the chief of staff, the director of nursing, and possibly other key administrative heads, while still retaining a majority of community representatives.

In Type D, administrators play down their executive role in order to serve as integrators and leaders for consensus management by a team to deal with increasing external demands and more limited resources. The management team may vary from a limited partnership between the chief of staff and administrator to a larger team that might include the administrator, chief of the medical staff, the director of nursing, possibly the financial officer (who becomes increasingly important under a regulated system), and/or others. The team would have responsibility for determining objectives, establishing priorities and allocating resources, formulating policies, and setting standards, all of which would be submitted to the board for approval. The board has to ensure that they fulfill these responsibilities; it also holds the team accountable for measurable agreed-upon results. The administrator still has the leadership role of seeing that decisions are based on the best available information, and that they are executed. Staff specialists, while reporting to the administrator, would function in a more collegial relationship to health professionals providing information directly to departments and to the management team as in a matrix organizational structure (Neuhauser, 1972). It is important to repeat that while these are collegial involvements in problem solving and the development of decisions under Type D, implementation of decisions and accountability for results are still centralized under appropriate administrative heads, e.g., the director of nursing is accountable to the team and board for nursing.

One might expect that under this arrangement the administrator would have less control over nurses, medical staff, and the fiscal area. However, experience with a number of hospitals has shown that in practice, except for budget control, many administrators exercise little effective control over the efficiency and effectiveness of nursing care (e.g., see Illinois Commission on Nursing Report 1971) or medical care. With a team approach and mutual trust, evaluation and accountability for results by each of the team members could increase the real influence of the administrator over quality and efficiency of professional services. The administrator should have responsibility for the management of patient care and we suggest it could be exercised most effectively in a team system.

Ansoff (1973) described the evolution of the concept of a manager; he was seen as an entrepreneur up to about the 1870s, became a functional specialist between then and 1920, and a generalist from the 1920s until today. For the future, he predicts that demands on managers of complex systems will exceed the capacity and comprehension of any single individual, and suggests that "such overload has been the major reason for the emergence of the concept of the corporate office which *replaces the chief executive officer with a team of co-equals*" (emphasis ours). He calls for a differentiated manager who would be what psychologists call a T-shaped individual. He would be a generalist (the top of the T) in the sense that he would share with all other managers a common understanding of the generic social guidance and control process called management. The stem of the T would be his or her special skills, personal traits, or unique perspective. While Ansoff is talking about industrial management, his model seems particularly appropriate to the hospital, which is already one of the most complex and divided organizations in our society.

A number of arguments can be put forth against a management team approach in addition to the expectation that some hospital administrators will fear it. For example, the training and orientation of physicians is the antithesis of training for management. Dennis (1968), the Chancellor of Health Services at the University of Arkansas, described how medical training develops physician behavior of independence rather than cooperation (see Chapter 5). However, it should be noted that many examples of effective physician managers can be found.

Other arguments against the management team concept are that the consensus management inherent in a management team approach fosters conformity, which is a barrier to creativity. However, a counterargument would be that heterogenous groups have proved they can develop creative solutions, although interpersonal cooperation is more likely with homogenous groups (Collins and Guetzkow, 1964). Moreover, research has shown groups are more willing to take risks than individual decision makers (Clark, 1971). Another argument against a team approach is that it may handicap cost control. Participation by physicians, nurses, or other professionals may result in higher expenditures for esoteric programs or unnecessarily high staffing. On the other hand, there appear to be few incentives for administrators or governing board members to control costs at the present time (Schulz and Rose, 1973). Other arguments against a Type D team is that it is like a committee. Who really is in control, who will accept accountability and responsibility, can all, or will it be none of the team?

Looking at these four roles we conclude there is no "role for all seasons," but that each is appropriate for a certain time and environmental interaction. The Type A role was appropriate for the laissez faire era of the past or, at present, for certain governmental and other hospitals where there is close board supervision of operations. Type B was and still is appropriate in community hospitals where there is a balance of power and need for coordination by a boundary spanner. The Type C role appears viable in a rapid growth situation where resources are abundant and the administrator can negotiate for them in order to build a larger and higher quality institution meeting most of the desires of physicians, nurses, and board members. Moreover, a type C role is common in a highly regulated bureaucratic environment, one in which hospitals are increasingly finding themselves (see Perrow, 1972 for a review and evaluation of bureaucratic and other models). We believe, however, that a Type D administrator would also be appropriate in growth situations; more importantly we suggest that it may be an effective alternative for the era of scarcity of resources and increasing external regulation projected for the foreseeable future.

There have been a few examples of the Type D model in recent years. Danielson (1966) described a management advisory council used in one hospital that appears to operate as a Type D model. He stated that "this is a council where the only criterion for adoption of an idea is its own validity. No dictate but consensus—no pecking order to threaten assigned official prerogatives, or votes to cause division." The management advisory council consisted of the chairmen of the three major clinical departments and the senior executive officer of the hospital. According to Danielson (1975) the arrangement works. The Mayo Clinic in Rochester, Minnesota is another example of a successful organization that has used a management committee approach. The management team concept appears to be working well in Great Britain even though the British system has serious troubles; but these problems are primarily due to other factors (Schulz and Chester, forthcoming.)

CONCLUSIONS

What may be the most effective role for the administrator in the future as needs of society and environmental resources and values change? It has previously been suggested, and will be elaborated on further in Chapters 14 and 15, that external forces will increasingly set expectations and impose constraints on the hospital. Hospitals are likely to have less influence over their external environment than at any time in the past. If such a situation comes to pass, it will require increasing managerial control over internal affairs. This would suggest an increasing need for:

More effective management of and accountability from the medical staff, which is a primary influence on the hospital and essentially controls 87 cents of the hospital dollar (Knowles, 1966).

More effective management of the nursing area, since there appears to be little relationship between patient needs and nurse staffing. Nursing is the highest single cost item in a hospital (Illinois Commission on Nursing, 1971). More effective management of other professional services is also needed.

More managerial expertise and more effective management information systems and use of such systems.

A generally more efficient operation that conserves increasingly scarce resources and establishes priorities that will achieve hospital goals more effectively.

More effective integration of services both internally and with external agencies.

More knowledgeable decisions regarding objectives, plans, policies, and organizational arrangements, and more effective and efficient implementation of decisions in relationship to hospital programs and activities.

In order to meet these increasing needs more, not less, hospital leadership is needed. The Type A model in which the administrator does not have a major external role and does not participate in the management of patient care does not appear appropriate for the future for most hospitals. The Type B role is more reactive and does not appear to provide the necessary leadership expectations for the future. The Type C role, if implemented in practice and not just with a change of title, calls for strong leadership. However, we suggest it could result in negotiations and confrontations rather than cooperation and medical staff and nursing accountability A Type C administrator who tries to use participative techniques may be looked upon by employees and physicians as a manipulator.

In most situations, it would appear that the Type D role may meet the needs or criteria suggested above more effectively than the other types, but it has a number of requirements in order to be effective. An administrator in a Type D role will need to be much more of a "star" than in any other role model He or she will have to earn status through knowledge, attitudes, and skills rather than through just legitimate authority in holding information and controlling funds. He or she will have to be confident enough to work as an equal with other team members. The administrator will have to be extremely objective and sensitive to changing needs and expectations in order to expedite accomplishment of proper goals efficiently and effectively. This places a considerable burden on health administration programs to select students who have the requisite personal and intellectual capacities, and to help them obtain the required knowledge, attitudes, and skills. Without this administrators are likely to revert from a D to an A role—if their institutions survive.

The Type D role also requires other strong members on the management team. The nursing head will need considerable confidence and knowledge, and appropriate attitudes and skills to be an equal partner on the team. This places additional burdens on the training of nursing administrators at a time when there is a deemphasis on nursing administration education.

Functional specialists will have a more important role in hospitals, and it is important that they be able to understand and communicate effectively in the health setting (see Gustafson et al., 1975). Moreover, in order to attract more competent individuals to the health industry, it should be possible for them to reach top administration jobs as members of the management team. Finally, a Type D arrangement requires effective physician participation in decision activities (see Perkins 1974 and Schulz and Chester, forthcoming).

Physicians will have to be more aware of the needs and opportunities for more effective and efficient health services and of the social, economic, political, and managerial aspects of health care. To develop such attitudes within the present medical education system will not be easy. However, there have been some successful examples, and continuing education programs such as those run by Wesley Eisele, M.D., in Colorado have been influential. Educational programs in England for nurse administration, physicians, and other members of the health team appear to go a long way toward providing the necessary knowledge, attitudes, and skills.

It is our recommendation that the training of health administrators be integrated wherever possible with the training of nursing administrators, functional specialists for health institutions, and medical students or house staff who are likely to end up in leadership roles. This is being attempted in a few settings and it appears to have considerable potential for payoffs. On a shorter-range basis, administrators should remember that they, too, are role senders and can have an important influence on changing the role behavior of nursing and medical administrators and functional specialists so that they become more effective members of at least an informal management team.

In conclusion, roles have been changing and are likely to change more dramatically in the future. Rather than fearing changes and attempting to solidify the status quo with more formal authority, we suggest that administrators and governing board members carefully examine changing environmental and institutional ground rules and study alternative organizational and role models for meeting societal and institutional objectives. While we suggest that a Type D management team role model may be a better way to run the hospital of the future, we must caution administrators that a move to such a role would probably be irreversible during their tenure of administration. It is a role that would probably take time to develop, but a gradual transition can be made from a Type B to a Type D, or a Type C to a Type D.

REFERENCES

ACHA: *Principles of Appointment and Tenure of Executive Officers,* American College of Hospital Administrators Task Force V, Chicago, 1973.

Anderson, Betty Jane: "Hospital Governing Board and Medical Staff Relations," *Milwaukee Medical Society Times,* vol. 47, no. 4, p. 4, April 1974.

Ansoff, H. Igor: "The Next Twenty Years in Management Education," *The Library Quarterly,* vol. 43, no. 4, pp. 293-328, Oct. 1973.

Battistella, Roger M. and Theodore E. Chester: "The 1974 Reorganization of the British National Health Service—Aims and Issues," *New England Journal of Medicine,* pp. 610-615, Sept. 20, 1973.

Bennis, Warren: "Beyond Bureaucracy," *Transactions,* July-Aug. 1965.

Clark, Russell D. III: "Group-Induced Shift toward Risk," *Psychological Bulletin,* vol. 76, no. 4, pp. 251-270, 1971.

Collins, B. E. and H. Guetzkow: *A Social Psychology of Group Processes for Decision Making,* Wiley, 1964.

Connors, Edward J. and Joseph C. Hutts: "How Administrators Spend Their Day," *Hospitals, J.A.H.A.,* vol. 41, Feb. 16, 1967.

Danielson, John M.: "Organized Action: Management Advisory Councils," *JAMA,* pp. 1062-1063, June 20, 1966.

Danielson, John M.: personal communications, 1975.

Davis, R. C.: *The Fundamental of Top Management,* Harper and Row, New York, 1951.

Davis, Samuel and Stanley Henshaw: *Decision Analysis in Hospital Administration* (monograph), Association of University Programs in Health Administration, Washington, D.C., April 1974.

Dennis, James L.: Speech delivered in 1968 while Dean, University of Oklahoma School of Medicine. Currently, Dr. Dennis is Vice President for Health Sciences, University of Arkansas Medical Center, Little Rock, Arkansas.

Dolson, Miriam T.: "How Administrators Rate Different Tasks of Importance," *The Modern Hospital,* June 1965.

Fayol, Henri: *Industrial and General Administration,* Pitman, London, 1930.

Fielder, Fred E.: *A Theory of Leadership Effectiveness,* McGraw-Hill, New York, 1967.

Filley, Allan C. and Robert House: *Managerial Process and Organization Behavior,* Scott Foresman, Glenview, Illinois, 1969, pp. 60-64.

Gustafson, David, Glenwood Rowse, and Nancy J. Howes: "Roles and Training for Future Health Systems Engineers," in *Education for Health Administration,* vol. 2, Health Administration Press, Ann Arbor, Mich., 1975.

Illinois Commission on Nursing: *Nurse Utilization, Illinois: A Study in Thirty-One Hospitals, 1966-1970,* vol. 3, Illinois Study Commission on Nursing sponsored by the Illinois League for Nursing, Illinois Nurses Association and Illinois Hospital Association, Chicago, 1971.

Katz, Daniel and Robert L. Kahn: *The Social Psychology of Organizations,* Wiley, New York, 1966.

Knowles, John: *The Teaching Hospital,* Harvard University Press, Cambridge, Mass., 1966.

Likert, Rensis: *New Patterns in Management,* McGraw-Hill, New York, 1961.

Likert, Rensis: *The Human Organization, Its Management and Value*, McGraw-Hill, New York, 1967.

Mulder, M.: "Power Equalization Through Participation," *Administrative Science Quarterly*, vol. 16, pp. 31-38, March 1971.

Murray, R. T.: "How Administrators Spend Their Time," *Hospital Progress*, vol. 49, pp. 49-58, 1968.

National Industrial Conference Board: "The Chief Executive and His Job," *Studies in Personnel Policy*, no. 214, 1969.

Neuhauser, Duncan: "The Hospital as a Matrix Organization'" *Hospital Administration*, Fall 1972.

Parsons, Talcott: *Structure and Process in Modern Societies*, Free Press, New York, 1960.

Perkins, Roy S.: "The Perspective of the Medical Staff," in *Evaluating the Contemporary Hospital: Report of the 1974 National Forum on Hospital and Health Affairs*, Department of Health Administration, Duke University, Durham, N.C., 1974.

Perrow, Charles: "The Analysis of Goals in Complex Organizations," *American Sociological Review*, vol. 26, pp. 854-866, 1961.

Perrow, Charles: *Complex Organizations: A Critical Essay*, Scott Foresman, Glenview, Ill., 1972.

Petit, Thomas: "A Behavioral Theory of Management," *Academy of Management*, pp. 341-350, Dec. 1967.

Pfeffer, Jeffrey: "Size and Composition of Corporate Boards of Directors Organization and Environment," *Administrative Sciences Quarterly*, vol. 17, no. 2, pp. 218-228, 1972.

Pfeffer, Jeffrey: "Size Composition and Function of Hospital Boards of Directors: A Study of Organization–Environment Linkage," *Administrative Sciences Quarterly*, vol. 18, no. 3, pp. 349-363, 1973.

Rowbottom, Ralph et al.: *Hospital Organization*, Heinemann Books, London, 1973.

Schulz, Rockwell and Alton C. Johnson: "Conflict in Administration," *Hospital Administration*, vol. 16, Summer 1971.

Schulz, Rockwell and T. E. Chester: "Physician Participation in Management Decision Activities in England and Implications for the U.S." (forthcoming).

Schulz, Rockwell and Jerry Rose: "Can Hospitals Be Expected to Control Costs?" *Inquiry*, June 1973.

Vance, Stanley: *Boards of Directors: Structure and Performance*, University of Oregon Press, Eugene, 1964.

Vroom, Victor H. and Philip W. Yetton: *Leadership and Decision Making*, Pittsburgh University Press, Pittsburgh, 1973.

Weber, Max: *Theory of Social and Economic Organization*, 1921, ed. and trans. A. M. Henderson and T. Parsons, Oxford University Press, 1947.

Wren, George: "Titles of Hospital Administrators," *Hospital Administration*, pp..68-82, Spring 1974.

Zald, Mayer N.: "The Power and Function of Boards of Directors: A Theoretical Synthesis," *American Journal of Sociology*, vol. 75, pp. 97-111, 1969.

Chapter 10

Managerial Functional Specialists

"Hospitals do not utilize managerial tools commonly found in industry; no wonder costs of hospital care are so high." This frequently heard invective against hospitals is a simplistic response to certain truths. However, there is considerable evidence that few hospitals utilize modern accounting systems, operations research techniques, industrial engineering processes, and other quantitative methods that have been applied in other industries (Stimson and Stimson, 1972; Kovner and Lusk, 1973; Gustafson et al., 1975; and personal experiences and communications). Moreover, in those cases where managerial tools, especially computers, have been used, the results have sometimes been questionable and have frequently contributed to increases in hospital costs.

In this chapter we will suggest ways to improve the use of managerial tools by functional specialists such as accountants, industrial engineers, and planners. We will not attempt to review the body of knowledge of these disciplines since they are described in a number of basic texts. Among those that relate directly to hospitals are Berman and Weeks (1971), Silvers and Prahelad (1974), Griffith (1972), Koza (1973), Levy and Loomba (1973), and Stimson and Stimson (1972).

Moreover, further consideration is given to some of these issues in later chapters on management of quality, costs, and conflict. In addition to managerial specialists concerned with quantitative methods, this chapter also briefly considers specialists for personnel, public relations, planning, and the employment of consultants. Other important managerial specialists, e.g., material management specialists, are not considered due to limitations of space.

The first section of this chapter presents definitions for quantitative methods, their use and functional specialties. The second looks at hospital financial managers, systems (industrial) engineers, data processing, and planners, and brielfy considers personnel management and public relations. The final section discusses factors that might improve the effectiveness of functional specialists and the use of consultants.

APPLICATIONS OF QUANTITATIVE METHODS AND MANAGEMENT SPECIALISTS IN HOSPITALS

The knowledge and skills of functional specialists are becoming increasingly important in the management of hospitals for a number of reasons:

The increasing size and complexity of hospital operations require more formal procedures than have been necessary in the past. Informal contacts between the medical staff, nursing, and other departments and the administration are no longer frequent and communication problems are increasing.

It is difficult for the administrator to keep informed about internal operations since he or she spends more time on external affairs important to the hospital.

Assuming that everything is satisfactory unless the administrator or governing board hears complaints is no longer an acceptable method of management because the environment in which a hospital operates is changing so fast. Moreover, complaints seem to be increasing, and continually putting out fires is not effective managerial control.

Hospitals are coming under increasing scrutiny. Administrators and trustees need measures of hospital effectiveness in order to have better control over institutional destiny.

Resources with which to operate the hospital are becoming increasingly scarce. In years past hospitals could raise rates or increase volume almost at will to obtain additional resources. Today more mileage must be obtained from very limited resources.

Administrators and governing boards have less authority today. Employees, public agencies, and consumers must be convinced to act in certain ways and administrators and trustees must back up their requests with proof.

Managerial knowledge and skills have advanced to a point where specialists are needed to cope with and apply them.

In other words administrators, governing board members, and others involved in the management of hospitals need both a great deal of information and experts who are qualified to analyze it.

Management information systems, operations research (OR), systems analysis, econometrics, financial management, institutional research, data processing, computer sciences, systems and procedures, methods improvement, scientific management, and many more terms are used in describing the application of quantitative methods in management. The confusion and overlap are not only in the terminology, but also in the characteristics of the functional specialists who work with quantitative methods and those who do not; in the educational programs (disciplines) in which they receive the training; and within respective professional associations.

Table 10-1 attempts to summarize the functions of a number of managerial specialists, listing some of their tools and the university disciplines that supply their training. It is important to stress that these are only examples; there are many other titles, combinations of functions, and disciplines of training that may be found in larger hospitals. Clearly there is a need for better definition of tools and their uses, in addition to more team work among specialists.

FUNCTIONAL SPECIALISTS

In this section the functions of fiscal management, systems engineering, computer applications, planning, personnel management and public relations, and volunteer services will be considered primarily on the basis of applications of the body of knowledge.

Fiscal Management

Specialists in accounting functions have been present in hospitals for many years. However, theirs has been (and in some institutions still is) mainly a bookkeeping and an accounts and collections function. Incentives for accounting functions in the past have been to meet the requirements of Internal Revenue Services, public accounting, and the needs of trustees who were primarily concerned with the solvency of the institution. Incentives for cost accounting came from the requirements for participation in the Medicare program in the late 1960s. Incentives for more effective budgeting have come from price controls, social security amendments (P.L. 92-603), certificate-of-need legislation, and rate review programs in the early 1970s (these are described in later chapters).

Recently there has been a trend away from the narrower concept of hospital accounting and toward broader concerns of hospital financial management. This reflects increasing needs for managerial decisions based on a quantitative analysis of the cost-effectiveness implications of alternative actions. For example, the discipline of finance can provide the administration and the governing board with data on the cost implications of various capital investment opportunities through the use of finance tools such as present value and internal rate of return analysis.

In spite of the benefits of better control they offer, accounting and finance tools have not been widely used. For example, Blue Cross officials in one state reported that 70 percent of the hospitals in that state either were not familiar with appropriate

Table 10-1 Examples of Management Specialties, Tools, and Training

Functional specialty	Tools	University discipline as a site of training
Financial management or controller, accountant, business office, etc.	Accounting reports, budgets, responsibility accounting, cost volume analysis, cost accounting, OR tools, credit extension, management of cash, inventory and capital structure, etc.	Business (accounting and/or finance)
Systems engineering or industrial engineering, methods improvement, systems design, etc.	Design, implementation, control and evaluation techniques, time and motion, facility layouts, OR techniques, etc.	Industrial engineering (IE), production management
Data processing or computer services, information systems, etc.	Computers, OR techniques, etc.	Accounting, IE, computer sciences, economics, statistics, etc.
Planning or institutional research, R&D, etc.	Statistical analysis, computers, group process techniques, OR, systems, marketing, etc.	Generalist background in health administration or planning or almost any specialized department
Personnel management	Job design, position descriptions and controls, training, etc.	Business (personnel management)
Public relations	Surveys, communications devices	Generalist or journalism, etc.
Materials management or purchasing agent, etc.	Inventory control techniques	Business, pharmacy, nursing, IE, etc.

budgeting techniques or were just beginning to establish budget systems. There appear to be a number of reasons for this, including the following:

The primary goals of hospitals involve service rather than the profit maximization of the typical business firm, which has more sophisticated accounting and finance methods.

Many hospital financial managers have had minimal training. While data on the qualifications of hospital financial managers are sparse, a survey of registrants of Hospital Financial Management Association (HFMA) educational programs suggests that large numbers of hopsital financial departments are headed by individuals without a college education. Presumably, most of those without a college education are in small hospitals.

Many hospital administrators lack knowledge of good accounting and finance practices. The majority of hospital administrators in the nation have not had formal training in hospital management.[1] Moreover, until recently, some programs in hospital administration provided little training in fiscal management.

Participative accounting practices such as responsibility accounting are not utilized.

There is considerable evidence of communication difficulties between hospital financial managers and heads of professional departments because of language barriers caused by technical terminology and mistaken perception of motives. For example, many professionals believed financial managers were not interested in patient care— only in money. And financial managers believed professionals had no interest in costs.

Incentives for financial management were lacking because of the ease of obtaining higher income until recently by raising rates and increasing volume of service. There have been more incentives for income maximization and larger facilities than for cost containment (Schulz and Rose, 1973).

The personal characteristics of some financial managers—their attitudes, skills, knowledge, and behavior—limit their effectiveness.

Financial managers need to be particularly skillful in communicating with nurses, physicians, and other health professionals who lack the knowledge of, and motives for financial control (unlike managers in industry with whom financial managers work).

Most financial managers have been hired from commercial enterprises and are unfamiliar with hospital objectives, dealing with professionals, patient care programs, and so forth.

Some financial managers have gone into hospitals after unsuccessful careers in industry.

Financial managers who serve in hospitals where the administrator fills a Type A or B role (see Chapter 9) will probably find their role similarly diminished. Delbecq suggests that one reason why functional specialists are used less in hospitals than in other industries of similar size is their inability to influence the organizational elite (personal communications). In industrial concerns the president clearly has the most influence and he relies on the advice of functional specialists, particularly the financial vice president.

---

[1] Hospital association directors in three midwestern states estimated in 1970 that the number of hospitals in their states headed by formally trained administrators ranged from 20 percent to 45 percent (personal communications).

In professional organizations such as hospitals, formal recognition of professional competency is a sought-after goal. Professional recognition of the financial manager as a C.P.A. is deemed by administrators to be an ideal qualification for a hospital setting. Financial managers are usually in the top echelon of administration reporting directly to the administrator or chief executive officer as would the director of nursing service. As we suggested above and in Chapter 9, the effective role of the financial manager will depend upon the role of the administrator.

In the last section of this chapter we will discuss some ways of improving the role of financial management in hospitals.

Hospital Systems Engineering

Hospital systems or management engineering has its basis primarily in the discipline of industrial engineering. This discipline had its origins with Frederick W. Taylor and Frank Gilbreth around the turn of the century and utilized tools of time and motion studies. While this traditional "efficiency expert" approach is still prevalent in some hospital programs, the role of the industrial engineer has broadened in many others.

The American Institute of Industrial Engineering (AIIE) has adopted the following definition, which indicates a broadened role for industrial engineering: "Industrial Engineering is concerned with the design, improvement and installation of integrated systems of men, materials and equipment. It draws upon specialized knowledge and skill in mathematical, physical and social sciences together with the principles and methods of engineering analysis and design to specify, predict and evaluate the results to be obtained from such systems" (AHA, 1970, p. 4). This definition has also been adopted by the Hospital Management Systems Society.

A unique aspect of systems engineering is its emphasis upon improvements; in contrast, administrators, physicians, and others are frequently more concerned with maintenance. It is apparent that improvements, like maintenance, require teamwork. Good relationships between the engineer and administrators, physicians, nurses, and other professionals are crucial to success.

Gustafson et al. (1975) suggest that systems engineers can have an important role in meeting the following kinds of problems in hospitals:

Facilitating and obtaining agreement on goals, and plans to achieve goals
Organizing and coordinating services to reduce costs and improve accessibility of care
Setting up more effective ways of evaluating and improving the quality of care provided
Improving personnel utilization
Improving work methods

They suggest that, to accomplish the above, the engineer would work in a multi-disciplinary team as a specialist in technical facilitation, designing and changing strategies during the design, implementation, and evaluation phases of a hospital project. The engineer should be able to set up, obtain, and analyze measurements for the above with help from others in the hospital team and build conceptual design and mathematical models for decision making with assistance from content experts such as administrators and physicians. Some variation in training is needed depending upon which of the above problems the engineer is going to handle.

The AHA Committee on Management Engineering (AHA, 1970) suggests three major functions for systems engineers: (1) providing staff services to hospital administration by improving work systems, establishing standards, developing job descriptions, determining layouts, conducting cost/benefit analysis, improving organizational arrangements, establishing information systems, etc.; (2) providing staff education to establish receptivity to change, facilitate communications, and improve capabilities of personnel; and (3) conducting research for improvement in the delivery of hospital services. Systems engineers can be employed as staff by hospitals; in smaller institutions a group of hospitals could share engineering personnel or a hospital might employ consultant engineers. Each alternative has advantages and disadvantages, and there is no clear-cut formula for choosing the best one in a given situation. In many hospitals the systems engineer is located on the third level of management, usually reporting to an assistant or associate administrator, and consequently conducting the lower-return projects.

As was true of other functional specialists, Gustafson et al. (1975) found that in only a few instances were systems engineers fulfilling the theoretical roles described above, or having a major impact on hospital problems. This is interesting when the AHA (1975) reports that 55 percent of 6,079 hospitals responding to their survey report they employ industrial engineers on a full-time, shared, or consulting basis.

In personal experience we have found that administrators give only lip service to systems engineering, apparently believing that as long as they had appointed someone to improve productivity and control costs they were meeting responsibilities to their community for this function. Gustafson et al. found administrators who had little conception of what constitutes a modern engineering program. On the other hand, he found social and political failures to be more prevalent than inadequacy of engineering technical skills. Conflict among the overlapping functional specialties of financial management, data processing, engineering, and others was not uncommon. An appropriate team approach among these closely related functions was lacking in a number of cases, to the detriment of the potential of each. Chapter 13 presents some suggestions for ways to reduce such conflict.

While many hospital engineering programs seemed to have little impact, in a few significant results were found. In one large hospital that one of the authors surveyed, the administrator documented *real* savings of over $1 million annually due in large part to the efforts of a systems engineering program. Four major characteristics of this program that were lacking in others surveyed were:

1 Top management was committed to cost reduction, knowledgeable about industrial engineering practices, and very supportive of engineers.
2 Engineers were knowledgeable about hospital objectives, operations, and problems.

3 Engineers were not only competent in their field, but had personal stature and elan. They communicated well with professionals and would be found at coffee or lunch with nurses, physicians, and others rather than clustering as a group by themselves, as was evident in other hospitals.

4 The hospital appeared to fit into a Type D model (see Chapter 9). It was not hierarchically organized, that is, communication was generally across the organization between individuals rather than vertical as in traditional lines of authority. Physicians, nurses, and others would contact or be contacted directly by the engineers rather than go through formal lines of authority. There were good relations and respect among various functional specialists all of whom appeared to be very strong.

5 Engineers were technical facilitators in designing, implementing, and evaluating rather than traditional work measurement engineers.

We suggest that many of these findings for systems engineering regarding the important ingredients for success might apply equally to other functional specialty programs.

Computer Systems

In the late 1950s and early 1960s computerization and automation were hailed as the solution to the rising costs of a labor-intensive industry and to the problems of coordinating increasingly complex hospital services. Jydstrup and Gross (1966) found that information handling accounted for approximately 25 percent of each hospital's total operating costs. Many hospitals were eager to install computer systems. A few hospitals as small as 100 beds have rather elaborate computers. Trustees, administrators, and physicians have been proud of their computers, seeing them as an indication of their hospital's sophistication and progress. A 1968 survey of all hospitals in the United States indicated that 578 had computer installations, and nearly 20 percent of all hospitals over 100 beds had them (Mariner, 1971). Mariner noted that only 283 of the hospitals with computers employed operations researchers or systems analysts, suggesting a "dangerous tendency toward installing equipment today and worrying about its use tomorrow."[2]

Management information systems is a commonly used term to describe the total data gathering and analysis system of the hospital. Gillette et al. (1970) suggest that there are eight information subsystems in a hospital:

1 *Patient diagnosis and treatment system,* which would include information derived from such hospital departments as clinical laboratories, pathology, electrocardiology, diagnostic radiology, pharmacy, rehabilitation services, and nursing services
2 *Patient record system,* which would involve medical records, admissions insurance, etc., in addition to the above departments
3 *Patient scheduling and order system,* which would include all patient care departments and support services such as dietary and housekeeping

[2]It is important to note that while computers are important *tools* of operation researchers and system analysts, they are by no means synonomous with operations research and systems analysis, which have many other tools.

4 *Patient accounting system,* which involves most of the above plus accounting, credit and collection offices, etc.

5 *Expenditure and general accounting system,* which includes budgeting, payroll, materials, and plant systems in addition to patient service departments

6 *Personnel system of* employee and position information

7 *General supportive services system,* which include industrial engineering, data processing, plant management, etc.

8 *Management control system,* which runs through all systems for effective and efficient management

Most computer applications in hospitals are in routine accounting functions such as payroll and patient billing. The clinical laboratory and hospital pharmacy have also been areas of computer application in a number of hospitals. Automated history taking, diagnosis, and patient records have been subjects of considerable research as have menu planning, employee staffing, patient scheduling, and so forth. A number of companies, e.g., aerospace companies and computer manufacturers, are currently marketing total hospital information systems.

Rigorous evaluation of computer applications has been lacking. However, the little evaluation that has been done suggests that it is difficult to justify computer usage in patient-oriented services on the basis of cost savings (Stimson and Stimson, 1972). Singer (1970) in his survey found that "justification for introducing computerized systems in hospitals was not well documented nor were evaluations based on adequate before-and-after comparisons." Some hospitals share computer services, which would appear to be a logical way of increasing capabilities and sharing costs. However, there is reluctance in many other hospitals to share patient and institutional information that may be confidential with other institutions, Blue Cross, or planning agencies. Moreover, the prestige of owning one's own computer is no small deterrent to sharing.

Although applications of computer technology in hospitals have not as yet lived up to expectations, few will refute their potential for automating medical, patient care, and support systems. Stimson and Stimson's (1972) analysis of some of the reasons why operations research has not been implemented in hospitals seems pertinent to the application of computer technology:

1 Tendency to view the hospital as a separable system

2 Tendency to view the hospital as a mechanistic system

3 Failure to foresee the dysfunctional consequences of introducing computer-based technology in the hospital

4 Failure to assess the complexities involved in applying computer-based technology in the hospital

5 Lack of attention to model building and the way data for models are generated

6 Omission of variables that are difficult to quantify

7 Failure to include detailed information on the costs and benefits of proposed changes

8 Failure to recognize limitations on the power of the administrator

9 Neglect of the literature on implementation

One might add other factors such as a general resistance to change. It is also important to note that these factors reflect the complexity of the task of effectively utilizing computer technology.

Organizationally, computer systems may be found in the fiscal management area (especially if computer applications are primarily in accounting systems) or they may be in a separate unit, in systems engineering, or in another location. The head of the unit may have received his training in any one of a number of disciplines or received on-the-job training from a computer manufacturer or a software consulting service.

In site visits to a number of institutions we found the same sort of problems with computer services as we did with other functional specialties, e.g., poor communications and jurisdictional disputes, and inability to evaluate current operations or potential for computers among top administrators. In the institutions we visited, computer services did appear to be a more aggressive operation than some other staff services and to enjoy more organizational support.

Planning

Planning is generally considered to be one of the most important functions of hospital administration. The dynamics of health care, the need to improve the delivery of health services, and the increasing pressures on hospitals all argue for long-range planning. Some may say that things are changing so fast that it is fruitless to plan, yet rapid change and the hospitals' increasing difficulty in controlling their own destiny are precisely why planning is so important. Long-range plans are a blueprint for hospital decisions and are preferable to making decisions in a vacuum or not making them at all, which usually results in the worst kinds of decisions. Plans provide an opportunity for the hospital to be proactive and a leader, rather than reactive, and if they are developed and understood by the hospital community, they can help unify diverse interests and goals.

There are a number of important criteria for effective long-range planning:

Plans should be based on a thorough study of the needs the hospital is established to serve. This is not an easy task. It requires study of community needs and advice from consumer representatives and scholars of community needs.

Broad participation is important to effective planning and implementation of plans. In addition to consumers (whose participation can be accomplished through group process techniques such as nominal groups [Delbecq and Van de Ven, 1972]), the medical staff and other members of the hospital family should be included.

Plans should be comprehensive and developed in a continuum from:
    Definition of community needs
    Definition of objectives
    Programs to achieve objectives
    Organizational arrangement for fulfilling programs
    Staffing required
    Facilities needed
    Financial requirements (this is likely to result in revisions of objectives programs, staffing, etc.)

Relationships with others

Return to start cycle again as needs and other factors continually change

Plans should be flexible, action-oriented, and continually updated consistent with other changes.

Plans should strive for higher levels of achievement.

Plans should be realistic within constraints of resources.

Plans should be time-phased from long-range back to the forthcoming year.

Plans should be a basis for hospital operation e.g., decisions, budget systems, and evaluations.

In spite of the importance of planning, but possibly because of its magnitude, few hospitals have plans that meet the above criteria. Many hospitals have long-range facility plans, but these are only means to ends. Some hospitals plan facilities, then must attempt to fit programs into facilities rather than designing facilities to meet the programs.

Many hospitals have planning committees as a part of their governing board and occasionally they include operating personnel as well. Staff services so essential to the planning process are usually left to the administrator or someone else who is committed to many other tasks. Consultants frequently provide planning services, but usually on a one-shot basis so that plans become outdated rapidly.

Institutional research and development (R&D) aimed at improving hospital services is another function usually neglected by all but the largest hospitals. Anyone with the title of head of hospital development is usually a fund raiser. Research and development are important functions of the more progressive industrial corporations, but it is more difficult for hospitals than for industries to demonstrate tangible returns on R&D investments. Most hospitals depend upon universities for research in the delivery of health services, but they could do a great deal of R&D either in association with universities or on their own.

Funding for R&D can be obtained from both federal and private sources. Local industries may be willing to support a hospital research and demonstration project even when they would not support other hospital activities. In Chapter 7 we suggested a number of opportunities for hospital R&D.

Personnel Management

Personnel management is an increasingly important, specialized function in the modern hospital. The principal objective of personnel management is to enable administrators and department heads to integrate organizational and employee needs. In a labor-intensive organization such as a hospital, this indeed is a significant function.

Of the many activities performed by the personnel department, the procurement of employees is the most basic. The range of responsibility ranges from the recruiting and initial screening of employees to the actual hiring of some employees. The basic personnel management philosophy is for personnel to perform actual recruiting and initial screening but for the department head to make the final decision to hire. In practice, it appears that the personnel department often does the hiring because department heads have confidence in the ability of the personnel staff and accept their recommendations regarding potential employees.

In the procurement activity, the members of the personnel department should be proficient in developing labor market information, carrying out recruitment campaigns, developing job descriptions, evaluating and validating selection instruments such as tests, administering selection tools such as application blanks, maintaining files of accepted as well as rejected applicants, and aiding in the orientation of new employees to the hospital.

A second activity or function performed by the personnel department is assisting department heads and administrators in the evaluation of employee performance. This may involve developing evaluation instruments, training management personnel to evaluate employees, and discussing results with them, as well as auditing promotions, transfers. salary increases, dismissals, and resignations.

Wage and salary administration is a third function assigned to personnel specialists. The purpose is to develop and maintain equity in wage and salary payments as well as to evaluate the overall labor budget.

Because of the increasing importance attached to training and development, personnel specialists have been appointed as training directors. The general objective is to enable department heads and administrators to meet their employee development responsibilities by utilizing training techniques and general educational programs. In larger hospitals, the training function may be established as a separate unit or department.

As hospital employees become unionized, specialists in labor relations to aid in contract negotiation and administration are hired by hospitals and are usually affiliated with the personnel department.

With the passage of the federal Occupational Safety and Health Act and the development of standards for hospitals, the safety function is frequently made a part of the personnel department's responsibility.

Personnel records may or may not be the responsibility of the personnel department, but auditing the personnel function and assisting in developing effective personnel policies should be. The auditing function includes examining such indicators as turnover records and grievances. Policy recommendations are concerned with equity concepts and changing employee needs and expectations, as well as organizational needs. Thus, the personnel specialist usually has direct access to the chief executive officer, even if he does not report to him directly.

Public Relations and Volunteer Services

Public relations is usually conceived of as a publicity or fund raising function in hospitals. We would like to suggest that its functions could be considerably broader, particularly in this era of consumer activism. Market analysis, use of ombudsmen, and evaluation of patient and community needs and satisfactions are functions that are often neglected by hospitals even though they are critical to the two-way communications so important to effective relations. Most hospital public relations programs, recognizing the importance of employee relationships with the public and patients, consider this an important part of their responsibility.

Volunteer service (relationships with the women's auxiliary) is a common staff service in hospitals. It is usually a separate department run by a paid woman employee who has good rapport with the volunteers. Hospital volunteers provide important services in the hospital such as transporting patients and providing recreational and social services. They can be effective spokespersons for both the hospital and a large segment of the public (usually the middle and upper class), and aid in raising funds for the hospital.

FACTORS THAT MIGHT IMPROVE EFFECTIVENESS
OF FUNCTIONAL SPECIALISTS

In previous sections we have discussed a number of problems associated with functional specialties and specialists. Because of advancing knowledge and the need for more effective management of costs and quality of service, there will be increasing emphasis on most of these specialties. We would like to suggest a number of conditions that might improve the effectiveness of functional specialists:

Administrators, trustees, medical staff, and heads of professional departments should be more knowledgeable about the contributions functional specialists could offer for improved patient care and hospital efficiency.

Functional specialists should be able to relate more effectively with providers of care and administrators.

Administrators should be oriented toward more participative management. Line department heads such as nurses and chiefs of professional services should have responsibility and accountability for management of their departments, and seek help and information directly from functional specialists.

Functional specialists should have the capability and opportunity to move up on the administrative ladder. Without more general administrative and health care knowledge—a calling card of masters in health administration and communication skills—most functional specialists will be locked into their jobs. In industry functional specialists have the opportunity to move up to the chief executive position.

We suggest that most of these conditions can be promoted by educational programs in health administration. Such programs can give potential administrators, and in many cases health providers as well, better knowledge of the skills of functional specialists. This can be done through both formal learning experiences in the classroom and informal learning experiences providing for associations among administrative, provider, and functional specialty students. Many medical, nursing, and other health professional schools are loosening their curricula, and many of their students are interested in the socioeconomics of health care, computer technology, finances, etc.; therefore survey courses or other learning experiences in these areas might be introduced.

Programs in health administration and/or training programs for functional specialists could provide learning experiences for the specialists to enable them to communicate and relate more effectively with providers of health care. Programs should select students carefully and help to give them the knowledge, skills, and attitudes needed to move up the administrative ladder. This should help to attract top functional specialists to the health field, rather than those who cannot be high achievers in industry.

With increasing emphasis on equal opportunities for women, hospital functional specialties appear to be roles for which more women might be recruited. Hospital professionals are predominantly women, but few women have been recruited for managerial roles in financial management, systems engineering, and other functional specialties.

A Type D administrative organization with a matrix rather than a hierarchical organization would foster communications between functional specialists and health providers and increase managerial responsibility among specialists.

Programs in health administration might consider giving students training as specialists, in order to qualify them for first-job opportunities as functional specialists, in addition to training for the chief executive role. Many business schools have moved away from generalist training (that is, training students to be presidents of corporations) and toward giving them first-job skills in marketing, production management, etc. Ansoff (1973) suggests that the differentiated specialist will be the manager of the future. Such an approach would seem to be particularly relevant for hospitals, because few hospitals can offer management training comparable to that provided by large corporations for MBA or baccalaureate graduates. This is not to suggest that functional specialists should not have "star" status in their own right. On the contrary, in the Type D organization we suggest that the functional specialist could have a status similar to that of the administrator. As we have noted previously, status is related to expertise in professional organizations. Indeed, a number of studies suggest that administrative line authority does not have much status among physician and nursing professionals.

Making changes through educational programs in health services administration is, however, a slow way of solving problems. Some more immediate ways are through continuing and in-service education programs, and changing administrative roles toward Type C and, more ideally, D. External pressures for cost controls are also likely make the role of the functional specialists more influential. It is important to note that specialists have a major influence on quality improvements and control as well as on costs.

We believe that more effective application of specialty skills is one of the best ways of improving the management of hospitals. It deserves concern and effort from trustees, administrators, and providers and from their training programs. Some of the more exciting opportunities for hospital administration are likely to be related to these management specialties. This is discussed further in later chapters on management of quality, costs, and conflict.

Consultants

Increasingly, hospitals are employing consultants for a variety of reasons. There are a number of different types of consultants. For example, there are diversified and large general management consultant firms that have different specialists and serve a variety of industries including health services. Their professional organization is The Association of Consulting Management Engineers (ACME) and a listing of such firms can be obtained from ACME. There are firms and individuals that specialize only in hospitals and their professional organization is the American Association of Hospital Consultants (AAHC). Architects are consultants, and there are consultants that specialize in systems engineering, finance, laundries, etc. Consulting psychologists are utilized for conflict resolution, screening candidates for top management positions, and other services. University professors will frequently act as consultants to health institutions providing scholarly expertise or possibly group process assistance to help the institution use its expertise more effectively. Well-known practitioners, e.g., hospital administrators, directors of nursing, medical record librarians, will also serve as consultants to other hospitals. All have certain advantages and disadvantages.

Consultants can be helpful to hospitals by providing:

Time so that hospital personnel may not have to work uninterruptedly and quickly to solve a problem, plan, etc.
Knowledge and experience from other settings
Objectivity and understanding to approach a problem from an independent perspective
Analytical skills from experience
Perspective to see facets that an organization may not see

They are useful when an institution needs one or more of the following:

One-time assistance
Help with internal communications
Outside appraisal
Reasons (e.g., tension) for change to take the onus off people inside the organization
Help with conflict resolution
Long-range plans
Expert advice, time, etc.

In selecting consultants it is important to carefully define the problem and scope of work required. It is also important to interview several firms when a large assignment is involved, to check on previous work they have done, and to find out who will actually do the work. To ensure that results will be accepted, it is essential that all who will be concerned with recommendations approve of the consultant selected.

A number of factors can be helpful in using consultants most effectively. For example, for a major consulting assignment, it is important that the consultants develop a work plan and schedule, and specify expectations for the assignment at various stages of the project. All concerned with the project should agree on expectations in advance in order to avoid misunderstanding of the expected results in relation to costs of the project. Financial arrangements on a time and expense basis with a definite ceiling hold a consultant accountable for the time put into the assignment as well as for results. Consultants' rates will range from $100 a day to over $500 a day depending upon their experience and reputation.

The consultant and client should work as a team during the project, for example agreeing on objectives, alternative solutions, criteria for evaluating alternatives, and recommendations. Wherever possible recommendations should start to be implemented while consultants are still working. A plan of action with identified responsibilities and a mechanism for continual updating should also be developed. Evaluation is essential and should be based on expectations agreed on at the outset.

In the light of the increasing complexities, challenges, and opportunities facing health services, the use of consultants should continue to increase. Somewhat surprisingly however, when harder times fall on organizations, they frequently drop the use of consultants first, much as corporations with falling sales may cut their advertising budgets first in order to cut costs. We have found that it is usually the stronger and leading organizations that use consultants; for example, most of the 500 largest corporations in the United States use consultants while many smaller companies who need them most will not seek outside help. Using consultants can be a good investment and should not be looked upon as a sign of weakness.

REFERENCES

AHA: *Management Engineering for Hospitals,* American Hospital Association, 1970.

AHA: "Research Capsule No. 15: Hospital Use of Industrial Engineers," *Hospitals, J.A.H.A.,* pp. 186-188, Feb. 1, 1975.

Ansoff, H. Igor: "The Next Twenty Years in Management Education," *The Library Quarterly,* vol. 43, no. 4, 1973.

Berman, Howard J. and Lewis E. Weeks: *The Financial Management of Hospitals,* Bureau of Hospital Administration, School of Public Health, University of Michigan, Ann Arbor, 1971.

Delbecq, Andre L. and Andrew H. Van de Ven: "A Group Process Model for Problem Identification and Program Planning," *Journal of Applied Behavioral Science,* vol. 7, no. 4, 1972.

Gillette, Philip J., Philip W. Rathbun, and Harry B. Wolfe: "Hospital Information Systems—Part 2," *Hospitals, J.A.M.A.,* vol. 44, pp. 45ff., Sept. 1, 1970.

Gustafson, David, Glenwood Rowse, and Nancy Howes: "Roles and Training for Future Health Systems Engineering" in *Education for Health Administration,* vol. II, Health Administration Press, Ann Arbor, Mich. 1975.

Griffith, John R.: *Quantitative Techniques for Hospital Planning and Control,* D.C. Heath, Lexington, Mass., 1972.

IE News Bulletin, p. 6, Oct. 1974.

Jydstrup, Ronald A. and Malvern Gross: "Cost of Information Handling in a Hospital," *Health Services Research,* vol. 1, pp. 235-271, Winter 1966.

Kovner, Anthony R. and Edward J. Lusk: "Effective Hospital Budgeting," *Hospital Administration,* pp. 44-64, Fall 1973.

Koza, Russell C.: *Mathematical and Operations Research Techniques in Health Administration,* Colorado Associated University Press, Boulder, 1973.

Levey, Samuel and N. Paul Loomba: *Health Care Administration,* J. B. Lippincott, Philadelphia, 1973.

Mariner, E. T.: "Hospitals Haven't Realized Potential of Data Processing," *Hospital Financial Management Journal,* pp. 3-5, Feb. 1971.

Silvers, J. B., and C. K. Prahalad: *Financial Management of Health Institutions,* Spectrum Publications, Flushing, N.Y., 1974.

Singer, J. Peter: "Hospital Computer Systems: Myths and Realities," *Hospital Financial Management Journal,* pp. 3-7, June 1970.

Stimson, David H. and Ruth H. Stimson: *Operations Research in Hospitals,* Hospital Research and Educational Trust, Chicago, 1972.

Administrative Functions: Transformation of Inputs to Outputs

In Part Two we described the hospital as a system composed of medical staff, nursing, and other services, and the coordination of these services with governing boards, administrators, and functional specialists. These elements, together with patients and their problems, are inputs into the system. As such they must provide high-quality and efficient service in order to transform the ill patient into one who is on the road to recovery. This is the output. It is also important for these inputs to function compatibly in trying to transform the ill patient into one on the road to recovery. In Part Three we examine the transformation of inputs to outputs through management of quality (Chapter 11), management of costs (Chapter 12), and management of conflict (Chapter 13). The diagram on the following page illustrates this transformation.

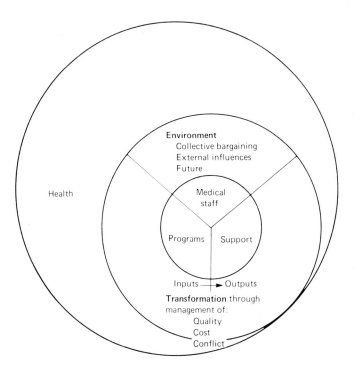

Management of Quality

What is quality? Attempting to define quality is like the proverbial blind men trying to describe an elephant from their limited vantage points. *Webster's New Collegiate Dictionary* defines quality as "excellence of character; an acquired trait; accomplishment." Such a definition is of little help in examining the quality of hospital service. If one were to ask a patient what hospital quality is, the response might be "to be treated with empathy, respect and concern" (Chewning, 1974). If one were to ask a physician, he might respond with "delivering the most advanced knowledge and skills of medical science to serve the patient." The hospital trustee might respond, "having the best people and facilities to deliver service." The hospital administrator would probably agree with the trustee but also add that "the professionals who provide the service continually evaluate their efforts and provide education for continuing improvements." Donabedian (1969) has attempted a fairly broad definition suggesting that "good" medical care is based on articles of faith, which he states as follows:

    1 Good medical care is limited to the practice of rational medicine based on medical science.

2 Good medical care emphasizes prevention.

3 Good medical care requires intelligent cooperation between lay public and the practitioners of scientific medicine.

4 Good medical care treats the individual as a whole.

5 Good medical care maintains a close and continuing personal relation between the physician and the patient.

6 Good medical care is coordinated with social welfare work.

7 Good medical care coordinates all types of medical services.

8 Good medical care implies the application of all necessary services of modern scientific medicine to the needs of all the people.

We suggest that hospital governing board members, administrators, and physicians must look at quality not just from one perspective, but from the perspective of all who are concerned.

In the past, quality control was the sole prerogative of the profession that had the knowledge and skills to evaluate quality, control licensure, and educate for improvement of quality, namely, the medical profession. Health care was not generally considered a right until very recently. Consumers usually obtain medical services on recommendations of friends who have limited technical knowledge, and therefore base their recommendations on personal relationships with the physician and/or what they can afford. However, responsibility for quality service no longer rests only with the professions that have the knowledge and skills; it is now shared by the governors, managers, and payers of health services. The Darling Case and other court interpretations confirm the "obligation of a hospital and its medical staff to oversee the quality of professional services rendered by individual medical staff members" (Hedgepeth, 1972). Recent Social Security amendments (P.L. 92-603) confirm the government's concern for quality as a major payer of health care through Professional Standards Review Organization (PSRO) requirements. Furthermore, consumer groups are becoming increasingly concerned about the management of quality. For example, Ralph Nader's study group report on the medical profession's self-regulation concluded (McCleery, 1971):

Our study set out to discover what systems of quality control the profession has established to monitor each physician's service to his patients, to evaluate how well these systems perform, and to determine whether the profession merits the trust which society has placed itself into the hands, and relied on the hearts, of all its physicians. We have had to conclude that the medical profession has failed to meet that trust.

. . . The study asked only whether or not a patient being treated by any physician in his office or hospital can be *reasonably sure:* that his physician is reasonably competent to treat that ailment (or that he will refer him to another whom the first believes to be reasonably competent); that his physician is reasonably up-to-date on diagnostic and treatment techniques, and on drug therapy information; that his physician will keep such records as to afford reasonable assurance that his work can later be effectively evaluated; that his physician's performance, no matter where given, will be monitored with reasonable frequency, objectivity and expertness by his peers.

. . . We are forced to conclude that the patient cannot be reasonably sure (p. 153).

Whether or not one agrees, it is significant that these conclusions have been reached, and stated publicly. A few years ago, such questions were seldom raised outside the profession. Historically, it was organized medicine that raised questions about the quality of medical education and clinical problems such as ghost surgery (where the patient believed his family doctor did the surgery, but in fact a surgeon did it after the patient was anesthetized), fee splitting (where the family physician referred to a surgeon for a kickback on the surgical fee), and itinerant surgery (where a surgeon would go to a small rural hospital and do surgery without being available for proper follow-up). One hears little about these problems today.

Just as different groups might look at the definition of quality from varying perspectives, so too might they look at quality controls. The middle- and upper-class consumers might respond that quality can be obtained if they have enough funds to select the kind of service they want when they want it, and if the supply of physicians and hospital services is large enough for them to make a choice and get a response. Consumers of lower socioeconomic status might argue for more patient advocates who are part of the health team, but represent only the patient's interests. Physicians might argue for continued peer review. (Peer review is the prevalent method of professional quality control in hospitals. It refers to an organized system in which some physicians review the quality of work done by others, e.g., through tissue committees and currently through PSROs.) The government is looking for quantifiable standards it can use to evaluate and manage quality. And administrators and trustees look to accreditation review and the diligence of the medical staff in peer review. Methods of managing quality are considered further in a later section of this chapter.

It is important to note that the quality of medical care in the United States is recognized throughout the world as generally outstanding (see Schwartz, 1973, *The Case for American Medicine*). Nevertheless, there is room for improvement when studies show medical mismanagement contributes significantly to deaths from trauma (Gertner et al., 1972) and chances for survival appear to be greater in larger and particularly teaching hospitals than in smaller rural hospitals (Peterson, 1973).

In the spring and summer of 1973 a study was made of the barriers to quality, access, and cost containment in the health field by the Commission on the Education of Health Administrators (Gustafson et al., 1975). Selected experts in the delivery of health services representing administrators, policy makers, and researchers developed a list of barriers and ranked them using a "Delphi Technique" (Gordon and Helmer, 1966). A study team then developed solution components to these barriers. Table 11-1 lists the barriers and their rankings by the 90 respondents. A review of this list shows the complexity of the problems and underscores the need for integrated efforts to find and implement solutions.

Table 11-1   Overall Major Barriers to the Quality of Health Care

No. of groups that agree (N = 6)*	Item description
6	Consumers lack understanding of preventive measures
6	Consumers lack understanding of when services are needed
6	Third-party payment policies do not adequately discriminate between poor- and good-quality care
5	Organization and coordination of all health services is inadequate
5	Consumers and providers view service as a reactive rather than a preventive function
5	Incentives for quality care provided by competitors, governing boards, third-party payers, and consumers are minimal
5	Lack of quality of care standards
4	Information and measures causally relating treatment interventions to outcomes are largely absent
4	Fee-for-service system encourages an increase in the volume of services provided but not in the quality of services
4	Consumers lack means of providing incentives to improve quality
4	Inability to agree on health goals
3	Needed services are not accessible when needed
3	Consumers lack understanding of availability of services
3	Communication between providers and consumers is inadequate

*90 respondents, 15 from each of the following 6 groups: experienced researchers, new researchers, planners and administrators, systems engineers, physicians, and nurses.

Source: David Gustafson, Glenwood Rowse, and Nancy Howes, from working papers from full report of "Roles and Training for Future Health Systems Engineers," in Education for Health Administration, vol. II, Health Administration Press, Ann Arbor, Mich., 1975.

APPROACHES TO EVALUATING QUALITY CARE

The American Public Health Association offers the following conceptual and operational definition for evaluation (APHA, 1960):

It is the process of determining the value or amount of success in achieving a predetermined objective. It includes at least the following steps: Formulation of the objective, identification of the proper criteria to be used in measuring success, determination and explanation of degree of success, recommendation for further program activity.

Few hospitals appear to have taken the first step of formulating explicit objectives against which the quality of hospital care can be evaluated. Formulating explicit objectives is not easy, as we have previously suggested. As Suchman (1967) suggests, there is a hierarchy of objectives in evaluation. For example, at the top, is the hospital attempting to improve the *health* of the community; that is, "complete physical, mental and social well-being" as defined by the World Health Organization? While measurements are difficult, health status indices are being developed that can be used operationally to measure changes in health (Patrick, Bush, and Chen, 1973). Is the hospital attempting to return the sick and injured to maximum potential healthfulness? Measurement of "outcomes" of care (Rosser and Watts, 1972) would help to evaluate success in achieving this objective. Objectives for providing the latest and most comprehensive care to patients would be at a lower end of objective hierarchy and would use "process" of care type measures.

Who should be evaluated to control quality of care? Pellegrino (1972, p. 309) suggests three types of functional classification of the team concerned with care: the *health care team*, which consists of all who are engaged in providing or planning for some service to improve the general or community health, without necessarily being in direct or indirect contact with the specific needs of a specific patient (this would include administrators, office personnel etc., in addition to physicians, nurses, etc.); the *medical care team*, which consists of those professionals, semiprofessionals and nonprofessionals who provide some service for the patient without any direct or personal contact, e.g., central supply personnel and laundry workers; and the *patient care team*, which comprises any group of professionals, semi- and nonprofessionals who jointly provide services that bring them into direct personal and physical contact with the patient, and that are part of a program of management for the patient. In this chapter, we will focus on the more restrictive level of the patient care team because that is where most of quality control efforts have been made; nevertheless, we believe the broader considerations deserve much more attention than they have received.

Three approaches to evaluation of quality have been identified by Donabedian (1969) as: (1) structure, (2) process, and (3) outcome or end results. These are currently the most frequently used classifications although others have been proposed, for example, by DeGeyndt (1970). Donabedian defines the three approaches as:

> *Appraisal of structure* involves the evaluation of the settings and instrumentalities available and used for the provision of care. While including the physical aspects of facilities and equipment, structural appraisal goes far beyond to encompass the characteristics of the administrative organization and qualifications of health professionals. The term structure as used here also signifies the properties and resources used to provide care and the manner in which they are organized.
>
> Two major assumptions are made when structure is taken as an indicator of quality: first, that better care is more likely to be provided when better qualified staff, improved physical facilities and sounder fiscal and administrative organization are employed. Second, that we know enough to identify what is "good" in terms

of staff, physical structure and formal organization. That staff qualifications, physical structure and formal organization are not equaled with quality must be emphasized. It is only expected that there be a relationship between these structural elements and the quality of care, so that given good structural properties, good care is more likely (though not certain to occur). Devices like licensure, certification of facilities, and accreditation are based largely on these assumptions.

It appears that most informed consumers, hospital governing board members, and probably many administrators appraise quality of hospitals on a structural basis. Hospitals with teaching programs and medical school affiliations, the most modern facilities, the highest percentage of board certified specialists, and a strong financial and organizational structure are assumed to have the highest quality services. Such assumptions are not without foundation. For example, Goss (1970) and Roemer (1971) found a relationship between a hospital's commitment to teaching and its quality of care. Neuhauser (1971) found evidence to suggest a relationship between quality of administration and quality of care. However, structure is not a sufficient indicator of quality. Moreover, assumptions equating structural quality such as size, scope of services, and facility with quality of care have also contributed to the rising cost of hospital care (Schulz and Rose, 1973).

Donabedian goes on to define:

> . . . *assessment of process* as the evaluation of activities of physicians and other health professionals in the management of patients. The criterion generally used is the degree to which management of patients conforms with the standards and expectations of the respective professions. . . . When evaluation of process is the basis for judgments concerning quality . . . there is the explicit or implicit assumption that particular elements and aspects of care are known to be specifically related to successful or unsuccessful outcomes or end results.

Assessment of process is the basis of quality review techniques utilized by hospital medical staffs through medical records committees and other medical audit or quality review committees that review the process of patient care by reviewing patient charts. Process techniques rely on generally accepted norms or defined criteria, on subjective judgments, and on the diligence of reviewers.

> *Assessment of outcomes* is the evaluation of end results in terms of health and satisfaction. That this evaluation in many ways provides the final evidence of whether care has been good, bad, or indifferent is so because of broad fundamental social and professional agreement on what results are brought about, at least to a significant degree, by good care.

While outcome would seem to be the ideal appraisal of quality, it is also the most difficult to measure. Blood pressure, for example, is a single measure of outcome for hypertension, but for most illnesses there is no single sign. Mortality can of course be measured, but morbidity, i.e., the state of being diseased, and survival time are difficult to measure. Moreover, even when outcome can be measured effectively, there are problems correlating it with diagnosis and treatment. Psychological and social factors also can confound the outcomes of appropriate care.

In a study of five different methods of process and outcome evaluation, Brook and Appel (1973) found the evaluation of care depended upon the method used. For 296 patients reviewed in a major city hospital, from 1.4 percent to 63.2 percent of the patients were judged to have received adequate care depending upon the method used to evaluate the quality of patient care. Judgment of *process* using explicit criteria yielded the fewest acceptable cases (1.4 percent). Brook (1973, p. 37) states:

> The method currently in vogue, assessment of quality of care based upon explicit process criteria is likely to produce the most stringent judgment of quality of care. The use and acceptance of this method is likely to double if not triple the number of personal health services provided without substantially improving the health of the American people. Thus, the result of the admirable intention of both physicians and general public to raise the quality of care by assessing the process of that care may have dire economic consequences and actually lower the health level of the population by directing money away from other social needs such as housing into medical care processes which are only thought to have an effect on health level.

The ultimate goal is a decrease in disease, death, disability, discomfort, and disaffection. Outcome measures are receiving more attention and progress is being made toward the development of effective indicators by investigators at a number of universities. Lewis (1974) notes that in a fifty-year period quality of care activities have gone a full cycle from original emphasis on outcomes to structure, then to process, and now back to outcomes. He suggests that "perhaps only individual consumer involvement/control in the process of care will result in improved outcomes."

METHODS FOR MANAGING QUALITY
OF PHYSICIANS' SERVICES

Peer review, medical audit, quality assurance, and utilization review are terms commonly associated with the management of the quality of medical care. Peer review refers to some physicians reviewing the quality of work done by other physicians. It can be done on a prospective, retrospective, and/or concurrent basis. Prospective review could be a consultation from another physician before a procedure is done. The medical audit is usually a retrospective review of patient medical records. In medical audit, quality is defined as degree of conformity with standards of accepted principles and practices. The medical audit was initially promoted by the American College of Surgeons and has been continued through efforts of the Joint Commission on Accreditation of Hospitals (JCAH). Quality Assurance Program (QAP) was initiated by the American Hospital Association as a utilization review to be performed while the patient is in the hospital. It was prompted by concerns of Blue Cross, and subsequently of the Social Security Administration in connection with Medicare and

Medicaid, about unnecessary utilization of hospital services. Medical audit and utilization review now go hand in hand.

Peer review can be on an implicit or explicit basis (Brook 1973). Implicit review is based upon overall physician judgment of the quality care rendered by another physician. Explicit review refers to a specification of criteria and/or standards.

A number of different peer review programs are used by health institutions. The JCAH has concerned itself with several quality assurance measures for medical care in the hospital (*Perspectives on Accreditation,* 1973):

Effective performance of medical staff credentials function

Adjunctive protective devices through activity of infection control and pharmacy and therapeutic policy functions

Medical care evaluation through both retrospective (medical audit) and concurrent (utilization review) programs

Tailored programs of continuing medical education shaped by demonstrated current needs especially those revealed in medical audit and utilization review

The JCAH suggests that the critical requirements of an acceptable medical care evaluation system are as follows:

1 It must be *objective,* stable, and not capricious. Criteria must be established as measuring devices.

2 It must be *efficient,* specifically in terms of physician time. Nonmedical personnel should be utilized for the time-consuming tasks which do not themselves require clinical judgment.

3 It must be *documented,* with all critical decisions in writing and signed by the responsible person.

4 It must be *clinically sound.* Thus, all clinical criteria must be subject to justifiable local amendment.

5 It must be *flexible.* There must be allowance for variation from criteria for good cause which is shown in the record.

6 The system must be *action-oriented.* There must be a logical action resulting, suited to the need, whether this be education, counseling, policy amendment, sanctions, or intervention.

Figure 11-1 portrays the JCAH retrospective medical audit procedure.

As of July 1975, JCAH requires continuous evaluation through reliable and valid measures of physicians' performance and if studies uncover "less than optional" care the hospital must "show that it did something to correct the situation—even if that requires lifting or curtailing doctors' staff privileges." (*Medical World News,* Jan. 13, 1975). By July 1976, each major service (e.g., medicine, surgery, etc.) must be doing at least one audit a month. Hospitals can use Physician Evaluation Procedure (PEP) developed by the JCAH, which is a peer review based on criteria set by the staff stressing "outcome" of care rather than "process," or they can use their own system, or MAP.

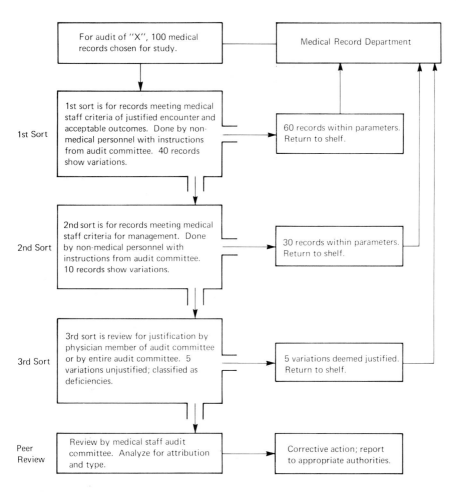

Figure 11-1   Retrospective medical audit procedure

The Commission on Professional and Hospital Activities in Ann Arbor, Michigan, under a grant from the W. K. Kellogg Foundation, pioneered mechanisms called Professional Activities Studies (PAS) and Medical Audit Program (MAP) to aid hospitals in peer review activities (Slee, 1969). The mechanisms use norms that allow peer review groups to review the practices of individual physicians and the hospital medical staff as a whole against the averages of physicians of all hospitals participating in the program. In essence, it is management by exception in which deviations from norms are singled out for more thorough individual review. While these mechanisms are used by audit and utilization committees, they do not appear to have been actively used by administrators and trustees in their overall evaluation of hospital effectiveness (Schulz and Rose, 1973). In a PAS-type program the hospital medical record librarian takes data from all charts and feeds them into the program's central computer. The program returns information summarizing the experiences of each physician in treating diseases in relation to the norms of all other physicians' experiences for treating similar diseases.

Another approach has been pioneered by Beverly Payne, M.D., for the Michigan State Medical Society and Hawaii Medical Association, Robert Evans, M.D., at York (Pennsylvania) Hospital, and Clement Brown, M.D., at Chestnut Hill Hospital in Philadelphia. It is based on developing criteria for the diagnosis and treatment of specific diseases—a process review. The development of criteria for patient management of specific diseases provides an important learning experience for hospital medical staff members as well as a basis on which to evaluate quality of care. In addition, Payne (1973) utilized nurses and others in his work, resulting in improved teamwork. Perhaps most important is that a review based on criteria also provides for concurrent review while the patient is in the hospital and expedites the use of nonphysicians in concurrent quality care review.

The Experimental Medical Care Review Organization (EMCRO) established on a pilot basis in eight different locations in the early 1970s is another example of a criteria-based review program. In this type of program criteria, norms, and standards are developed for processes and/or outcomes for specific diseases, usually by physicians in the program. Then a sample of cases is audited against the criteria, and exceptions are noted and discussed with the physician involved. The education of physicians and sanctions when necessary are the outputs of the review (HEW, 1973).

Another program utilizing concurrent procedures (and some nonphysician reviewers) is the Quality Assurance Program (OAP) developed by the American Hospital Association (Brown and Sale, 1974). It is interesting to note that the American Medical Association House of Delegates voted in June 1973 to "express grave concern to the AHA about QAP because of its potential for lay control of medical practice." However, the legal as well as moral responsibility of the hospital's board, medical staff, and administration to control quality is well documented (for example, see Musser, 1973, and Bernstein, 1974).

A. L. Cochrane (1972) in Great Britain advocates a randomized control trial (RCT) of evaluating the effectiveness and efficiency of different treatment groups to which patients are randomly assigned. This approach raises a number of questions not the least of which are ethical questions.

A tool to help improve the quality of patient care that has gained wide acclaim is the Problem-Oriented Medical Record (POMR) developed by Lawrence Weed, M.D. As the name implies the POMR highlights rather than obscures the patient's problems as is frequently the case with traditional medical records (Weed, 1971). It aids the physician in identifying problems, and in planning and evaluating the course of treatment. It focuses on the whole patient, helps to coordinate various health skills through their communication in the medical record, and encourages the patient to become a participant in the solution of the problems. Elements of the POMR are:

Data base: A carefully defined standardized and rigorously observed comprehensive data base on the patient.

Problems list: A complete list of the patient's problems, titled and numbered.

Plans: Titled and numbered plans for each problem with a plan for collecting more data, a plan for treatment, and a plan for educating the patient about the nature of the problem and his role in management. This latter step in particular is often neglected under traditional patient management approaches.

Follow-up: Titled and numbered progress notes on each problem, structured to include subjective data, objective data, and assessment, as well as a plan for the diagnosis, treatment, and education of the patient, and a goal for each patient.

A 1973 amendment to the Social Security Act (P.L. 92-603) directs physicians to establish and operate Professional Standards Review Organizations (PSROs). This portion of the law has three major objectives: to certify (1) that health services are necessary; (2) that quality of services meets professionally recognized standards of care; and (3) that the type of facilities used is the most economical in keeping with the medical needs of patients whose health care is paid for by the government under Medicare and Medicaid.

While a variety of administrative *forms* are possible, all PSROs are required to adhere to a number of criteria *(Medical World News,* March 30, 1973):

They must during the course of the review operation develop and maintain profiles for each patient, practitioner, and provider.

They are responsible for determining whether various aspects of existing in-house review procedures at health institutions meet standards acceptable to the PSRO.

There must be broad physician participation in the review process on a rotating basis, rather than simple delegation of the review responsibility to a few doctors.

It is the intent of the law that PSROs be established on the basis of the doctor population to be served. Number of physicians covered might run between 300 and 1,000.

Data accumulated by each organization must be maintained in such a fashion that performance of PSROs can be compared and evaluated.

Senator Bennett, author of the legislation, believes that PSROs can save the government and public substantial funds. Brook (1973) and others doubt such savings, citing research on other quality assurance programs that shows that they improve the style of care but also increase costs *(Medical World News,* March 30, 1973).

The number of proposals, techniques, and outside pressures is confusing, to say nothing of the myriad of acronyms. Clearly, though, the medical profession is trying to respond to current pressures. A key question is: Will the critics of physicians' self-regulation accept these efforts? And, more importantly, how will the evaluation procedures themselves be evaluated, if at all? It is also important to ask about the role of the governing board member and administrator in the evaluation of physicians' services. Is it sufficient to be sure that the medical staff is actively evaluating quality care? It would seem that the APHA conceptual and operational definition of evaluation, which includes the steps of formulating objectives (in terms of broad community health needs), identifying proper criteria to be used in measuring success, determining and explaining the degree of success, and recommending further action, is the most appropriate for answering these questions. If these steps are followed and associated actions exposed, then administrators, trustees, and consumer advocates should be satisfied. If not, then each has the right and obligation to intervene in peer review to ensure that they *are* followed. It is disturbing to note, however, that one hospital that publicly exposed its quality assessment results was criticized and placed on the defensive rather than rewarded for its honesty and its willingness to make the results of quality assessment public (Brook, 1973).

METHODS FOR MANAGING QUALITY OF OTHER SERVICES

Although the quality of patient care receives primary attention in an institution the quality of health care it provides is obviously also important. Considerations for evaluating the quality of other services are basically the same as those used to evaluate physician services. They concern structure, process, and outcome approaches, but usually include more patient satisfaction indicators. The principles of evaluation defined by the APHA or those proposed by Suchman (1967), Schulberg et al. (1969), and others are also appropriate for evaluating quality of other services. We do not consider licensure in this chapter since it is generally believed to be an ineffective control of quality. We will briefly consider quality care in nursing, indicators in other services, and patient satisfaction.

Quality of Nursing Services

Quality control in nursing service is a key factor in hospital and physician effectiveness and patient welfare. Principal control is usually an informal one—the evaluation made by physicians in the process of patient management and by the patient. Obviously, if the medical staff see problems in the quality of nursing service, they will let it be known. The formal organizational method is through the patient care committee described in Chapter 5. The informal mechanism is when physicians pound on the desks of nursing and hospital administrators and/or trustees or when they apply the sanctions of taking their patients elsewhere.

Patients, too, have a role in evaluating and controlling the quality of nursing service. Patients are capable of evaluating, through their own observations and experiences, how well nurses perform the functions of improving patients' adjustments to hospitalization or illness, and of promoting patient comfort and hygiene. Patient reactions are an important dimension of nursing service. However, patients may not be as well equipped to evaluate treatment services. This, of course, is where physician evaluation is important.

Formal evaluation and control of nursing service can be managed through nursing audit techniques; these may include expert observation of nursing services or review of patient charts *by nurses* as is done in a medical audit by physicians. Gorham (1963) provides an example of the expert observation approach, but he notes a great deal of concern on the part of nurses about its effects on interpersonal relationships. Phaneuf (1963, 1966, 1968) provides an example on a nursing audit based on review of charts, and suggests it leads to innovations and other improvements in addition to a method of evaluating quality. Zimmer (1974) suggests a nursing peer review based on outcome criteria for nursing care. The Commission for Administrative Services in Hospitals (CASH) developed a quality control method for nursing that provides for setting nursing service objectives, an organization, and an index for managing quality (Alexander, 1972).

The Joint Commission on Accreditation of Hospitals has established standards for quality of nursing care. They are largely measures of structure rather than of process or outcome. The general standards on which JCAH surveyors base their evaluations are:

1　The nursing service shall be under the direction of a legally and professionally qualified registered nurse. There shall also be a sufficient number of duly licensed registered nurses on duty at all times to plan, assign, supervise, and evaluate nursing care as well as to give patients the nursing care that requires the judgment and specialized skills of a registered nurse.

2　The nursing service shall have a current written organizational plan that delineates its functional structure and its mechanisms for cooperative planning and decision making.

3　Written nursing care and administrative policies and procedures shall be developed to provide the nursing staff with acceptable methods of meeting its responsibilities and achieving projected goals.

4　There shall be evidence that the nursing service provides safe, efficient, and therapeutically effective implementation of the plans.

5　There shall be continuing training programs and educational opportunities for the development of nursing personnel.

While the JCAH interprets these standards in their accreditation manual, they are nevertheless subjective standards. Reportedly, the JCAH is currently discussing establishing interdisciplinary (including nursing and medical care) criteria for the total care of specific diseases.

Other Indicators and Methods of Quality Control

There are a number of indicators of quality that can be developed to measure other hospital services. For example, waiting time is an appropriate indicator for a number of services such as admitting office, x-ray, and laboratory. Errors are another, although reporting of errors has not proved to be particularly reliable and it is, of course, a negative indicator. However, many hospitals do keep records of medication errors, hospital-based infections, and other exceptions to expectations of quality.

Patient care committees consisting of medical staff members, nurses, other professionals, and administrators function actively in many hospitals to help control for quality.

Mechanic (1970) suggests that the satisfaction of health professionals (British GPs in his study) is related to providing quality service. Employee and physician satisfaction can, of course, be measured through attitude surveys, indicators of turnover, absenteeism, and so forth.

In addition to evaluation and information systems, a program of Management By Objectives (MBO) incorporates quality control as a basic premise. In an MBO program the worker and his or her superior establish mutually agreed-upon objectives which should include objectives for quality. Such a program should aid in evaluation in addition to establishing more appropriate objectives.

As we have urged throughout this book, the hospital should take a greater role in improving the health of its community in its broadest sense. Health status indicators, e.g., infant mortality and work-limiting disabilities and proxy measures of health, e.g., social and economic indicators, can be extremely valuable in determining what the hospital might do to improve the health of the community. Consumer education programs and the occupational and environmental health activities discussed previously should have impact on these health status indicators. The quality or value of hospital programs to the community might be measured through such indicators.

Patient Satisfaction

Increasing interest is being shown in studying patient satisfaction; this is an obvious, but frequently ignored, indicator of quality. Many hospitals survey patients to determine their general satisfaction and to detect problem areas such as cold food, noise, and other discomforts or obstacles to effective patient care. Patient surveys have inherent problems such as controlling for illness, and the cultural, social, and economic differences of patients and visitors (Chewning 1974). Nevertheless, while improvements in instruments are needed, such surveys are of value.

CONCLUSIONS

At the beginning of this chapter we noted that Ralph Nader's study group concluded that "patients cannot be reasonably sure" of the quality care they receive and that the medical profession has failed to meet the trust of society for quality control. Yet in this and other chapters we have described just a few of the many efforts made by hospitals, physicians, and others to control quality. The obvious conclusion is that quality care controls are not uniformly applied. Moreover, it is generally recognized that evaluation techniques and measurements can and will be improved. It is equally clear that the days when quality control efforts were left to the professionals themselves are gone. Trustees, administrators, and professionals will have to work with health policy makers and consumers to control quality. What does this mean?

At the national level most of the current activities center on the Social Security Administration's Medicare program, which has required PSROs. These efforts really relate to concerns about cost and utilization of services within a framework of acceptable minimum levels of quality. With an impending national health insurance program, greater concern and effort can be expected from the government, which will be a major source of funding programs. Other agencies are also concerned with the quality of delivery of health services and a central Bureau of Quality Assurance has been recently established within the U.S. Department of Health, Education and Welfare.

In spite of trends toward regional health planning and national controls, the hospital still has a legal and moral responsibility for controlling quality. Through its medical staff and other quality control methods it is able to detect early signs of problems in physicians, e.g., senility or alcoholism. Through its board and administrator it can curtail practices that endanger patients. Hospitals face unpleasant and tough decisions in such cases. For example, should a hospital admit a physician of questionable competence to its staff, but restrict and supervise his privileges and hope that his staff activities will improve his qualifications, or should it bar him from the staff to protect hospital patients? Since the physician is rarely controlled outside the hospital (except possibly in the treatment of Medicare cases under PSRO scrutiny) barring him or her from the staff may not be in the community's best interests.

The hospital is also the place of appeal or redress for the patient who feels that he or she has not received quality assurances. The hospital administrator has responsibility to examine and help control total technical and personal care to the patient including medical nursing, dietary, employee services, and physical surroundings, etc. The governing board has the ultimate responsibility for total quality of care and, through the administrator and medical staff organization, for quality assurance activities. Quality control is a team effort, and explicit objectives for quality need to be established. There are numerous tools and aids for controlling and promoting quality including accreditation, PAS, MAP, improving methods of measurement, and the other methods we have suggested in this chapter.

Just how far governmental agencies will go in controlling quality will depend on how well hospitals and PSROs meet their responsibilities and how effective they are in convincing consumers that they can trust the quality assurance efforts of hospitals and PSROs.

REFERENCES

Alexander, Edythe L.: *Nursing Administration in the Hospital Health Care System,* Mosby, St. Louis, 1972, pp. 253-360.

APHA: "Glossary of Administrative Terms in Public Health," *American Journal of Public Health,* vol. 50, pp. 225-226, Feb. 1960.

Bernstein, Arthur: "More on Medical Staff Privileges," *Hospitals, J.A.H.A.,* vol. 48, pp. 116-121, Mar. 1, 1974.

Brook, Robert: "Quality of Care Assessment: What Is the Most Appropriate Method?" in *The Hospital's Role in Assessing the Quality of Medical Care,* Proceedings of the Fifteenth Annual Symposium on Hospital Affairs, Center for Health Administration Studies, University of Chicago, May 1973.

Brook, Robert H. and Francis A. Appel: "Quality-of-Care Assessment: Choosing a Method for Peer Review," *New England Journal of Medicine,* vol. 288, no. 25, pp. 1323-1329, June 21, 1973.

Brown, Madison B. and William B. Sale "QAP: The AHA's Program: Preparing for PSRO Implementation," *Hospitals, J.A.H.A.,* vol. 48, no. 5, 1974.

Cochrane, A. L.: *Effectiveness and Efficiency,* The Nuffield Provincial Hospitals Trust, London, 1972.

Chewning, Betty: Unpublished findings from a survey of factors consumers found to be important in their satisfaction of medical care, University of Wisconsin, Madison, 1974.

DeGeyndt, Willy: "Five Approaches for Assessing the Quality of Care," *Hospital Administration*, pp. 21-42, Winter 1970.

Donabedian, Avedis: *A Guide to Medical Care Administration Vol. II, Medical Care Appraisal–Quality and Utilization*, American Public Health Association, Washington, D.C., 1969.

Gertner, Harold R., Jr. et al.: "Evaluation of the Management of Vehicular Fatalities Secondary to Abdominal Injury," *The Journal of Trauma*, vol. 12, no. 5, pp. 425-431, 1972.

Gordon, Theodore and Olaf Helmer: *Social Technology*, Rand Corporation, Santa Monica, Calif., 1966.

Gorham, William: "Methods for Measuring Staff Nursing Performance," *Nursing Research*, vol. 12, no. 1, pp. 4-11, Winter 1963.

Goss, Mary E.: "Organizational Goals and Quality of Medical Care: Evidence from Comparative Research on Hospitals," *Journal of Health & Social Behavior*, vol. II, p. 255-68, Dec. 1970.

Gustafson, David, Glenwood Rouse and Nancy Howes: "Roles and Training for Future Health Systems Engineers" in *Education for Health Administration, Vol. II*, Health Administration Press, Ann Arbor, Mich., 1975.

Hedgepeth, Jay H.: "Darling Revisited," *Hospitals, J.A.H.A.*, no. 46, pp. 58-60, Aug. 16, 1972.

Lewis, Charles: "The State of the Art of Quality Assessment–1973," *Medical Care*, vol. 12, no. 10, pp. 799-806, Oct. 1974.

McCleary, Robert: *One Life–One Physician: Ralph Nader's Study Group Report on the Medical Profession's Performance in Self Regulation*, Public Affairs Press, Washington, D.C., 1971.

Mechanic, David: "Correlates of Frustration among British General Practitioners," *Journal of Health & Social Behavior*, vols. I & II, pp. 87-104, June 1970.

Medical Care: "The PSRO Hospital Review System," vol. 13, no. 4, pp. 1-33, April 1975.

Medical World News: "PSRO's: Here They Come – Ready or Not," pp. 15–17, Mar. 30, 1973.

Medical World News: "Here Comes PEP, Broader Than PSRO," pp. 28-31, Jan. 13, 1975.

Musser, Wendell: "The Administrator's Role in Quality Assessment," in *The Hospital's Role in Assessing the Quality of Medical Care*, Proceedings of the Fifteenth Annual Symposium on Hospital Affairs, University of Chicago, May 1973.

Neuhauser, Duncan: *The Relationship Between Administrative Activities and Hospital Performance*, Center for Health Administration Studies, Research Series 28, University of Chicago, 1971.

Patrick, Donald L., J. W. Bush, and Milton Chen: "Toward an Operational Definition of Health," *Journal of Health and Social Behavior*, pp. 6-23, Mar. 1973.

Payne, Beverly: Speech to Madison (Wisconsin) General Hospital Medical Staff, Mar. 1973. See also Payne, "Continued Evolution of a System of Medical Care Appraisal," *Journal of American Medical Association*, vol. 201, no. 7, Aug. 14, 1967 and other publications of his.

Pellegrino, Edmund: "The Changing Matrix of Clinical Decision Making in the Hospital," in Basil Georgopoulos (ed.), *Organization Research on Health Institutions*. Institute for Social Research, University of Michigan, Ann Arbor, 1972.

Pellegrino, Edmund: "Quality Assurance of Medical Care: Analysis and Reflection," *Quality Assurance of Medical Care*, DHEW HSM 73-7021, Feb. 1973, pp. 461-483.

Perspectives on Accreditation: Joint Commission on Accreditation of Hospitals, Chicago, Mar. 1973.

Peterson, Osler: "The Importance of Obtaining High Quality Medical Care," in *The Hospital's Role in Assessing the Quality of Medical Care*, Proceedings of the Fifteenth Annual Symposium on Hospital Affairs, University of Chicago, May 1973.

Phaneuf, Maria C.: "A Nursing Audit Method," *Nursing Outlook*, pp. 42-45, May 1964.

Phaneuf, Maria C.: "The Nursing Audit for Evaluation of Patient Care," *Nursing Outlook,* pp. 51-54, June 1966.

Phaneuf, Maria C.: "Analysis of a Nursing Audit," *Nursing Outlook,* pp. 57-60, Jan. 1968.

Roemer, Milton I. and Jay W. Friedman: *Doctors in Hospitals: Medical Staff Organization and Hospital Performance*, Johns Hopkins Press, Baltimore, Md., 1971.

Rosser, R. M. and V. C. Watts: "The Measurement of Hospital Output," *International Journal of Epidemiology,* vol. 1, pp. 361-368, 1972.

Schulberg, Herbert C., Alan Sheldon, and Frank Baker (eds.): *Program Evaluation in the Health Field,* Behavioral Publications, New York, 1969.

Schulz, Rockwell and Jerry Rose: "Can Hospitals Be Expected to Control Costs?" *Inquiry,* pp. 3-8, June 1973.

Schwartz, Harry: *The Case for American Medicine,* David McKay, New York, 1972.

Slee, Virgil: "Measuring Hospital Effectiveness: Patterns of Medical Practice," *University of Michigan Medical Center Journal,* vol. 35, pp. 112-115, Apr.-June, 1969.

Suchman, Edward A.: *Evaluative Research,* Russell Sage Foundation, New York, 1967.

U.S. Department of Health, Education and Welfare: *Experimental Medical Care Review Organization (EMCRO) Programs.* National Center for Health Services R&D DHEW HSM 73-3017, Mar. 1973.

Weed, Lawrence L.: "Quality Control and the Medical Record," *Archives of Internal Medicine,* vol. 127, pp. 101-105, Jan. 1971. Copyright 1971, American Medical Association.

Zimmer, Marie: "A Model for Evaluating Nursing Care," *Hospitals, J.A.H.A.,* vol. 48, pp. 65ff., Mar. 1, 1973.

Chapter 12

Management of Costs

Most Americans apparently believe there is a crisis in health care, and much of their discontent is focused on rising costs. Ronald Anderson et al. (1971), in their household survey, found that three-quarters of the heads of families surveyed believed there was a crisis in health, and high costs were one of the greatest sources of dissatisfaction; however, only 38 percent were dissatisfied with out-of-pocket costs of medical care. Concerns over rising costs of health and particularly hospital costs are resulting in increasing controls over hospitals. Since World War II priority has been given to expanding hospital services and improving quality. In the 1970s priorities appear to be switching toward cost containment. In the first section of this chapter we will briefly review the rising costs of hospital service; the following sections deal with institutional factors related to costs, barriers to containing costs, incentives and rewards for controlling costs, and opportunities for internal cost control.[1]

[1] Major portions of the first two sections appeared in Rockwell Schulz and Jerry Rose, "Can Hospitals Be Expected to Control Costs?", *Inquiry,* pp. 3-8, June 1973.

RISING COSTS

National expenditures for health care have increased from $12 billion, or $82 per person in 1950 to about $100 billion, or $463 per person, in 1973 (DHEW 1975). Moreover, we are spending a significantly greater portion of our gross national product (GNP) on health rising from 4.5 percent to 7.7 percent over the 1950-1973 period. However, to put this in another perspective, in 1969 we spent nearly $27 billion on alcohol and tobacco—two items that cause some of our health problems— compared with $32 billion for hospital, physician, and drug services. Nevertheless, money spent on medical treatment services means that much less to be spent for other goods and services including environmental factors such as education that can have a great impact on improving health. Are current expenditures too much or too little? Answers to that complex question relate to tradeoffs on other expenditures, social priorities, and what appear to be individual preferences.

By far the largest component in the price rise was increasing hospital costs per patient-day. The average cost per patient-day in 1950 was less than $16; by 1973 it exceeded $102 (*Hospital Statistics*, 1974). Moreover, in terms of total annual expenditures for hospital service per person in the nation it increased from $25 per person in 1950 to $179 per person in 1973 (DHEW, 1975). The rate of increase was slowed after price controls were implemented in 1971, but the rate increased again after controls were lifted. Hospital service charges increased 15.7 percent in calendar year 1974 while the consumer price index rose 11.7 percent (*Hospital Week*, 1975).

Factors Contributing to the Rise in Hospital Costs

In their analysis of rising hospital costs between 1950 and 1970, Anderson and May (1972) suggest that increased use of hospitals was not a major factor in the last five years of the period; it accounted for only 12 percent of the increase while rising prices accounted for 86 percent. Factors contributing to price increases include the following:

Rising Wage Rates Hospitals are a labor-intensive industry with employee salaries representing 60 to 75 percent of total costs

Hospital employees have had a catch-up in wages. In 1960 the average hourly wage of hospital employees was 68 percent of that of production workers in manufacturing industries. By 1965, it had increased to 74 percent, and by 1969 to 81 percent.

Advancing technologies and increasing specialization have expanded the hospital work force. Employees per patient in nongovernmental not-for-profit short-term hospitals increased from 1.91 in 1950 to 3.14 by 1973 (*Hospital Statistics*, 1974). Massachusetts General Hospital estimated 52.2 percent of its costs in 1970 were for medical technology, 29.9 percent for nursing, 7.4 percent for food and special diet, 5.7 percent for business office, and 4.8 percent for utilities, housekeeping, maintenance, laundry, etc. (Kovner and Lusk, 1973).

Larger and More Elaborate Facilities Coronary intensive care units and monitoring devices, autoanalyzers in laboratories, air conditioning, television, electric beds, cobalt and other radiation therapy devices, and so forth have added to facilities resulting in higher depreciation charges or amortization on construction loans.

Advancing technologies requiring more expensive equipment increase operating costs and lead to higher depreciation costs. In fiscal 1973 nonpayroll expenses increased over 12 percent while payroll costs increased just over 7 percent.

Insurance Has Reimbursed Hospitals on the Basis of Their Costs There have been few incentives to contain costs, since any increases can be passed on to third-party payers. Indeed, it has been easier to obtain financial success by maximizing income than by minimizing costs.

The Increased Scope of Services Has Led to More Services per Patient This has been a major factor in improving the quality of care according to most hospitals spokespersons.

General Inflation Has Caused an Increase in Supply Cost at the same time hospitals are using more disposable items in order to conserve labor.

Many of these factors are beyond the control of hospital governing board members and administrators given the expectations of society that the quality and scope of hospital service be improved.

Institutional Factors Related to Costs

Do costs vary by type of organization? For example, are costs in governmentally operated hospitals at one end of the spectrum lower than those in community hospitals at the other? Some say the profit incentive found in for-profit hospitals can help to contain costs. What about costs in teaching hospitals or not-for-profit hospital chains? Does size of hospital affect costs? In this section we examine some of the limited information available on costs in these various types of institutions.

Comparisons with Governmentally Operated Hospitals

Figures on costs per patient-day in federal governmental hospitals (VA, Armed Forces, and Public Health Service) usually indicate that they are lower than in community general hospitals. However, length of stay is usually considerably longer: therefore, costs per day should be less. One of the authors of this book found when serving as a consultant to one of the federal hospitals systems that central administrative costs such as purchasing and personnel were not or could not be properly allocated to the individual hospitals; therefore, cost comparisons could not be made with community hospitals in the same area.

A comparison of health costs in the United States, a system dominated by non-governmental services, with those in Sweden and England where the systems are dominated by government, shows no clear conclusions about the effect of government control on rising costs. Anderson (1972) shows the total cost of health services in the three countries as a percent of national income increase for 1950 and 1968 (see Table 12-1).

Anderson concludes: "The United States falls midway between the two more socialized systems in its increase in health care expenditures using the most comparative measures possible. There is, then, no clear relationship between extent of governmental control of the health care system and control of health costs (p. 139)." However, he also notes that "All health systems [are] moving into greater organization and bureaucratization in order to control cost against the last reservoir of real or imagined ills (in health services administration both are real in their consequences). This move will be rationalized by claims to spurious efficiency. . . . Thus we continue to revert to political power to force change . . ." (p. 208).

Chester (1972) compares hospital costs in the United States, England, Sweden, and West Germany for the year 1970 as shown in Table 12-2.

He notes that in all countries except the United States the patient paid little if any of the cost whereas in the United States federal, state, and local governments paid only 48 percent of total hospital costs in the nation.

For-Profit Hospitals

Some argue that for-profit or proprietary hospitals that have profit incentives will control costs more effectively. Approximately 13 percent of the hospitals in the United States are for-profit with 21 percent of them, or 3 percent of the total, operated by large hospital chains. Most of the non-chain-operated hospitals are small (nearly two-thirds have less than 50 beds) whereas most of the chain-operated hospitals (86 percent) are over 50 beds. For-profit hospitals represent an even smaller portion of the hospital beds having only 6 percent of the beds in the nation. The large hospital chains such as American Medical International and Hospital Corporation of America have grown rapidly. They claim their corporate management skills and incentives foster savings.

Critics of the development of for-profit chains suggest that such hospitals do not contribute needed services such as nursing and physician education; moreover, they accept only the high revenue cases, leaving the nonprofit hospitals with the expensive and nonpaying patients. Critics also imply that cost-cutting techniques used by for-profit hospitals may sacrifice quality. Spokesmen for

Table 12-1 Cost of Health Services as a Percent of National Income in United States, Sweden and England

	1958	1968
United States	5.3%	7.5%
Sweden	3.2	8.1
England	5.4	5.2

Source: Odin Anderson, *Health Care: Can There Be Equity?* Wiley, New York, 1972.

Table 12-2 Cost Per Day, Average Length of Stay, and Average Cost per Case in United States, England, Sweden, and West Germany, 1970

	Cost per day	Average length of stay	Average cost per case
United States	$80	8 days	$640
England	$20	12 days	$240
Sweden	$50	12 days	$600
West Germany	$30	18 days	$540

Adapted from Theodore Chester, "United States Hospital Costs in International Perspective," *The Annals,* pp. 79-80, Jan. 1972.

the chains are quick to point out, however, that the JCAH has approved 77 percent of chain hospitals compared with only 73 percent of nonprofit hospitals (Thomas, 1972). Ferber (1971), Director of Bureau of Research Services of the AHA, in his analysis of chain-operated for-profit hospitals, found some evidence to suggest they are "better able to realize economics of scale [than nonprofit hospitals]" and there are "tentative indications that chain hospitals serve a somewhat different patient mix, and that they tend to use personnel more efficiently." He concludes that "Few will disagree with the philosophy of the chains that socially responsive capitalism, given a reasonable profit incentive, has the potential of making a vital contribution to the improvement of the hospital and medical care system." It is apparent, however, that more data are needed before chain-operated for-profit hospitals can be properly evaluated against non-profit hospitals and non-profit chains. Non-profit chains are discussed in a later section.

Teaching Hospitals

Teaching hospitals, that is, those with education programs for interns and residents (including nursing schools), are generally conceded to have higher costs than non-teaching hospitals today. In years past when interns were paid $25 per month or when student nurses spent most of their time in service, these "donated" services resulted in savings to the hospital. Today, when intern wages are about $10,000 annually, and educational time, space, and support services are required for effective learning, it is generally believed that educational programs are costly to both hospitals and their patients. The Association of American Medical Colleges (AAMC) and others are attempting to determine teaching costs, but because of the problems involved in separating teaching and service costs, determining appropriate patient loads for training, etc., no widely accepted cost allocation methodology has emerged (Wing, 1972). A study by the Commission on Professional and Hospital Activities found that for similar cases the teaching effect in teaching hospitals accounted for a 10 percent longer stay (*PAS Reporter,* 1968).

In recent years there has been a major national debate over funding for teaching programs in hospitals. In most institutions it is the patient who pays most of the educational costs. Teaching hospitals and some third-party payers argue that educational institutions and/or the federal government should pay such costs. But medical schools and other educational institutions seldom have resources to cover all the costs of student or house staff clinical experiences. There is evidence that teaching hospitals provide higher quality service (for example, see Peterson, 1973; Roemer and Friedman, 1971). Freymann and Springer (1973) concluded from their study at Hartford (Connecticut) Hospital that, if all education programs (intern, resident, nursing, and allied health) were abolished, it would cost more to provide the same quality services at that hospital.

Johnsen and Eady (1972) found in a study of nine hospitals that the elimination of nursing diploma schools would save those institutions from $.91 to $2.45 per patient-day or less than 2 percent of total hospital costs. They reported that hospitals that have eliminated diploma nursing schools have usually continued with other nursing education programs. In other words, the cost of nursing education to patients is considerable, particularly under a step-down cost analysis that includes direct and indirect expenses such as a portion of the hospital administrator's salary. However, in view of the need to train personnel and the influence of training on quality care, the cost of nursing education is not excessive, particularly on the basis of cost differential to patients with and without a nursing school.

Not-for-Profit Chains

One might assume that hospitals in not-for-profit chains, i.e., hospital conglomerates or hospitals with satellite operations (see Platou and Rice, 1972; HRET, 1972; Starkweather, 1970) have lower costs due to less duplication of services and economies of scale. HRET (1972), for example, concluded that the Good Samaritan Hospital chain in Phoenix, Arizona, resulted in savings and improvement in quality as compared to previous hospitals of independent and competitive status. However, Motorola, one of the largest employers in Phoenix, has had a running battle with the Good Samaritan chain charging it with waste and unnecessarily high costs (Piper, 1972).

Economies of Scale?

A question that has been the subject of considerable research is whether or not costs vary by size or other classifications such as whether the system is profit or nonprofit. One would assume that there are increasing returns to scale. Larger hospitals should be more economical than smaller ones. A number of economists suggest that there are economies of scale in most cases, suggesting that the long-run average cost curve is U-shaped. However, there is considerable disagreement regarding the point or range of minimum long-run average cost. Carr and P. Feldstein (1967) suggest that the minimum is about 190 beds; M. Feldstein (1968) thinks it is between 300 and 900 beds.

There are several principles to be considered in applying returns to scale in the production of hospital services:

Principle of bulk transactions: The cost of dealing in large quantities is sometimes no greater than the cost of dealing in small quantities.

Principle of massed reserves: A larger hospital would be required to keep a smaller percentage of its beds unoccupied than two smaller hospitals keeping the same number of beds in reserve for varying weekly and seasonal demands on beds.

Principle of multiples: Since capacities of different types of machines and labor involve different scales of output, a hospital large enough to employ several of each variety is more likely to use them at a high level of efficiency.

Ingbar and Taylor (1968) in their study of hospital costs in Massachusetts suggest that economies of scale do not exist; indeed, they found the highest cost point to be around 150 to 200 beds, the point that Carr and Feldstein found to be the minimum. A major problem in determining returns to scale is that there are vast differences in measures of hospital output (patient-days, bed-days, etc.), case mix (referral and teaching institutions versus primary care facilities), size (beds, beds and outpatients), and so forth. Until these are properly controlled and measured it is likely that the arguments regarding economies of scale in hospitals will continue.

In summary, costs can be reduced by cutting services, reducing quality, or increasing efficiency. Reducing unnecessary services is a goal of utilization review activities. Reduction of services and quality is believed to be unacceptable to most people; however, a 1971 survey of a cross section of the population in northern California found that the majority wanted financing of health care turned over to the government even though they believed the quality of care would suffer (*Hospitals,* 1974). The question, of course, is What is *necessary* service and quality of care?

Efficiency, not merely cutting costs, is the objective sought. Pauly (1972) defines *technical efficiency* as follows:

> Standards of "high-quality" or "good" medical care are set in the light of current medical practice, and inefficiency exists when care in excess of or in any way differing from these standards is provided . . . waste therefore occur[s] when current methods are not used. Little reference is made to individual demands or tastes for various types of care, and there is no attempt to compare the costs of such care with the evaluations its recipients make of it (pp. 3-4).

Current standards may demand that a board-certified obstetrician assist a mother in her delivery. In that case, it would be technically inefficient to use a midwife even though the cost would be less. "The *economically efficient* production process is that which, for a given value of output, minimizes the cost of inputs used to produce that output" (Berki, p. 53, 1972). In other words, the best technical combination of inputs may not be economically the most efficient. In the above example, if the value of the output were the same, it might be economically efficient to use a midwife. The problem in determining an efficient hospital service lies in the differences in standards of appropriate output, the utilities (values) to the patient, institution, and community, and the various combinations of inputs. No wonder there is little agreement on economies of scale or on many other characteristics of hospital systems.

BARRIERS TO COST CONTAINMENT

The rising costs of hospital care can be contained or reduced, everyone will agree. However, how to do this without compromising expectations for the safety, convenience, and comfort of the consumers and indeed while effecting improvements remains the major question. Before exploring alternatives for cost containment we will review some of the barriers to containing costs.

The 1973 survey of national experts on barriers to improved quality of health services that we described in the last chapter also examined cost barriers. Table 12-3 lists the barriers and the number of groups of experts who ranked them as the most important. It is interesting that organization, coordination, and evaluation barriers were ranked high by all groups of respondents. Other barriers are those of problems of standards and measurements, lack of incentives, current systems, the economy, and consumer attitudes and education.

A review of this list would imply that cost containment is beyond the control of administrators and governing board members. Indeed, we suggest below that hospitals should not be expected to control costs given present conditions.

Variables influencing the cost of hospital care include (Dowling 1974):

Number of cases treated
Length of stay of patients
Case mix (types and severity of illnesses treated)
Intensity of service
Scope of service
Amenity level (e.g., television, carpeting, and personal service amenities)
Quality level
Efficiency
Input price levels (e.g., wages and supply costs)
Investment in human resources (e.g., programs to improve staff morale and skills)
Teaching programs

Many of these variables relate to utilization of hospitals.

Anderson and Sheatsley (1967) state, "There is an appreciable proportion of hospital use that can be reduced if circumstances really demand it." However, they go on to note that "The function of hospitals is far beyond life saving and it would seem that hospital care now adds comfort, safety and convenience."

Prepaid health plans have demonstrated opportunities for lowering hospital utilization from 10 to 40 percent (Klarman, 1969). Altman (1965), Duff (1972), and Gertman and Bucher (1971) report problems of unnecessary bed-days. Others raise questions about excessive use of laboratory and x-ray procedures (Griner, 1967; Rourke, 1972; Russe, 1969); and unnecessary surgery has been identified as an increasing problem (Bunker, 1970; Knowles, 1971). It is also questionable that productivity is being managed effectively. Inefficient staffing patterns, particularly in nursing services, are suggested in several studies (Connor, 1961; Harris, 1970; Illinois Study Commission on Nursing, 1971). It is frequently observed that under the

Table 12-3 Top 15 Indicated Barriers to Containing Costs of Health Care

No. of groups that agree out of 5*	Item description
5	Organization and coordination of health services is inadequate
5	Evaluation skills of providers for proposed innovations are lacking
4	Consumers lack understanding of when services are needed
4	Information and measures causally relating treatment interventions to outcomes are largely absent
4	Incentives for efficiency provided by competitors, governing boards, third-party payers, and consumers are minimal
4	Consumers lack means of providing incentives to reduce costs
3	Inflation
3	The increasing and changing nature of demand for services
3	Consumers lack understanding of preventive measures
3	The "medical mystique" causes consumers and trustees to hesitate to take issue with the physician
2	Fee for service system encourages overtreatment
2	Needed cost/benefit information does not exist
2	Cost reduction projects have had the wrong focus
2	Implementation skills needed for cost reduction projects are not present
2	Management skills of physicians are lacking

*75 respondents, $\cong$ fifteen from each of the following five groups: experienced researchers, new researchers, planners and administrators, systems engineers, and nurses. Response rates were too low to include the data from physicians. It is important to note that in totaling rankings from all respondents the ordering would not be the same as shown above. These are, however, the top 15 barriers indicated by all respondents.

Source: David Gustafson, Glenwood Rouse, and Nancy Howes, from working papers from the full report of "Roles and Training for Future Health Systems Engineers," in *Education for Health Administration,* vol. II, Health Administration Press, Ann Arbor, Mich., 1975.

fee-for-service mechanism, physicians have few incentives to minimize hospital utilization. Indeed, patient safety, patients' hospitalization benefits, and physician productivity and convenience are incentives for physicians to increase utilization of hospital services. Utilization peer review procedures are in operation in most hospitals to counteract these incentives for unnecessary utilization, but their effectiveness has been questioned (Somers, 1972).

The hospital governing board, on the other hand, holds the hospital in trust for the community, and implicit in its trusteeship is conservation of scarce community resources. The administrator is employed with the charge of managing the hospital to provide highest quality service at lowest possible cost; usually the charge is not spelled out more explicitly than this. When trustees of a community voluntary hospital judge the effectiveness of the hospital's administrator, it is likely they will do so on the basis of the success or lack of problems related to: (1) solvency of the institution; (2) indicators of quality of services; (3) harmony within the institution; and (4) growth of services and facilities. It is suggested that these criteria serve as operating goals for hospital administrators. Given the environment in which hospitals function today, it appears that these criteria or goals contribute to the rapid rise in hospital costs.

While there is overlap between the four suggested criteria of managerial success, they appear to be related hierarchically.

Solvency

The first or base-level criterion of success of almost any enterprise is solvency. In not-for-profit enterprises such as hospitals, unless income and expenses at least meet over a period of time, the enterprise cannot continue to exist, let alone provide services. Financial condition is also the most easily measured criterion of success.

Until the last couple of decades, the demand and the ability to pay for hospital services were severely limited; therefore, operating income was severely limited. Administrators struggled to keep costs in line with income ceilings. In the 1950s, 1960s and early 1970s, however, with a rising standard of living and the emergence of third-party payers, hospitals could meet solvency goals and improve their financial position by increasing services and, within federal guidelines, raising prices. The demand for hospital services, at least until the last year or two, appeared insatiable. One way to increase hospital income is to expand the scope of services and improve the comfort and esthetics of hospital facilities in order to attract more patients in competition with other hospitals. As Pauly (1970) suggests, hospitals are income maximizers. Moreover, Pauly and Redisch (1973) suggest that hospitals try to maximize physicians' incomes.

Except for regulatory requirements, there are few incentives—and in most hospitals no rewards—for administrators, trustees, and medical staff members to reduce unnecessary hospital admission, length of stay, and overutilization of laboratory, x-ray, and other ancillary services, particularly in the growing number of hospitals with excess capacity. Even though length of stay has been declining, a study found no evidence to suggest that administrators and trustees of community voluntary hospitals were actively attempting to reduce hospital utilization (Schulz, 1972).

Quality of Service

Assuming an institution has achieved the solvency necessary for it to exist, it will obviously attempt to improve the quality of its services to patients. Quality is much more difficult to measure than financial success. While there are some indicators of quality, many of them are not likely to be discussed publicly by trustees, volunteers, physicians, administrators, and other members of the hospital family. Examples of quality indicators are improved autopsy, infection, or medication error rates. Hospital officials are more likely to discuss adding more sophisticated equipment and services catering to the comfort and esthetic ideals of patients, and adding teaching and research programs. While all of these probably improve "quality," they also increase costs. As Bugbee (1971) has stated, "There is no administrator worth his salt who doesn't wish for additional money to improve services."

Institutional Harmony

In order to achieve solvency and correct any obvious problems in quality of services, the administrator may be required to endure conflict and confrontation. However, once the criteria of solvency and quality are essentially met, the administrator will be marked as successful if the medical staff and employees are generally satisfied. At this point, a happy ship is more important than a tight one.

Inquiries to a number of administrators suggest that methods engineering activities in hospitals are meeting with little success in terms of increasing hospital employee productivity by reducing staffing. Hardwick and Wolfe (1971) also reported on problems in achieving projected savings from industrial engineering efforts, and the crucial role of the administrator in achieving real cost reductions. There is some evidence to suggest that staffing could be reduced in most hospitals without sacrificing patient safety. However, for most administrators and hospital department heads, there are few rewards and many risks to harmony in reducing staffing.

Institutional Growth

Increasing services and beds are usually considered a mark of success and prestige by communities, trustees, and the medical staff, as well as by the administrator. All point with pride to bigger and better facilities. Growth is used as a measure of success by the trustee and hospital administrator, just as it is by their counterparts in for-profit industries. A promotion for an administrator, other than a change in title and board membership, consists of becoming the administrator of a larger and more prestigious hospital. Increasing size and improving hospital status help to promote administrators in the community in the eyes of their colleagues, and enhance their credentials for new jobs in larger and more prestigious hospitals. Larger facilities and a broader scope of services contribute to increased utilization. They also result in higher fixed hospital costs such as depreciation, interest, and building maintenance, thereby reducing opportunities for control over total hospital costs.

Unless community health needs have been carefully assessed and hospital objectives clearly defined in terms of meeting those needs, institutional objectives may take priority over community objectives. Gross and Grambsch (1969) found evidence in major American universities that institutional goals took precedence over output goals. Student discontent and current legislative reactions against universities might have been predicted from the findings of their study. It is possible that, in the age of prosperity, community hospitals subconsciously gave priority to institutional rather than community goals and objectives—as some consumer groups charge.

Between 1971 and 1974 hospitals were subjected to price and wage controls under the Economic Stabilization Program (ESP), which allowed price increases of approximately 6 percent per year. This was well below increases in previous years. The AHA complained loudly that ESP was unfair to hospitals, that hospitals had been operating efficiently and that ESP handicapped quality improvements. They noted that during ESP operating margins of community hospitals declined to 1.2 percent of total revenue down from over 3 percent in a number of years prior to ESP (AHA, 1973). However, in working with a number of hospitals on a goal-setting study (unpublished) during and just after ESP, the authors found that cost containment goals had a low priority in relationship to quality and satisfaction goals.

Prospective reimbursement schemes have been proposed and tried, since it is recognized that traditional cost reimbursement provides no incentive to cost containment. Prospective reimbursement is a method by which a third party (e.g., Blue Cross or Social Security Administration) reimburses hospitals on amounts or rates established in advance. Hospitals are paid these amounts or rates regardless of the costs they actually incur. Consequently, if costs are less than projected, the hospital keeps the savings; if costs are greater, the hospital must absorb the loss. Payment plans based on amounts, e.g., total hospital budgets or capitation units, places financial incentives on reducing cases treated, length of stay, complexity of case-mix, intensity of service, scope of service, amenity and quality levels, input prices, investment in resources and teaching programs, and incentives for improving efficiency. Payment plans based on prospective rate reimbursement, e.g., specified rate per service or per patient-day, usually does not put incentives on reducing utilization of services. While there has been some evidence of modest cost savings from some of the experimental prospective reimbursement schemes, other factors must be considered, such as administrative feasibility and evaluating their effectiveness (Dowling 1974). Prospective rate review activities are discussed further in the next chapter.

INCENTIVES AND REWARDS TO CONTROL HOSPITAL COSTS

Three general ways to establish incentives and rewards for controlling costs are: (1) government controls; (2) market controls; and (3) institutional voluntary cost controls.

Government Controls

There is growing concern over the rising costs of hospital care on the part of federal, state, and local governments. Given the fact that the financing of hospital care is increasingly centralized in the federal government through Medicare and Medicaid, and the possibility of an overall national health insurance plan, it is likely that cost controls will be exerted from the national rather than the institutional level. If the federal government severely limits hospital utilization and prices, the first criterion of institutional solvency will again predominate in the establishment of administrative rewards. If income is relatively fixed, control over costs will be the only way to attain solvency. Government rate controls will certainly emphasize controls over the utilization of services as well. Setting appropriate and equitable standards is a problem—but information systems such as Medicare Analysis of Days of Care (MADOC), Professional

Activities Study (PAS), Medical Audit Program (MAP), and Hospital Administrative Service (HAS) from which standards might be established are being improved.

While stringent government controls can reduce utilization and force greater operational efficiencies on hospitals, this alternative of bureaucratic interference is repugnant to most providers of health services. Moreover, general governmental regulations or standards tend to compromise the needs and expectations of individual consumers.

Market Controls

Market controls such as prepaid health plans have been proposed and widely discussed as an alternative to federal cost controls. Prepaid health programs such as the Kaiser Health Plan are designed to provide financial incentives for the lower utilization of costly services and facilities by maintaining personal health. Moreover, purchasers of prepaid health care can be informed of the costs of comprehensive health care by providers, which enables them to shop for lower-cost services. Providers then must meet competitive prices, which will limit the use of expensive services and focus more attention on control of costs. A variable-cost insurance plan to pressure hospitals to minimize "lavish" services has also been proposed (Kaplan and Lave, 1971), but this does not seem feasible.

Closed-panel prepaid programs like Kaiser have not grown rapidly, primarily due to provider resistance, but consumer resistance is also evident. Open-panel or foundation-type plans such as the San Joaquin Foundation plan are being developed, but there is not yet enough evidence on which to judge their effectiveness in controlling hospital cost.

Institutional Voluntary Cost Controls

It appears possible for hospitals to voluntarily establish and achieve objectives for containing the rising costs of hospital care. In a follow-up of a recent survey of hospital employee productivity and utilization, administrators of comparable hospitals that had lower nursing hours per-patient day were interviewed (Schulz, 1972). One of these administrators, whose hospital had high nursing productivity, had clearly defined goals, and knew exactly what experience was in relation to goals. This administrator identified cost and quality problem areas, and described what was being done to correct them. Productivity in most of the other professional and nonprofessional departments in the hospital was consistently higher than in comparable hospitals in the area; moreover, length-of-stay by age and diagnosis was lower. Occupancy and other factors that could affect productivity and utilization did not appear to vary significantly from other hospitals, and the hospital had a reputation for high-quality service.

However, the other administrators with low nursing hours per patient-day attributed productivity solely to occupancy; moreover, unlike the case described above, there was little consistency in relative productivity among other professional and non-professional departments in their hospitals. Some administrators did not really know how they compared with other hospitals in productivity and length of stay, even though they received HAS, MADOC and, in a few cases, PAS and MAP length-of-stay reports. It is not suggested that these findings are conclusive. Research is continuing regarding hospital goals, the influence an administrator can exercise over costs, and managerial methods for controlling costs (for example, see Neuhauser, 1971).

A number of steps, consistent with those suggested previously, are recommended for an overall voluntary cost containment hospital management program:

1 Study community service needs and quality and cost expectations that the hospital is expected to meet. Needs should be defined in measurable terms based on data and opinions outside the hospital.

2 Identify the purposes of the hospital in relation to meeting needs.

3 Establish measurable objectives and goals with priorities and schedules. These should be stated explicitly so that at the end of a specified period it is known whether or not they have been achieved. For example, length-of-stay as reported from PAS should be reduced to x amount, or nursing hours per patient-day be reduced by x amount. Quality goals can be measured by satisfaction and opinion surveys, in addition to other structure, process, and outcome measures.

Perrow (1967) suggests that the goals pursued by individuals in an organization (operational goals) may be quite different from official or stated institutional goals. It is important that official and operational goals be the same.

4 Establish programs to achieve goals. Management methods and tools to help achieve goals are available, e.g., program, planning, and budgeting systems. Management methods and tools are also improving—for example, operations research techniques can be used to reduce a hospital's bed needs as demonstrated by Griffith (1973).

5 Establish administrative evaluation and rewards based on the achievement of goals. In essence, it is suggested that management-by-objectives principles be applied to trustees, medical staff, and the administration of the hospital (Odiorne, 1965).

The major problem with institutional voluntary cost controls is that there is currently little incentive for hospital administrators, trustees, and medical staff to expand the time and effort needed. A number of voluntary incentive systems have been proposed and/or tried, for example, target rate, departmental efficiency, and capitation payment approaches based on sharing savings between hospitals and third-party payers (Hill, 1970). However, none has proven to be very effective.

Can hospitals be expected to control costs voluntarily? At the present time, administrators of fee-for-service hospitals receive few rewards for containing costs and should not therefore be expected to do so aggressively. It is easier for hospitals to contain costs if controls are established externally by regulatory agencies or by the market through prepaid plans. Externally established cost controls provide administrators and trustees with authority (and a scapegoat) for instituting hard line measures to evaluate utilization and productivity. The Joint Commission on Accreditation of Hospitals has given this kind of leverage to administrators, trustees, and medical staff members to improve control over quality of service.

If the voluntary fee-for-service system is to be retained while costs are to be controlled more effectively, it is recommended that hospitals establish operational goals and utilize information systems that evaluate quality, cost, and service effectiveness in relation to these goals. The government, the market, or voluntary groups such as JCAH or Blue Cross could provide the necessary incentives without imposing monetary or operational standards on hospitals. For example, JCAH could require hospitals to establish and publicized *explicit* goals for efficiency and effectiveness. A hospital might then set a target of, say, a 90 percent annual occupancy rate in medicine and surgery, together with a target to eliminate a certain number of beds and reduce staffing per patient-day to a specified number. Section 234 of P.L. 92-603 requires hospitals to have a three-year plan and budget.

Explicit goals should go hand in hand with the development and utilization of appropriate management information systems and participative management techniques. This means that standards would be developed by each institution rather than imposed by government or other external groups. Emphasis on processes and peer controls is consistent with current JCAH and government philosophies. Moreover, publicized objectives and measurements of success provide for market controls through better-informed consumers. More importantly, such goals and measurements could revise expectations on which administrative trustee and medical staff rewards are based. In Figure 9-1 (Chapter 9) we presented a model for role behavior. If containing costs is a major role purpose of the administrator then values and rewards to that effect will need to be made explicit through environmental factors, i.e., governmental or market incentives, and/or through organizational factors, i.e., institutional voluntary controls, or through personal values of the administrator.

We will know we have reached the millennium of controlling hospital costs when trustees and administrators *proudly* report at their annual meeting: "Home care patients have increased, inpatient days per population declined, and total employees have been reduced, while occupancy rate has increased in accordance with our target for the year to close at least one more nursing unit."

OPPORTUNITIES FOR INTERNAL COST CONTROLS

If there are incentives to contain costs and clearly established goals, targets, and management commitment to do so, a number of internal cost containment tactics might be employed.

Shared Services

Aside from the advantages related to economies of scale, it would seem obvious that sharing of services, merging of institutions, forming conglomerates, or whatever form of association you wish to call it, would help reduce duplication of services. One high-volume obstetrical unit, emergency service, cobalt unit, or similar high-cost marginal volume service can be more economical than two or more low-volume units, as many hospitals have found. Without profit or solvency incentives many hospitals still continue to support prestigious but losing services duplicated elsewhere in the community. Shared services are discussed further in Chapter 16.

Systems Engineering and Operations Research While systems engineering and operations techniques (referred to as industrial engineering, methods improvement, scientific management, etc.) have not been particularly effective in hospitals, they have been successful in private industry. Systems engineering has been used in hospitals over a number of years (see Chapter 10). Operations research is developing and Griffith (1973) reports success with such applications as in patient and personnel scheduling systems to improve utilization and productivity. Again, the effectiveness of such approaches appears to depend primarily on the commitment of top management.

Employee Incentive Systems

Gustafson et al. (1972) reviewed a number of incentive systems designed to reward hospital employees in direct relation to increases in productivity. They reviewed the few incentive systems that have been utilized in hospitals, and evaluated those more widely used in industry on the basis of their applicability to hospitals. Ranges of employee incentive systems from which a hospital can develop its own plan include:

Individual incentive plans related to standards based on work measurement techniques.

Team incentive systems based on productivity of the team.

Large group incentive systems based on the productivity of a department or whole hospital such as:

A profit sharing plan, which is not applicable in a pure sense, but of which variations are possible.

Cost savings sharing, which is more appropriate in hospitals because it is based on cutting costs rather than increasing revenue and profits (Jehring, 1967).

A labor savings (Scanlon) plan, whereby payoff to the employee is based on a reduction in the percentage of total product revenue involved in paying labor costs. Usually employee management committees review suggestions for improvements.

A value added (Rucker) plan in which payoff is based upon the ratio:

$$\frac{\text{Revenue Material Cost}}{\text{Labor Cost}}$$

where the numerator is an estimate of the value added by the hospital to the service provided.

While most of these systems appear to have limited application to nonprofit service industries, a few hospitals have reported significant results (Jehring, 1967). In the early days of Medicare, the Social Security Administration sought innovative incentive systems as a way of containing costs. There were few proposals for such innovative systems and even fewer reports of successful results.

Ambulatory and Outreach Services as Alternatives to Inpatient Services

We have already suggested that outreach services such as home care, consumer health education, and environmental and occupational health services could have a major impact on improving the health of the community. They can also help to obviate the expensive inpatient hospital services.

Mather (1971) reports from a small but well-controlled study that there was no difference in the results of home treatment of myocardial infarction (heart attacks) and of care in a hospital intensive care unit, which can cost as much as $200 per day. Peace of mind through the availability of hospital services is important to most people, but it is expensive (though the expense is of little concern to those with insurance). Davis and Detmer (1972) and others report that a number of surgical procedures normally done on an inpatient basis can be performed as effectively and at considerably less cost on an outpatient basis. And diagnostic work-ups and other procedures are still being done on an inpatient basis merely because the patient has inpatient insurance coverage. The Comptroller General of the United States Study of Health Facility Construction Costs (1972) suggests additional alternatives to expensive inpatient services.

Physician Accountability for Costs

It has been commonly suggested that physicians in effect control 87 percent of hospital operating costs, and yet are not held accountable (Knowles, 1966). As we noted in Chapter 5, a number of national commissions and individual writers have suggested that the way to control hospital costs is to involve the physician. Etzioni (1974) suggests that "gains in efficiency achieved through the use of lay administrators [and decreasing participation of physicians] might be cancelled out by the decreasing-cost consciousness of physicians (p. 23)." Schulz (1972), however, found no relationship between physician membership on hospital governing boards and participation in management decision activities and hospital costs. A major problem is the feasibility of involving physicians and holding them accountable under current organizational arrangements.

Financial Control Systems

Advanced financial control systems can be important tools for containing costs. However, budgets, cost accounting systems, and so forth can be developed and applied most effectively if there is involvement of and accountability by those who are responsible for costs, e.g., hospital department heads. As noted previously, we have heard a number of administrators confess that they do not share financial reports and systems with their department heads for fear the latter will not understand them and will just ask for more money. However, hospitals can no longer raise rates easily and with external pressures for containing costs it is likely that financial information systems will involve department heads and other personnel. We have noted an increasing willingness on the part of administrators to expose their financial records. (See Chapter 10 for a more detailed discussion of financial and information systems.)

CONCLUSIONS

We conclude there are many ways to contain hospital costs more effectively than is done in most hospitals today. Moreover, costs can be contained at no sacrifice to patient safety and probably at little, if any, sacrifice to patient comfort and convenience. The main ingredient to success is to offer incentives and rewards. With increasing federal controls and growing concern about hospital solvency, the incentives and rewards appear to be developing. We hope that the proper approaches to cost containment will be taken and that patient safety, comfort, and convenience will not suffer to any great extent.

REFERENCES

AHA: Guide Issues of *Hospitals, J.A.H.A.,* Aug. 16, 1973.

Altman, Isidore: "Some Factors Affecting Hospital Length of Stay," *Hospitals, J.A.H.A.,* vol. 39, no. 68, 1965.

Anderson, Odin W.: *Health Care: Can There Be Equity?* Wiley, New York, 1972.

Anderson, Odin W. and Paul Sheatsley: *Hospital Use: A Survey of Patient and Physician Decisions,* Center for Health Administration Studies Research Series 24, University of Chicago, 1967.

Anderson, Ronald and J. Joel May: "Factors Associated with Increasing Costs of Crisis in Medical Care: An Impetus for Changing the Delivery Systems?" *Economics and Business Bulletin,* Temple University, pp. 41-52, 1971.

Anderson, Ronald and J. Joel May: "Factors Associated with Increasing Cost of Hospital Care," *The Annals,* vol. 399, pp. 62-72, Jan. 1972.

Berki, Sylvester E.: *Hospital Economics,* Lexington Books, Lexington, Mass., 1972.

Bugbee, George: "Good Care is Worth the Cost," *Hospitals, J.A.H.A.,* vol. 45, p. 15, 1971.

Bunker, John P.: "Surgical Manpower, A Comparison of Operations and Surgeons in United States, England and Wales," *New England Journal of Medicine,* vol. 20, pp. 135-144, 1970.

Carr, W. J. and P. J. Feldstein: "The Relationship of Cost to Hospital Size," *Inquiry,* pp. 45-65, June 1967.

Chester, Theodore E.: "United States Hospital Costs in International Perspective," *The Annals,* pp. 73-81, Jan. 1972.

Comptroller General of United States: *Study of Health Facilities Construction Costs,* B-164031 (3), Washington, D.C., 1972.

Connor, Robert J.: "A Work Sampling Study of Variations in Nursing Work Load," *Hospitals, J.A.H.A.,* vol. 35, no. 40, 1961.

Davis, James E. and Don E. Detmer: "The Ambulatory Surgical Unit." *Annals of Surgery,* vol. 175, no. 6, pp. 856-862, June 1972.

Dowling, William L.: "Prospective Reimbursement of Hospitals," *Inquiry,* vol. 11, pp. 163-180, Sept. 1974.

Duff, R. S.: "Use of Utilization Review to Assess the Quality of Pediatric Inpatient Care," *Pediatrics,* vol. 49, pp. 169-176, 1972.

Etzioni, Amitai: "Cost Consciousness in Hospitals: Sociological Factors," *Center for Policy Research: First Five Years, 1968-1973,* Center for Policy Research, 475 Riverside Drive, New York, 1974.

Feldstein, Martin S.: *Economic Analysis for Health Services Efficiency,* Markham, Chicago, 1968.

Ferber, Bernard: "An Analysis of Chain Operated For-Profit Hospitals," *Health Service Research,* pp. 49-60, Spring 1971.

Freymann, John G. and John K. Springer: "Cost of Hospital Based Education," *Hospitals, J.A.H.A.,* pp. 65ff., Mar. 1, 1973.

Gertman, Paul and Bruce Bucher: "Inappropriate Hospital-Bed Days and Their Relationship to Length of Stay Parameters," paper presented at the 99th Annual Meeting, American Public Health Association, Minneapolis, Minnesota, 1971.

Golladay, Fredrick L. and Kenneth R. Smith: *Regulating the Health Industry* (monograph), study prepared for the Health Policy Council (of Wisconsin) by the Wisconsin Regional Medical Program, Madison, 1974.

Griffith, John, Walton Hancock, and Fred C. Munson: "Practical Ways to Contain Hospital Costs," *Harvard Business Review,* pp. 131-139, Nov.-Dec. 1973.

Griner, Paul F. and Benjamin Lipzin: "Use of the Laboratory in a Teaching Hospital," *Annals of Internal Medicine,* vol. 75, pp. 157-163, 1971.

Gross, Edward and Paul Grambsch: *University Goals and Academic Power,* American Council on Education, Washington, D.C., 1968.

Gustafson, David, John Doyle, and J. Joel May: *Employee Incentive System of Hospitals,* GPO, Stock #1726-0026, Washington, D.C., 1972.

Hardwick, Patrick C. and Harvey Wolfe: *An Incentive Reimbursement/Industrial Engineering Experiment,* Department of Health, Education and Welfare, Publication no. (HSM) 72-3003, p. 31, 1971.

Harris, David H.: "Nursing Staffing Requirements," *Hospitals, J.A.H.A.,* vol. 44, no. 64, 1970.

Hill, Lawrence A.: "Internal Control," *Hospitals, J.A.H.A.,* vol. 44, 1970.

Hospitals Statistics 1974 Edition, American Hospital Association, Chicago.

Hospital Week, American Hospital Association, Chicago, Feb. 28, 1975.

Hospitals, J.A.H.A.: "Respect Is First Demand [of Consumers]," pp. 57-61, Aug. 16, 1974.

HRET: *Final Report Demonstration and Evaluation of Integrated Health Care Facilities,* vol. IV (technical version), Chicago Hospital Research and Educational Trust and Northwestern University, 1972.

Illinois Study Commission on Nursing: "Nurse Utilization: Illinois—A Study in Thirty-One Hospitals, 1966-1970, Vol. III," 1971.

Ingbar, M. L. and L. D. Taylor: *Hospital Costs in Massachusetts,* Harvard University Press, Cambridge, Mass., 1968.

Jehring, J. J.: *The Use of Subsystem Incentives in Hospitals,* Center for Study of Productivity Motivation, University of Wisconsin, Madison, 1967.

Johnsen, Gordon and Carol Eady: "How Much Does Diploma Nursing Education Really Cost?" *Nursing Outlook,* vol. 20, no. 10, pp. 658-661, 1972.

Kaplan, Robert S. and Lester B. Lave: "Patient Incentives and Hospital Insurance," *Health Services Research,* pp. 288-300, Winter 1971.

Klarman, Herbert E.: "Approaches to Moderating the Increases in Medical Care Costs," *Medical Care,* vol. 7, pp. 175-190, 1969.

Klarman, Herbert E. (ed.): *Empirical Studies in Health Economics.* The Johns Hopkins Press, Baltimore, 1970.

Knowles, John: *The Teaching Hospital,* Harvard University Press, Cambridge, Mass., 1966.

Knowles, John: "Spellbinding and Spellbreaking in American Medicine," address delivered at the First Annual Meeting of the Institute of Medicine, National Academy of Sciences, Washington, D.C., Nov. 18, 1971.

Kovner, Anthony R. and Edward Lusk: "Effective Hospital Budgeting," *Hospital Administration,* vol. 18, no. 4, pp. 44-64, 1973.

Mather, H. G. et al.: "Acute Myocardial Infarction: Home and Hospital Treatment," *British Medical Journal,* vol. 3, pp. 334-338, 1971.

Neuhauser, Duncan: *The Relationship Between Administrative Activities and Hospital Performance,* Center for Health Administration Studies Research Series 28, University of Chicago, 1971.

Odiorne, George S.: *Management by Objectives,* Pitman, New York, 1965.

PAS Reporter: "How Much Longer Do Patients Stay in Teaching Hospitals?" vol. 6, no. 7, 1968.

Pauly, Mark V.: "Efficiency, Incentives and Reimbursement for Health Care," *Inquiry,* vol. 7, p. 117, 1970.

Pauly, Mark V.: *Medical Care at Public Expense,* Praeger, New York, 1972.

Pauly, Mark V. and Michael Redisch: "The Not-for-Profit Hospital as a Physicians' Cooperative," *American Economic Review,* vol. 63, no. 1, pp. 87-99, Mar. 1973.

Perrow, Charles: "The Analysis of Goals in Complex Organizations," in W. A. Hill and D. M. Egan (eds.), *Readings in Organization Theory,* Allyn and Bacon, Boston, 1967, p. 130.

Peterson, Osler: "The Importance of Obtaining High Quality Medical Care," in *Hospitals' Role in Assessing the Quality of Medical Care,* Proceedings of the Fifteenth Annual Symposium on Hospital Affairs, University of Chicago, May 1973.

Piper, Kenneth: Remarks at a Public Hearing of Maricopa County Comprehensive Health Planning Council, Dec. 12, 1972.

Platou, Carl N. and James A. Rice: "Multihospital Holding Companies," *Harvard Business Review,* pp. 14+, May-June 1972.

Roemer, Milton and Joy W. Friedman: *Doctors in Hospitals,* Johns Hopkins Press, Baltimore, Md., 1971.

Rourke, Anthony J. J.: "Are All Those X-Rays and Tests Really Necessary?" *Modern Hospital,* Jan. 1972.

Russe, Henry P.: "The Use and Abuse of Laboratory Tests," *Medical Clinics of North America,* vol. 53, pp. 223-231, Jan. 1969.

Schulz, Rockwell: *Relationship Between Medical Staff Participation in Hospital Management and Factors of Cost of Medical Care,* unpublished Ph.D. dissertation, University of Michigan, Ann Arbor, 1972, p. 144 (available from University Microfilms).

Schulz, Rockwell and Jerry Rose: "Can Hospitals Be Expected to Control Costs?" *Inquiry,* pp. 3-8, June, 1973.

Somers, Herman: "Hospital Utilization Controls: What Is the Way?" *New England Journal of Medicine,* vol. 22, p. 1362, 1972.

Starkweather, David B.: "Health Facility Combinations: Some Conceptualizations," Address Author at Program in Hospital Administration, School of Public Health, University of California, Berkeley, 1970.

Thomas, Dana L.: "Annual Check-Up: Proprietary Hospital Chains Continue to Thrive," *Barron's,* p. 3ff., July 31, 1972.

U.S. Department of Health, Education and Welfare: *Statistics Note,* Social Security Administration Publication No. (SSA) 75-11701, Feb. 19, 1975.

Wing, Paul: "Clinical Costs of Medical Education," *Inquiry,* vol. 9, pp. 36-43, 1972.

Chapter 13

The Management
of Conflict[1]

A certain amount of conflict is beneficial to organizations. For example, conflict creates tension that leads to change and innovation. However, the potential for excessive conflict in hospitals is readily apparent. It is doubtful that any other organization has such a wide range of specialized personnel gathered together in one work group. The administrator is continually faced with eruptions of personal or departmental conflict. Periodically, administrator-medical staff conflicts break into public view. Consumers of hospital services level charges of inefficiency, and inattention to consumer expectations, and employee strikes receive wide publicity. In addition, the unexpected and emergency nature of many of the treatments provides situations of stress that can lead to conflict.

In light of these considerations, it behooves the administrator of a hospital to be able to manage conflict. As a first step in this process, the administrator must identify

[1] This chapter was adapted from Rockwell Schulz and Alton C. Johnson, "Conflict in Hospitals," an article that originally appeared in *Hospital Administration,* published by the American Hospital Association, vol. 16, Summer 1971.

the underlying forces. The following section will review briefly the nature of individual, interpersonal, group, and client-hospital conflict. Conflict related to administrators, medical staff, and nursing groups will be discussed in some depth. In the second section, some mitigators of conflict will be presented.

THE NATURE OF CONFLICT

One might expect conflict to affect the quality of patient care adversely. This seems to be confirmed by the studies of Georgopoulos and Mann (1962), who found higher-quality care in hospitals where physicians and nurses had a greater understanding of each other's work, problems, and needs. Studies of mental hospitals report that patients are affected adversely by staff conflict (Stanton and Schwartz, 1954; Caudill, 1958; Blau and Scott, 1962). While conflict may foster institutional innovation and progress, the welfare of the individual patient is served more effectively by institutional stability and harmony. Moreover, conflict can be debilitating for participants, rigidify the social system in which it occurs, and lead to gross distortions of reality (Walton, 1969). Thus, we assume that controlling conflict is an important goal for most hospitals as we examine sources and mitigators of conflict.

Individual Conflict

Conflict can be intrapersonal, that is, within the individual himself. We sometimes hear of the employee whose standard of living exceeds the pay he receives from his job. If there is no change in this situation, he soon becomes in conflict with himself because his needs are not met. One reaction is for him to strike out at supervisors and fellow employees as an escape from his dilemma. We sometimes note this type of reaction when other needs such as security or self-esteem are not met. An individual employee in a hospital may also find the work situation frustrating because there are no promotional opportunities without more education. To complicate the situation even more, education is costly and means loss of income while pursued.

Referring back to the role behavior model in Chapter 9 (Figure 9-1, page 149), personal attributes can contribute to conflict. Kahn's studies relate personality variables to experiences of strain (Kahn, 1964). He found tension more pronounced for introverts, emotionally sensitive people, and individuals who were strongly achievement-oriented. Personality characteristics also affected the degree of individual conflict and tension. Individuals who were relatively flexible and those who were achievement-oriented were more susceptible to conflict pressures.

Interpersonal Conflict

A second type of conflict relates to interpersonal factors (see Figure 9-1). An individual's role in the hospital can have a major effect on the conflict to which he is subjected. His personal characteristics and past experiences will determine how well he can cope with role conflict. Role theory, including role conflict, has received considerable study, although little in a hospital setting. Katz and Kahn (1966) define *role conflict* as "the simultaneous occurrence of two or more role sendings such that compliance with one would make more difficult compliance with the other" (p. 184). It is easy to imagine the role conflicts faced by physicians, nurses, and administrators. Physicians, for example, function as agents for the individual patient, their own specialty, their profession, their staff, their institution, and their community as well as in the role of individual practitioners. The physicians' obligations to these individuals and groups, and their obligations to themselves, are peridiocally in conflict (defined as inter-role conflict by Katz and Kahn). The nurse is frequently caught between multiple lines of authority (intersender conflict). The administrator often functions in a boundary role, between nurse and physician, two physicians, patient and employee, and so on.

Role ambiguity is related to role conflict. It can be defined as uncertainty about the way one's work is evaluated by superiors, and about scope of responsibility, opportunities for advancement, and expectations of others for job performance. A variety of studies have demonstrated that there is frequently a wide disparity between what a superior expects of a subordinate and what the subordinate thinks is expected. In an industrial setting, Kahn (1964) found the individual consequences of role ambiguity generally comparable to the individual effects of role conflict. These consequences include "low job satisfaction, low self-confidence, a high sense of futility and a high score on the tension index" (p. 380). House and Rizzo (1972), however, suggest that on the basis of their research with business executives that more emphasis should be placed upon eliminating role ambiguity as an intervening variable between leadership behavior and organizational effectiveness.

Thus, interpersonal conflict is defined broadly to include both (1) interpersonal disagreements over substantive issues, such as policies and practices, and (2) interpersonal antagonisms, that is, the more personal and emotional differences that arise between independent human beings (Walton, 1969). Both forms are very common in the hospital setting, although interpersonal antagonisms would seem to be more prevalent because by nature they deal with emotions. However, no studies were found concerning the relative frequency, severity, or source of interpersonal conflict in hospitals.

Surveys in industrial enterprises found that tension and strain increased directly with occupational status. Individuals in professional and technical occupations experienced the most tension followed by managerial, then clerical, and sales (Kahn, 1964). However, Kahn found the medical administrator in the industrial plant who works under conditions of high role conflict scored low on tension. In a case study he found that administrators kept potential conflicts in a delicate balance by retreating into their own section of expertise; that is, statistical and financial management. The obvious implication is that administrators can minimize conflict by restricting their role. While this finding is based on a single case study in a nonhospital setting, one can logically assume that there will be a positive relationship between the scope of the administrators' roles and efforts to effect changes and the degree of administrative conflict. A coping mechanism that limits scope may aid the equanimity of administrators, but will not help fulfill their broader obligations and responsibilities.

Considerable basic conflict in nursing is evident from many studies (see Chapter 6). Most of these inquiries indicate that nurses are satisfied with their vocation, but dissatisfied with specific conditions of salary, workload, working hours, etc. (Corwin and Taves, 1963). However, Argyris (1965) suggests more basic problems such as frustration of the dominant predispositions of nurses. He reports that nurses in the hospital he studied were not able to fulfill effectively important predispositions, such as being self-controlled, indispensable, compatible, and expert.

Status may be a source of conflict among nurses. In years past, nursing was one of the few careers women could enter and attain some degree of professional prestige. Today, many more vocational opportunities are opening to women as sex discrimination continues to decline. Women can, or at least believe they can, gain greater recognition in fields such as business, government, medicine, and teaching (Corwin and Taves, 1963).

Whereas in the past nurses were virtually the only professionals in the hospital besides physicians, they are now receiving increasing competition for status from a proliferation of allied health professionals, many of whom have higher standards of education, pay, and autonomy.

Organizational forces present conflict for nurses. Nurses' career advancement has shifted from an individual to an organizational context in which a nurse must move through the bureaucratic hierarchy to gain recognition. In this hierarchy, however, rewards are not given for professional patient care, but rather for administrative skills. The development of clinical nurse specialization is a reaction to this "person-role conflict."

The nurse also has to contend with increasing numbers of technicians such as the clinical pharmacist. All these changes call for a new role and an examination of the professional position of the nurse. We reported on some of these struggles in Chapter 6.

Group Conflict

Certain internal characteristics inherent in the hospital organization foster conflict. For example, interdependence, specialization and heterogeneity of personnel, and levels of authority all appear to be correlated positively with conflict (Corwin, 1969). In fact, few organizations require as many diverse skills as the hospital, which has an average of about three employees for each patient, and uses a heterogeneous health team influenced by over 300 different professional societies and associations.

In industry, top executives usually enjoy both formal and informal power and status. In the hospital organization, however, power and status do not appear to be centered in the same individuals. This characteristic, probably unique to hospital organization, is a basic source of administration-medical staff conflict.

Power has been defined as the maximum ability of a person or group to influence individuals or groups. Influence is understood as the degree of change that may be effected in individuals or groups. Authority has been defined as legitimate power (Filley and House, 1969). From their review of a variety of authors, Filley and House have summarized the basis of power derived from (1) legitimacy; (2) control of rewards and sanctions, including money; (3) expertise; (4) personal liking; and (5) co-ercion. Observation tells us that the hospital administrator usually has (1) legitimacy from delegated authority for hospital affairs from the governing board; (2) effective control of funds, beds, and other resources; (3) increasing expertise, particularly as management information systems improve; (4) personal liking, and (5) the ability to coerce through the demands of outside agencies such as the Joint Commission on the Accreditation of Hospitals. The increasing dominance of the administrator has been discussed in previous chapters.

The Status Factor

The evidence from other studies is somewhat conflicting. For example, Georgopoulos and Mann (1962), after describing the administrators as the most influential persons, attribute their source of influence to delegated authority from trustees; the sources of physicians' influence are said to include their expertise, prestige, status, and power in relation to both patients and the community. On the other hand, a 1968 survey reported that "trustees and medical staffs do not view the administrator as a leader, but as a generally passive influence caught between the board and doctors" (*Modern Hospital,* 1968, p. 29). Goss (1963) suggests that physicians tend to view administra-tion as a less prestigious kind of work, and Bellin (1973) describes the administrator's need for status. Moreover, a University of Chicago (*Hospitals,* 1974) survey of patients and physicians in three Chicago hospitals found hospital administrators' prestige ranked behind the various physician specialists and behind the director of nursing service and the pharmacy profession.

Hospital administrators' drive for professionalism and their desire for more presti-gious titles such as president or executive vice-president suggest that they too feel a need to improve their status. Since physicians attempt to maintain or increase their power, and administrators to improve their status, both, presumably, feel threatened. Under such circumstances conflict increases.

Physicians and nurses, like professionals in other fields, give their first allegiance to professional rather than organizational status (Argyris, 1965). Hence, the potential for professional-institutional goal conflict is present.

The hospital organization is sometimes referred to as a duopoly with essentially autonomous administrative and medical staff organizations. Croog (1963) suggests that each system is oriented to a different set of values, one emphasizing provision of service, the other maintenance of operations of organization. The Barr report related hospital inefficiencies to this dual management authority (Secretary's Advisory Committee on Hospital Effectiveness, 1967).

Germane to our discussion of intergroup conflict is the concept of territory. (Ardrey 1966) points out that "territory" has both physical and psychological identification. When a territory has been staked out in terms of professional contact, education, or work interests, it will be defended. The higher the degree of commit-ment, the greater will be the defense against intrusion or change by an "outsider." In addition, if the "intruder" is considered to be a "threat" to the group's territory, the defense will be greater. According to this theory, when groups such as administrative personnel, medical staff, or newly created technical assistants begin to encroach upon what was once the exclusive territory of the specialist, conflict can be expected.

An interesting offset to the idea of territory is Barnard's (1938) "zone of indifference." Barnard believes that, within limits, people are indifferent to change or encroachment. This suggests that one way to reduce intergroup conflict where territorial concepts are involved is to increase the zone of indifference. This may be achieved through participation in decision making, improved communication, or change in status, to name only a few possibilities.

Client-Hospital Conflict

Hospitals have not been immune from conflict with consumers; however, few empirical studies have examined this problem. Patients have very little voice in hospital matters nor, until quite recently, have they seemed to desire one. We suspect this is largely due to their faith in the professionals' ability to decide what is best for them. Consumer activists apparently do not see current constituencies or activities of hospital governing boards as an effective voice for the client. The AHA (1973) Patient's Bill of Rights is an example of attempts to reduce conflicts and be more responsive to consumer expectations. In Chapter 4, other aspects of hospital-consumer conflict were discussed.

A lack of clearly defined community service goals may be an underlying factor in client-hospital conflict. Etzioni (1964) suggests that "sometimes an organizational goal becomes the servant of the organization rather than its master. . . . Goals can be distorted by frequent measuring of organizational efforts, because as a rule, some aspects of its output are more measurable than others" (pp. 4-11). Certainly, hospitals are susceptible to this inversion of ends and means as we suggested previously. The hospital financial statement, for example, is one of the few easily understood measurements available to trustees and administrators and it usually stresses institutional as opposed to patient goals.

Conflict or competition between hospitals is evident from the major programs, such as comprehensive health planning, designed to reduce it. However, there appears to be little empirical research into the seriousness, underlying sources, or measurable effects of such conflict. It can be assumed that the displacement of community service goals by institutional goals would have important consequences, since what is best for a particular hospital is not always best for the community it serves.

Regardless of the source, it is evident that a considerable degree of conflict exists in hospitals. The problem, then, is to find ways and means to mitigate, or at least control, conflict. The next section suggests some possible approaches.

MITIGATION OF CONFLICT

In the first section of this chapter we suggested that many policies, practices, and procedures in hospitals tend to reinforce conflict. In part this is a perceptual problem;

however, in hospitals, as in other organizations, there are certain traditional loyalties, and conflict may arise if these are challenged. If, for example, a situation is pushed to the point where employees must take a pro-union or pro-patient position, this may result in "person-role conflict." Such situations, and the work-flow patterns and pressures that result from emergency events, cannot be completely eliminated. However, the wise administrator will try to eliminate situations that tend to reinforce conflict behavior and the resulting lack of effectiveness.

Before presenting a decision model that we have found useful in diagnosing and mitigating conflict, we will review some general managerial approaches to the problem. Historically, one of the earliest approaches was to eliminate the opposition. In the animal world we see many examples of the stronger eliminating the weaker in the battle. The weaker member is not necessarily killed, but he is certainly excluded from the battlefield. The history of warfare certainly gives us sufficient examples of man's use of this approach.

Certainly we do not expect to see warfare situations in health service organizations. However, the tactic of dominating or eliminating the opposition is certainly used. Opposing people are transferred or fired, departments are reorganized or eliminated, salary increases are withheld, or boycotts conducted. Finally, we are all familiar with the "put-down" practiced by many individuals. In general, however, although the domineering approach may force conflict "underground," it is hardly a viable approach in this day and age.

A second general approach is the development of bureaucratic rationality with its resulting policies, rules, and procedures. In this situation, the concept of authority is contained either in documents or in informal procedures. Deviations are examined in the light of policy and a basis for eliminating the conflict-inducing practice is provided. This type of approach may seem very efficient, but is probably not effective, especially as far as employees or patients are concerned. We have all been refused a request for an explanation with the comment: "It's a policy." Again, conflict is probably not mitigated.

The third general approach involves bargaining. We have devoted an entire chapter to bargaining (Chapter 14). Suffice it to say at this point that it often results in a win-lose situation: "I gain what you give up." Probably if bargaining were thought of as a problem-solving process rather than in terms of balance of power, it would be more useful in settling conflict. In fact, it can be argued that bargaining cannot exist unless there is conflict.

These general approaches provide a basis for developing a more comprehensive but specific model. Figure 13-1 presents a decision model for diagnosing and mitigating hospital conflict. It lists conflict participants and some of the underlying sources of conflict covered in the first part of this chapter. A brief description of the mitigators listed in the exhibit follows.

Action Program for Mitigation of Conflict

Comprehensive Institutional Goal Setting Comprehensive institutional goal setting is a formalized program to define goals and objectives *explicitly*. Too often goals are

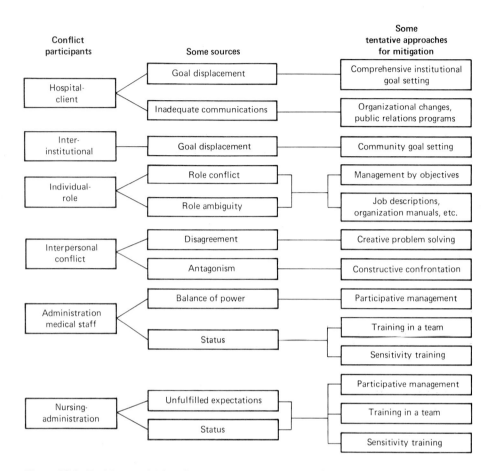

Figure 13-1 Decision model for diagnosing and mitigating hospital conflict

defined implicitly, e.g., "high-quality care at low cost." Explicit goals list measures that will affect quality and costs. Often goals can be stated in terms of specially attainable objectives.

As suggested in previous chapters, goal definition should begin with a study of the needs of the society the institution intends to serve in order to obviate displacement of goals. Medical staff members and employees, in addition to administrators and trustees, should participate. Sociologists, political scientists, and economists, as well as planners and citizens of the publics served, could provide appropriate resource personnel. Explicit institutional goals aid community understanding, assist internal and external evaluation of outputs by reducing overemphasis on inputs such as costs and facilities, help sublimate personal differences by focusing efforts on end results, and help to marshal required resources for attaining goals.

Organizational Changes, Public Relations Programs Communications can be improved by broadening the official lines of communication with the citizens served by the institution. Policies for governing board membership might be revised to represent more appropriately the constituencies served. Or, an advisory board might be established to review expressed needs of constituencies and hospital programs to meet needs. A public relations program based on appropriate client attitude surveys might be beneficial.

Community Goal Setting While many communities are beginning to prepare plans for community health services, some have not effectively articulated the explicit goals and objectives that the plans are meant to serve. Appropriate comprehensive health planning by the community should stimulate institutions to focus on community needs and objectives rather than just on institutional needs and objectives.

Management by Objectives and Role Definition Management by objectives (MBO) is the participation between the subordinate and his superior in setting the subordinate's goal (Odiorne, 1965; Brady, 1973; Mali, 1972; Carroll and Tosi, 1973). Through interaction and discussion, a subordinate can determine precisely what is expected of him, thus reducing the anxiety that results from ambiguity. MBO is designed to improve work independence in task performance while at the same time increasing accountability.

Role definition through job descriptions and administrative manuals can also help to reduce role conflict and ambiguity. These tools are familiar to most administrators.

Creative Problem Solving Creative problem solving utilizes techniques that sublimate antagonistic conflict and foster creativity. Maier (1964) notes the distinction between "choice behavior," which is an examination and a selection from the alternatives, and "problem-solving," which is a searching or idea-getting process. When choice situations are turned into problem-solving situations, participants are apt to focus on end results rather than on who is presenting or standing for what. This approach maximizes creativity and sublimates hostility, self-pity, and rigidity. Creative problem solving promotes end results in which everyone wins, rather than choice situations in which there is a winner and loser or compromises in which everyone loses.

Transactional analysis, the "I'm OK, you're OK" adult-to-adult communications, is another approach based on the philosophy of trying to avoid interpersonal conflict (Harris, 1969).

Constructive Confrontation Issues of conflict tend to proliferate when there are interpersonal antagonisms between individuals. A manager can take certain steps to avoid issues that may result in open interpersonal conflict. However, the indirect effects of interpersonal antagonism will frequently persist and in the long run may be more damaging than open confrontation. Walton (1969) suggests using constructive confrontation with third-party intervention, particularly by consultants from outside the institution. The components of confrontation include (1) clarifying the issues with parties, (2) expressing feelings descriptively, (3) expressing facts and fantasies, and (4) resolution and agreement. It would appear, however, that third-party intervention should be utilized sparingly.

Participative Management Participative management is a philosophy of management in which hospital employees and physicians participate in a meaningful way in the administration of the hospital. It is a philosophy espoused by our Type D administrator's role, by Rensis Likert (1961), and by the late Douglas McGregor (1960), who wrote of "Theory X and Theory Y." Studies by Coleman (1957), Corwin (1969), and others support the view that broad participation in authority systems minimizes major incidents of conflict, although minor incidents may be more frequent.

Management by objectives and comprehensive institutional goal setting are examples of participative management. As we suggested in Chapter 9, the administrators do not abdicate their responsibility, they share it. By sharing planning, coordination, control, and management information, administrators can actually gain more control over their responsibilities (Tannenbaum, 1962).

Sensitivity Training Sensitivity training, with emphasis on institutional social system development, can help to overcome "hang-ups" related to concerns over status (Buchanan, 1968; Lewin, 1948). Laboratory training based on the more traditional group dynamics training is suggested in preference to the individual self-awareness training that at times borders on therapy. It is the latter—personal development training—that has been criticized in recent years.

Training in a Team Health workers are expected to function as a team, yet they are seldom trained to do so. Since hospital administrators spend more time with physicians and nurses than with any other group, it would be beneficial if they had meaningful dialogues in the formative educational period as we suggested in Chapter 10. This could be arranged through seminars or research projects on subjects such as ethics, legal problems, group dynamics, or contemporary problems in health. Opportunities could be presented for informal as well as formal associations. Interdisciplinary study could also be arranged through the work environment.

Combined degree programs between medicine and hospital administration and/or nursing and hospital administration should be considered seriously. In addition to improving team associations at the educational level, such programs would help to improve the administrative skills of those who in fact administer a large part of health services.

SUMMARY

Conflict in hospitals is a complex issue. While it deserves considerably more research, much can be done to apply available knowledge of its sources and of mitigating activities. In general, increased demands for service and attempts to diagnose and lessen conflicts will result in new policies and procedures. Among these will be research studies to identify the impact of various conflict situations. In addition, one can expect to see changes in goal setting, planning, organizational relationships, and training programs.

REFERENCES

AHA: "Patients Bill of Rights Affirmed as Revised by the Board of Trustees, November 17, 1972," American Hospital Association, Chicago, Jan. 22, 1973.

Ardrey, R.: *The Territorial Imperative,* Atheneum, New York, 1966.

Argyris, Chris: *Diagnosing Human Relations in Organizations: A Case Study of a Hospital,* Yale University Labor and Management Center, New Haven, Conn., 1965.

Barnard, Chester: *The Functions of the Executive,* Harvard University Press, Cambridge, Mass., 1938.

Bellin, Lowell E.: "The Health Administrator as a Status Seeker," *Journal of Medical Education,* vol. 48, pp. 896-904, 1973.

Blau, Peter M. and Richard W. Scott: *Formal Organizations,* Chandler Publishing, New York, 1962.

Brady, Rodney H.: "MBO Goes to Work in the Public Sector," *Harvard Business Review,* pp. 65-74, Mar.-Apr. 1973.

Buchanan, Paul C.: "Laboratory Training and Organization Development," *Administrative Science Quarterly,* pp. 466-477, Sept. 1969.

Carroll, Stephen J., Jr. and Henry L. Tosi, Jr., *Management by Objectives Applications and Research,* Macmillan, New York, 1973.

Caudill, William A.: *The Psychiatric Hospital as a Small Society,* Harvard University Press, Cambridge, Mass., 1958.

Coleman, James S.: *Community Conflict,* Free Press, Glencoe, Ill., 1957.

Corwin, R. G. and Marvin J. Taves: "Nursing and Other Health Professions," in H. E. Freeman et al. (eds.), *Handbook of Medical Sociology,* Prentice-Hall, Englewood Cliffs, N.J., 1963.

Corwin, Robert: "Patterns of Organizational Conflict," *Administrative Science Quarterly,* pp. 507-520, Dec. 1969.

Croog, S. H.: "Interpersonal Relations in Medical Settings," in H. E. Freeman et al. (eds.), *Handbook of Medical Sociology,* Prentice-Hall, Englewood Cliffs, N.J., 1963.

Etzioni, Amitai: *Modern Organizations,* Prentice-Hall, Englewood Cliffs, N.J., 1964.

Filley, Alan C. and Robert J. House: *Managerial Process and Organization Behavior,* Scott, Foresman, New York, 1969.

Georgopoulos, Basil S. and Floyd C. Mann: *The Community General Hospital,* Macmillan, New York, 1962.

Goss, Mary E. W.: "Patterns of Bureaucracy Among Staff Physicians," in Eliot Friedson (ed.), *The Hospital in Modern Society,* Free Press, N.Y., 1963.

Harris, Thomas A.: *I'm OK — You're OK,* Harper and Row, New York, 1967.

Hospitals, J.A.H.A.: "Medical, Health Occupations Rated on Basis of Prestige," p. 115, Oct. 16, 1974.

House, Robert J. and John R. Rizzo: "Role Conflict and Ambiguity as Critical Variables in a Model of Organizational Behavior," *Organizational Behavior and Human Performance,* 7, 1972, pp. 467-505.

Kahn, R. L. et al.: *Organizational Stress: Studies in Role Conflict and Ambiguity,* John Wiley, New York, 1964.

Katz, Daniel and Robert L. Kahn: *The Social Psychology of Organizations,* Wiley, New York, 1966.

Lewin, Kurt: *Resolving Social Conflict: Selected Papers on Group Dynamics,* Harper and Row, New York, 1968.

Likert, R.: *New Patterns of Management,* McGraw-Hill, New York, 1961.

Maier, Norman F.: "Maximizing Personal Creativity Through Better Problem Solving," *Personnel Administration,* vol. 27, 1964.

Mali, Paul: *Management by Objectives,* Wiley, New York, 1972.

McGregor, D.: *The Human Side of Enterprise,* McGraw-Hill, New York, 1960.

Modern Hospital: "Trustee's View of Administrators Told," p. 20, Oct. 1968.

Odiorne, George: *Management by Objectives,* Pitman Brothers, New York, 1965.

Rx for Action, report of the Health Task Force of the Urban Coalition, John Gardner, Chairman, Washington, D.C., 1969.

Schulz, Rockwell and Alton C. Johnson: "Conflict in Hospitals," *Hospital Administration,* vol. 16, pp. 36-49, Summer 1971.

Scott, W. Richard: "Some Implications of Organizational Theory for Research on Health Services," *Milbank Memorial Fund Quarterly,* vol. 44, no. 4, Oct. 1966.

Secretary's Advisory Committee on Hospital Effectiveness, Department of Health, Education and Welfare, 1967.

Stanton, Alfred H. and Morris S. Schwartz: *The Mental Hospital,* Basic Books, New York, 1954.

Tannenbaum, A. S.: "Control in Organizations: Individual Adjustment and Organizational Performance," *Administrative Science Quarterly,* p. 236, Sept. 1962.

Walton, Richard E.: *Interpersonal Peacemaking: Confrontations and Third-Party Consultation,* Addison-Wesley, Reading, Mass., 1969.

Part Four

Environmental Influences and Constraints

Can administrators, governing boards, and medical staff really control the transformation of inputs into outputs now that environmental factors are having increasing influence and putting more constraints on operations? In this section we examine external influences such as collective bargaining (although one might argue that this is an internal influence), voluntary control agencies (e.g., the Joint Commission on Accreditation of Hospitals), areawide health planning agencies, and federal and governmental regulatory agencies. We conclude that environmental factors have increased, not decreased, the responsibilities and authority of hospital governance and administration. They have complicated the coordination involved in transforming inputs into outputs and expanded the external role of administration. External influences provide new opportunities as well as constraints for the administrator and governing board member.

In Chapter 14 we discuss collective bargaining as an important environmental influence affecting the internal operation of the hospital. External influences on the regulation of hospitals are considered in Chapter 15. Finally, we look to the future in Chapter 16 suggesting influences that environmental changes may have on hospital management.

Collective Bargaining

It is highly unlikely that a chapter on collective bargaining would have appeared in a book concerned with hospital administration 25 years ago. At that time there were very few hospital unions and the legal climate was unfavorable for union organization and growth. What has caused a change to come about? This question is the concern of the first part of this chapter. Later sections deal with collective bargaining in hospitals, the collective bargaining process, and contract administration.

CHANGING PHILOSOPHIES REGARDING UNIONS

A union is a group of employees who have joined together to seek common goals or objectives. The two "bread-and-butter" issues are wages and security. Other significant objectives are hours of work, working conditions, and work rules. In addition, unions are concerned about altering the arbitrary power of managers in decisions affecting layoffs, firing, changes in work assignments, and similar factors affecting the work environment.

Although the term *collective bargaining* was coined in approximately 1900 by Beatrice and Sidney Webb, the union itself is one of our early institutions. Unions of the early 1800s were local in membership and usually fraternal organizations. These unions had social aspects, but more importantly they were formed to give some measure of security to the out-of-work person or to the family of a disabled or diseased worker. Until the organization of the large industrial unions (those accepting all members regardless of job or occupation affiliation) in the 1930s, most associations were craft associations.

The major reasons for the inability of unions to organize industrial workers was that such workers were highly replaceable. They did not require a long educational or training period, and our immigration laws permitted a constant supply of labor. In the 1930s, the simple principle of controlling the plant gate (employee entrance) was hit upon by employees as an effective power measure. After all, if the replacements could not enter the plant, the company could not operate. We see the same principle followed today in the form of the picket line, which makes employees and others feel self-conscious about entering even if they are not actually prevented from doing so. An understanding of the significance of the picket line is important to the hospital administration, because most union members, whether employees, patients, or visitors, are reluctant to cross a picket line. Thus, a small union representing a very small proportion of employees in a hospital may have a significant effect on hospital operations.

It is likely that a union in a hospital or a related health services facility will be craft in nature. That is, it will be for employees with a given skill or from a given professional group, e.g., electricians, plumbers, medical technologists, or nurses.

The 1930s also saw a shift in the legal framework surrounding the rights of employees to join unions. The National Labor Relations (Wagner) Act of 1935 established the first national labor policy of protecting the rights of workers to organize and to elect their representatives for collective bargaining. The heart of the Act is contained in Section 7, which embodies the following enumeration of Findings and Policies contained in the introductory section of the Act:

> It is hereby declared to be the policy of the United States to eliminate the causes of certain substantial obstructions to the free flow of commerce and to mitigate and eliminate these obstructions when they have occurred by encouraging the practice and procedure of collective bargaining and by protecting the exercise by workers of full freedom of association, self-organization, and designation of representatives of their own choosing, for the purpose of negotiating the terms of their employment of other mutual aid or protection.

Section 7 states:

> Employees shall have the right to self-organization, to form, join, or assist labor organizations, to bargain collectively through representatives of their own choosing, and to engage in concerted activities, for the purpose of collective bargaining or other mutual aid or protection.

The Wagner Act apparently provided for hospitals to be unionized. In 1947, the Wagner Act was amended by the Labor Management Relations (Taft-Hartley) Act. Two of the more controversial additions were: (1) the inclusion of employee or union unfair labor practices, and (2) allowing the states to prohibit union security provisions (the right-to-work concept). Of more significance to our discussion is the fact that the Taft-Hartley Act removed hospitals from coverage under the law. However, in 1974, after years of lobbying by such groups as the ANA, not-for-profit hospitals were removed from exemption from coverage under the Labor Management Relations Act (Taft-Hartley). The legislation provides for a 10-day notification period before a strike (substantially less than the 60 days cooling-off period asked for by hospitals) to help hospitals make arrangements for patients who might be affected by a strike.

It is assumed that the 1974 legislation will lead to an increase in union activity in hospitals. However, it is interesting to note that the state of Wisconsin has had enabling legislation on the books since 1939 and nonprofit hospitals have been included. Despite the existence of enabling legislation over a long period of time, it was not until the 1960s that much organizing activity developed, and this was only in the larger metropolitan areas.

Governmental hospitals represent approximately one-third of all hospitals. It is this group of hospitals that has seen the highest rate of unionization. The union involved is usually the American Federation of State, County and Municipal Employees (AFSCME of the AFL-CIO). For federal employees, the Lloyd-LaFollette Act of 1912 is considered to be the basis of a general expression of congressional sentiment in favor of the right to organize. However, for various reasons, bargaining as performed in industry has not been considered to be feasible for most governmental agencies. President Franklin D. Roosevelt probably best expressed this in 1937 to the President of the National Federation of Employees when he said: "The very nature and purposes of Government make it impossible for administrative officials to represent fully or bind the employer in mutual discussion with Government employee organizations. The employer is the whole people, who speak by means of laws enacted by their representatives in Congress. Accordingly, administrative officials and employees alike are governed and guided, and in many instances restricted, by laws which establish policies, procedures, or rules in personnel matters."

Since this time, President Kennedy's executive order 10988 in 1962 established collective bargaining rights for federal employees, and President Nixon's 1969 executive order 11491 set forth Labor Management Relations in the Federal Service. In addition, enabling legislation setting forth collective bargaining procedures for state employees has been passed by many states, which resulted in the unionization of state-owned hospitals.

Based upon the growth of unions in industry, it appears that a favorable legal climate will promote the growth of hospital unions. This has been true for railroad, industrial, and government employees. As restrictions are lifted on the unionization of hospital and related health care facilities, one can anticipate a growth of unions even more rapid than that of the past 10 years.

In addition to these factors, there are other forces at work in the health industry that tend to favor unionism. For example, Kralewski (1974) suggests that:

> The rapid movement of the health care field toward large scale organizational settings, coupled with rapid change and expansion, both within these organizations and the field in general, has created, and continues to create, a great deal of anxiety among the various health professions. Roles are being challenged and changed, status hierarchies are shifting and power bases are crumbling under organizational pressures. As a consequence, health care professionals increasingly are turning toward collective bargaining as a means of developing a countervailing power to present their interests and to protect their territorial prerogatives (p. 40).

Oswald (1975), research director for the Service Employees International Union, is of the opinion that working conditions and the extension of the National Labor Relations Act to govern hospital workers will result in more unionized employees in hospitals, but that union organizers will have difficulties because hospitals will be expected to take strong antiunion postures. Nash (1974) takes a somewhat different posture in his case study of Montefiore Hospital and Medical Center. He concludes that "the value system in Montefiore facilitated the entrance of the union and now functions as a bond between the leadership of the union and the hospital" (p. 63). The basis or core of the value system in a hospital is patient care, which operates as an integrating force.

EMPLOYEES, ADMINISTRATORS, AND UNIONS

Matlock (1972) sums up the objectives of employee groups as:

> The (professional) groups have taken up the weapons of trade unionism not only to redress the balance of power between themselves and their employers, but also to give weight to the professional judgment on the standards, performance, and quality of the services that they themselves provide, and judgment that frequently conflicts with the bureaucracies that employ them (p. 11).

Hospital employees represent the largest group of unorganized employees in the United States. Osterhaus (1967) suggests that they "should be the easiest group to organize because of lower wages received, dictatorial administration procedures, lack of recognition, few, if any, grievance procedures, and lack of prestige" (p. 80). These are significant factors and will be more important when organization drives become more determined. We will briefly list some of the groups that are currently active in collective bargaining in hospitals and then return to the issues of the vulnerability of hospitals for collective bargaining.

A great deal of the organizing of nonprofessional workers in hospitals has been done by trade unions that have their base in the industrial sector. Of the total number of union contracts with hospitals, 36 percent are held by unions that have a solid membership base in such associations as The Service Employees' International Union, Hotel and Allied Services Union, Hotel Restaurant Employees' and Bartenders' Union, and the National Hospital and Nursing Home Employees Union (affiliated with the Retail, Wholesale Department Store Union) (Pointer and Metzger, 1972). The American Federation of State, County, and Municipal Employees (AFSCME of the AFL-CIO) has been very active—in 1965 about one-quarter of its total members were hospital employees (Osterhaus, 1967). Currently, local 1199 of the Drug and Hospital Union is particularly active and has coupled unionism with civil rights. The Building Service Employees International Union has concentrated on nongovernmental general acute hospitals and has been particularly active in such cities as San Francisco, Minneapolis–St. Paul, New York, Chicago, and Los Angeles. The Teamsters Union was also active, particularly in the late 1950s.

In the area of collective bargaining for and by professional groups, in 1946 the American Nurses' Association (ANA) adopted its economic security program, which called for collective bargaining. In 1968 the ANA dropped its 18-year-old no-strike policy, leaving this matter to individual state nurses' associations. Panosh (1973) reviewed the literature and concluded that the 1960s were marked by a number of examples of nursing dissatisfaction in the form of slowdowns, mass resignations, sick calls, and strikes.

Attempts are being made to organize other health professionals for collective bargaining. Nine international unions within the AFL-CIO set up a Council for Professional, Scientific, and Cultural Employees to facilitate organizing 10 million nonunion professional employees, with emphasis on the hospital sector (Pointer and Cannedy, 1972).

The professional associations are themselves becoming active. The American Society for Medical Technology (ASMT) is leading a drive to unite 17 organizations in a giant National Economic Council of Associations of Health Professionals to serve as a nationwide collective bargaining organization. The Council would be separate from the member organizations with its own staff and headquarters. Its purpose would be to prevent health professionals from being included in catch-all bargaining groups as organized by the trade unions. A committee was set up in April 1972 to begin working on a charter and by-laws. Seven groups have "fairly well decided on joining" the Council: American Medical Records Association, American Society for Microbiology, National Society of Clinical Laboratory Technologists, American Society for Medical Technologists, American Dietitic Association, American Association of Inhalation Therapy, American Society for Radiological Technicians.

Physician unions at the time of this writing center around the independent American Federation of Physicians and Dentists (AFPD) and the National Conference of Physicians Unions, AFL-CIO. In February 1973, the AFPD claimed to represent 8,000 professionals in six unions and guilds and predicted that 25,000 would come under the Federation's umbrella within a year (*Medical World News*, 1973). Physician strikes have taken place in Canada. Although technically not strikes, medical staff boycotts of hospitals over various issues appear to be increasing in the United States. House staffs, interns, and residents in teaching hospitals have formed collective bargaining units in a number of institutions. They struck New York City Hospitals in 1975. In the public hospitals "heal-ins" (that is, admitting large numbers of patients in order to strain facilities and raise costs in hospitals where patients do not pay directly for their services) have also been used as a means of coercion.

A key factor in the decision to join unions is the desire for better economic and working conditions. Most people want to increase their income. Seldom do you hear of a person refusing a wage or salary increase particularly if the wage or salary was low to begin with. Even more compelling is the *belief* that unions do help in getting increases in compensation and improved working conditions. Moreover, when the differential between lower- and upper-skill-level wages decreases, the higher-skill-level employees become more easily convinced that unionism is the answer, especially if there is a union present.

At the core of the compensation factor is the issue of perceived equity or inequity as the case may be. Unfortunately, in many situations, what might appear equitable to administration is far from equitable in the eyes of the wage earner. A little wisdom and understanding, and better communication on the part of the administrator can go far to alleviate situations in which the inequity is perceived rather than real. However, all too often no one cares, or takes the effort to make comparative studies or even to determine employee attitudes, until after the union points out such problems.

Employees today are also asking for increased control over their destinies. Generally, we do not like to be dependent upon others, nor do we want an adult-child relationship with out superiors. Immediate supervisors often appear (and often are) dictatorial, do not listen or try to understand, and enjoy their position of power. The union can bring group pressure on the recalcitrant supervisors, particularly by means of the grievance procedure.

Employees often believe that if only they could talk directly to the chief administrator, many problems could be redressed. However, it is very difficult for a lower-level employee to talk with the chief executive officer in a bureaucratic organization. Very few people have the necessary perserverance even if such a procedure were feasible. A union changes all this. Representatives from the union bargain directly with chief administrators. The employee believes that when the administrator "gets the word," working conditions will improve.

Related to this is the opinion of many that no one listens or cares about what goes on in the lower levels. As long as no major problems arise, it is assumed that all goes well. In this connection, one should point out that the chief executive officer (CEO) can and does become isolated from actual operating situations. Managers reporting to the CEO may want to look good and they are careful not to report problems which will reflect badly either on them or on the chief. Thus, the communication network that on paper looks good may, in fact, be quite ineffective.

A significant fact is that as more and more employees are unionized, joining a union becomes more the "in" thing to do. Of course, some employees have no choice. Where there is a union shop, the new employee must join the union in 30, 60, or 90 days, or whatever the probationary period may be.

Bennett (1972) has set forth reasons why unions have been successful in organizing employees. He includes the following:

1 Employees believed they received poor wages, and were dissatisfied with working conditions, e.g., supervision, food, and locker rooms.

2 Management was viewed as indifferent to employees' complaints about their working environment. There was no grievance procedure.

3 Generally, there was a failure to communicate.

Bennett (1972) also reported the results of an AFL-CIO study on why employees joined unions. The study pointed out the following advantages:

1 The assurance of better pay and job security through collective bargaining
2 Improved fringe benefits, pensions, holidays, and sick leave
3 Fair play, promotions, seniority rights
4 Grievance procedures
5 Better control of speed-up and production standards

Recently unions themselves have become more concerned with broader social issues. For example, the United Auto Workers are looking at job redesign and job enlargement in order to decrease fatigue and boredom in assembly line jobs. Also, the United Steel Workers have investigated alternatives to the strike, which causes loss of pay for workers and tends to encourage purchase from competitors including foreign steel companies.

While there are good reasons why employees may want to join a hospital union, there are some equally compelling reasons why they may not.

In the first place, unions are generally associated with blue-collar employees. To persons who have had considerable education and think of themselves as professionals, such an association is not always acceptable. After all, the blue-collar worker often has different interests, needs, and demands. In other words, professional employees are concerned with retaining their status and image. This is basically an individualistic attitude, and it tends to be present whenever professionals are engaged in a collective action.

The chance of advancement in terms of salary, title, and prestige is much greater for professional employees than for the majority of presently organized workers. Indeed, professionals can usually look forward to some kind of supervisory or managerial position if they so desire.

Another important factor that has mitigated against the unionization of hospitals is the concept of service. Many employees believe that their need to be of service is most certainly met through their work in a hospital. And, although the gratification of social needs will not offset lower economic renumeration, the union's emphasis on bread-and-butter issues often turns off the hospital employee. Although the concept of hospitals as charitable institutions is disappearing, the desire to be of service to mankind still remains and this cannot be satisfied by money. As Miller (1971) points out, many hospital employees lack the motivation to serve their own economic ends through collective bargaining.

Women make up a high percentage of employees in the health professions and, traditionally, they have been more difficult than men to organize. This may be due to short-term employment expectations, the fact that they are often supplementary breadwinners, or a concern for objectives other than those offered by unions. As attitudes change, these elements may become less significant in future years.

There is also the problem of union organization. Unions themselves have not had much experience in organizing hospitals. Also, hospitals have a multitude of skill and professional groups. The problem here is one of determining the proper bargaining unit. Just the thought of a solution raises some competitive issues among employee groups, and between employee groups and the unions. If representation is too fragmented, the union tends to lose power and the administration may find it difficult to negotiate an agreement with the union.

Thus, although gains have been made in employee unionization in hospitals, they have been modest. One survey (Kuby, 1972) noted that 7.7 percent of hospitals surveyed in 1967 were unionized; this figure increased to 14.7 percent in 1970. Non-governmental, not-for-profit hospitals with contracts increased from 8.2 to 12.4 percent during this same period. Needless to say, union organizers are not satisfied with these kinds of gains, and more attention to organization drives can be expected (see Table 14-1). Kuby also found larger hospitals to be more susceptible to organizing, which might be expected since most of them are in the larger urban centers.

It appears that administrators are often opposed to unions, especially militant ones. Their major concern is the disruption of service; they feel that (1) the recognition of a union is a direct invitation to strike; and (2) intolerable conditions would be created if critical hospital services were substantially curtailed or completely eliminated because of a strike (Golodner, 1970). Osterhaus (1967) identified four basic fears about unions in hospitals:

1 Unions bring the fear of strikes both during organizational campaigns and over contract negotiations. A strike can endanger the lives of patients and threatens the position of the hospital in the community.

2 Unionism costs money, especially in increased wage and benefit demands.

3 Unions cause management to lose control over the traditional management prerogatives.

4 Personnel management becomes more complicated.

Administrative fears concerning work stoppages are not without justification. One study found that 32.5 percent of all hospitals that received requests for union recognition were involved in work stoppages (see Table 14-2). This compares to 5.9 percent of hospitals that already had unions (Kuby, 1972).

The cost element is also crucial in a period of cost containment. Administrators are concerned that costs will be increased by union demands and that these will have to be passed on to the consumer in the form of increased payments. This is not so easily accomplished in a period of rate reviews and other controls.

Table 14-1   Extent of Collective Bargaining Contracts in Hospitals by Control of Hospital

Control	1961		1967		1970	
	Total number of registered hospitals	Percentage with contracts	Total number of registered hospitals	Percentage with contracts	Total number of registered hospitals	Percentage with contracts
All hospitals	6,923	3.0	7,172	7.7	7,123	14.7
Federal	437	0.0	416	22.6	408	52.0
Nonfederal	6,486	3.2	2,141	6.8	6,715	12.4
Nongovernmental not-for-profit	3,588	4.3	3,692	8.2	3,600	12.4
For-profit	973	4.3	923	4.9	858	8.0
State and local	1,925	1.0	2,141	5.3	2,257	14.1

Source: Reprinted, with permission, from *Hospitals, Journal of the American Hospital Association*, vol. 46, no. 7, Apr. 1, 1972, p. 217.

Table 14-2 Incidence of Work Stoppages by Type of Collective Bargaining Activity

Year	Hospitals with contract	Hospitals with requests	All registered hospitals
1967	12.8%	20.9%	2.0%
1970	5.9%	32.5%	2.1%

Source: Reprinted with permission, from *Hospitals, Journal of the American Hospital Association,* vol. 46, no. 7, Apr. 1, 1972, p. 218.

Goodfellow (1973, in a study of 329 companies, identified 12 items administrators should examine. If these items are neglected, employees are more likely to turn toward unionization. They are:

   1 Number of shifts. (The first shift is more loyal, the second and third less so in that order.)
   2 Female-male ratio. (Women are less interested in unions.)
   3 Housekeeping. (A dirty, poorly maintained hospital is more likely to be unionized.)
   4 Wage rates. (Are wage rates equitable in terms of length of service, well-developed appraisal systems, and fair differentials? Goodfellow's studies show that wages are rarely the real reason for joining a union.)
   5 Overtime practices. (Not all employees desire overtime. Overtime should be distributed fairly to all employees.)
   6 Seniority. (Employees prize seniority.)
   7 Promotion policy. (Employees should be given a chance on new jobs.)
   8 Job transfers. (Supervisors should not be allowed to sabotage the transfer requests of good employees.)
   9 Fringe benefits. (Employers tend to underestimate the significance of fringe benefits to employees.)
   10 Discipline and grievance procedures. (Employee handbooks should be developed to spell out conduct expected, standards, appeal procedures, and penalties.)
   11 Money. (The major desires of employees, all our studies found, are for three things: job security, company stability and money. That listing is also the order of importance; money ranks third.)
   12 Treatment. (In large hospitals this is generally measured by the administrator's efforts and the personnel directors contacts with employees.)

It is important to note that these issues generally concern personnel practices and have nothing to do with charity. Basically, they involve fair treatment for employees on the part of administrative people.

Zimmerman (1972) offers this conclusion: "It is important for management to realize that a union wins recognition because it *insures* improvements, many of which it could not deliver if it won, but improvements which it certainly could not deliver if the employee's economic, security, and participation needs were already satisfied."

Elkin (1975) adds that employees not only seek economic gains but also seek to develop a system of industrial jurisprudence designed to permit employees freedom from arbitrary decisions made by management.

COLLECTIVE BARGAINING PROCESS

As unions employ more highly trained and professional organizers, labor laws are extended, and changes in public opinion favoring unions and collective bargaining occur, we are likely to see more unions among hospital employees. Because of this, it is necessary that administrators in hospitals have an understanding and appreciation of the collective bargaining process. This is the objective of this section.

The first phase of the collective bargaining process involves negotiation. As Mintzberg (1973) points out in his study of executives, negotiation is one of the key roles of managers. The Random House *Dictionary of the English Language* (The Unabridged Edition, 1966) offers two definitions of negotiation that are useful to our discussion. To negotiate is "to deal or bargain with another or others as in the preparation of a treaty or in preliminaries to a business deal" and "to arrange for or bring about by discussion and settlement of terms." Note that these definitions suggest a *give and take* in order to reach a meeting of the minds, an agreement, or a decision. Also, there is nothing to preclude an individual or one-to-one negotiation as when an administrator "negotiates" his salary with the governing board.

Mintzberg (1973), in a further examination of the role of the manager (which includes the hospital administrator), suggests that the manager's work can be viewed as a programmed system. One of the programs he suggests is that of negotiation; that is, managers have several models or programs which they utilize in negotiating agreements either on an individual or a collective basis. For example, groups of employees do discuss through their representatives (department heads) requests (demands sometimes) for changes in hours of work, working conditions, salaries, procedures, etc. Indeed, the entire hospital may discuss (negotiate) with the board of directors an across-the-board, cost-of-living salary increase. Administrators may find themselves negotiating with the medical staff over such matters as arrangements with hospital-based specialists, emergency room service, house staff remuneration, or ethical issues. The medical staff boycotted hospitals in some instances when negotiations over issues of importance to both parties had broken down. In the future this kind of action may well increase, as medical staff-hospital interdependencies become more critical, particularly under a Type C administrative role as discussed in Chapter 9.

The role of negotiation is a common one for the manager. What is new for the administrator is bargaining with a union that represents employees, and has the power of work stoppage or arbitration to back up its demands. This bargaining process necessitates a programmed system that is different from the one that the administrator employed prior to unionization.

Some appreciation for the new programmed system can be achieved by reviewing the distinction the National Education Association has made between professional negotiation and collective bargaining. We use education rather than industry as a basis because there are so many professional employees in hospitals. Also, the unionization of teachers is at a more advanced stage than that of hospital professional employees. Hazard (1967) summarizes the definitions of professional negotiation as set forth in the National Educational Association's *Guidelines for Professional Negotiation.* These definitions are as follows:

> *Educational channels for mediation and appeal.* Advisory and fact-finding channels which are education-, not labor-oriented, which may be used to resolve an impasse.
>
> *Exclusive negotiation.* A right accorded solely to the majority organization to negotiate with the school board. Individuals and minority groups retain testimony rights.
>
> *Impasse.* Persistent disagreement between the parties requiring the use of mediation, fact finding, or appeal procedures for resolution.
>
> *Professional channels.* The administrative channels of a school system or institution.
>
> *Subjects of professional negotiation.* The topics of mutual concern to a local professional organization and a local school board. These subjects include, among other things, setting standards in employing professional personnel, community support for the school system, in-service training of personnel, class size, teacher turnover, personnel policies, salaries, working conditions, and communication within the school system (pp. 15 and 18).

The typical hospital administrator will probably respond by saying: Yes, there are professional negotiations in my hospital. Groups of employees do discuss through their representatives (department heads) requests (demands sometimes) for changing hours of work, working conditions, salaries, procedures, etc. Indeed, the entire hospital may discuss (negotiate) with the governing board an across-the-board, cost-of-living salary increase. In other words, rather than negotiating on an individual one-to-one basis, the administrator uses programmed systems for negotiating on a group basis.

If this is true, what is so unusual about a union? Isn't a union, after all, a group of employees joined together to bargain on wages, hours, and working conditions? The problem to management is that unions reduce the authority of administration in dealing with employees.

The hospital administrator may be very disturbed to discover that the union assumes a conflict of interest between it and management. This may indeed be an unhappy and unpleasant situation for administrators who firmly believe in a team approach. Needless to say, most team concepts or Theory Y propositions accommodate unions. Despite this, if there are a number of unions involved in a hospital there is bound to be some degree of rivalry between them. This will make the task of the administrator more difficult from time to time.

What may be even more disagreeable to the administrator is to find that the union wants to by-pass him and negotiate directly with the board. Whether or not this procedure is ever followed, the very possibility of it may make many administrators very dubious about unionization.

The key issue involved, however, is recognition and certification of the union as the exclusive bargaining representative of a group of employees. With hospitals now under the National Labor Management Relations Act, the actual election and certification is administered by the National Labor Relations Board. This is done through the General Council, which is appointed by the President of the United States. Reporting to the General Council are 31 regional directors for the 31 regions of the United States. Petitions for elections are filed in the regional office, which also processes complaints and holds initial hearings on unfair labor practices as outlined by law.

Regardless of the legal climate now or in the future, negotiation from a collective bargaining point of view must begin with the recognition of a union.

The first step in the recognition procedure is a petition filed by the prospective union or group of employees within a bargaining unit. This "show of interest" petition is filed with the National Labor Relations Board and must include 30 percent of the employees in the bargaining unit. If the governmental agency finds the petition in order, a copy is sent to the employer. At this time, if the hospital administrator has heard nothing about unionization in his hospital and/or has no expert on his staff, he would be well advised to call on a labor lawyer. The employer is also asked if he will submit to the election without a hearing. If a hearing is possible, an employer would be again advised to hold it so that details such as the nature of the bargaining unit (the employees to be covered) can be determined. When everything is in order, an election is held, supervised by the governmental agency. If a majority of the employees votes in favor of the union, the union is certified as the bargaining agent for all the employees in the bargaining unit.

A second possibility in union recognition may be voluntary recognition. Here the employer agrees to recognize the union as the bargaining unit without going through the election process. This may be a proper procedure in the interest of peaceful negotiations; however, management cannot expect preferential treatment or even more favorable treatment on the part of the union. Concern should be expressed that management not be threatened or coerced into union recognition, since either possibility may not be in the best interest of patients. However, voluntary recognition does take place and is usually viewed by the union as a real accomplishment.

When the union has been recognized by the National Labor Relations Board as the bargaining agent, the collective bargaining process begins in earnest. Usually the union makes its demands through a small number of members chosen to represent it. Management representatives may make a counter offer to the demands. At this time, the two groups of representatives sit down at the bargaining table and begin the give-and-take process of negotiation. There is no obligation by either party to agree to the demands or counteroffers made by the other. Eventually, agreement will result in a contract which will govern employee relations during the length of the contract period, usually one to three years. Both parties must "bargain in good faith." Bargaining in good faith is difficult to determine but may be described as bargaining willingly and conscientiously.

The union seeks to convince management that its demands are reasonable and realistic. Management is expected to remain cognizant of the many relationships and costs involved beyond the bargaining unit itself. When agreement is reached, the terms are reduced to writing in the form of the contract. Union members must then accept (ratify) the contract terms in its entirety by a majority vote. When the union has accepted, management signs the contract and it is officially in force. If no agreement is reached, a strike may result. Bargaining under strike conditions is a similar process but with added stress. Compulsory arbitration is an alternative in some states, as are contracts that have a no-strike clause.

Major areas included in the typical union-management contract are:

Preamble and purpose	Grievance procedure
Term, life, duration	Strikes
Bargaining unit	Holidays
Recognition	Vacations
Union security	Leaves of absence
Management rights	Shift differentials (wages)
Wages	Discharge
Reopening clause	Benefits
Hours of work	Safety

Most of these items are self-explanatory; we will discuss only two in detail.

Union security is very important to the union because it binds the members as well as outlining how new members join. Various forms of union security are as follows:

1 *Union shop.* An employee must join the union within a given period of time after he accepts employment in the hospital.

2 *Agency shop.* All employees in the bargaining unit must pay dues, but do not have to join the union. This form is often used with professional and technical employees.

3 *Exclusive bargaining agent.* The union is accepted as the bargaining agent for all employees but membership in the union is not required.

4 *Maintenance of membership.* Employees who are or become union members must maintain their membership during the life of the agreement.

5 *Closed shop.* In a closed shop, only union members are employed. With a few exceptions, this is illegal under the Taft-Hartley Act.

6 *Checkoff.* The employer agrees to deduct union dues from the employee's pay check.

Management rights (management prerogatives) refers to areas in which management maintains control. Such areas include who is to be hired, the nature of tasks to be performed, and any other item "not expressly covered in the contract." A reopening clause indicates when the contract may be renegotiated in part or in total due to unexpected circumstances such as high inflationary conditions during the life of the contract.

As Elkin (1974) points out, there are special provisions in the National Labor

Relations Act as it applies to a hopsital when a contract is already in effect. The party who desires to modify or terminate the contract must:

    1 Notify the other party to the contract in writing 90 days prior to contract expiration;

    2 Meet and confer with the other party about the contract changes;

    3 Notify the Federal Mediation and Conciliation Service (**FMCS**) and any state mediation agency 60 days prior to termination; and

    4 Continue the existing contract for 90 days or until termination, whichever is later (p. 53).

Obviously, these provisions are designed to prevent work stoppages interfering with the crucial nature of patient care.

It must be stressed that the first contract is usually the most difficult. There are no precedents and everything is new including the bargaining teams themselves. Needless to say, this often leads to some hard-to-live-with clauses that must be altered during the next negotiating session.

CONTRACT ADMINISTRATION

The fact that a contract has been signed by both parties does not mean that all relationships are terminated until the next bargaining session. To the contrary, the administration phase means the day-to-day living experiences under the contract, the phase in which both parties try to make it work. It is through these experiences that the soundness of the contract is determined. Naturally, there will be some problems. For example, parts of the contract may not be clear. Also, the sincerity of the parties is tested in this period. There is no logic to spending a great deal of time negotiating a contract only to have it sabotaged by one or both parties.

Generally, management assumes the responsibility for the administration of the contract. The union observes this operation, and is quick to point out significant (in the opinion of the union) deviations from the agreement.

Some parts of the contract require little administration, e.g., posting seniority lists or posting of job openings. Others tend to be very difficult and require great care in administration. Items such as seniority lists, layoffs, discipline, promotions, and wage rate changes can be very controversial. Great care should be taken in the establishment of procedures since they will set precedents for the future. Should there be items not specifically covered or not clear, it is good practice for management to sit down with the union and iron out these difficulties. Otherwise, management is usually courting a grievance.

Because department heads are likely to be most directly affected, particularly by a new contract, and to a lesser extent by renegotiated contracts, it is highly recommended that these people receive training designed to acquaint them with the union and the contract. All too often, department supervisors feel left out, especially if they do not understand union philosophy or the contract provisions. After all, a completely new relationship must be established, in which the union is a wedge between former management-employee relationships. Needless to say, department heads are often quite unhappy with the situation.

The greater the understanding of the department head, the easier the contract administration will be. A training session can clear up many potential problems. Otherwise, the informal grapevine will bring information, often faulty, to the department head. Management should be assured that the shop steward (the counterpart of the department head, who is elected by the employees to represent them at the department level) has received an in-depth briefing on the contract and on union procedures.

An important part of administration revolves around the grievance procedure. A grievance is usually considered to be any dissatisfaction or feeling of injustice regarding the work situation expressed by the employee. Some define a grievance more narrowly to refer only to those items stated in the contract. In this case, any dissatisfaction not related to the contract is not a formal grievance. This is usually likely to result in more dissatisfactions and poor employee-management relations, as well as items to be bargained for at the next negotiating session. Whatever definition management employs, it must find ways to get to the root of the problem and to acquire all salient facts, and must reach a decision with respect to its (management's) position.

The grievance procedure provides a system whereby the union and management can solve their problems jointly. All too often it is viewed as a win-lose situation as opposed to some sort of win-win mutual agreement. In a grievance situation, an employee believes he has a problem. He works out a potential solution and offers it to the department head. If the department head cannot accept the employee's position, or the employee is dissatisfied, the employee contacts the steward or committeeman. If the steward thinks the employee has a "case," or feels it is politically wise for the union to support the demand even if it is weak, a written grievance is filed with the employee's supervisor and usually the personnel department.

When a satisfactory solution to the problem is arrived at by the department head, employee, and steward with the assistance of personnel, the problem or grievance is ended. If there is a clear-cut case of contract violation, or if management clearly acted unfairly, the grievance is settled at this first level. When there is no settlement the grievance is passed on to the next level, which will involve administrators and the union president, and perhaps a representative from the national union office. The same clinical approaches are utilized to see if a settlement is possible. Where there is no agreement, a third party is called in. This final step is referred to as arbitration. However, there are some alternatives, e.g., calling in a fact-finder to investigate and make recommendations; these may or may not be acceptable to management and the union. Arbitration tends to be final, and both parties must abide by the decision, although it is possible in some cases, e.g., discrimination, to extend the controversy through the court system. The grievance system is often a key demand of employees in the contract negotiation, and is always protected by the union as a most significant right.

The role of the department head in the grievance procedure is a critical one. He must be aware of conditions in his department and understand the policies and procedures of administration. The more familiar he is with them, the more smoothly the grievance will be handled.

Grievances must be adjusted promptly and the grievance machinery (paper work and contacts) must be well understood and simple in process. Appeals from the first level (department decisions) must be readily available. Care must be taken in the selection of the arbitrator so that he understands the unique features of hospitals. Again, when administrators have questions about contract administration, especially grievances, they are well advised to seek expert advice.

An important addendum to contract administration is the interpretation of the contract in terms of changing laws. In addition, the period of time between the contract signing and the next negotiating session is one in which problems are brought to light, which may result in new demands by the union. Wise administrators will warn their managerial staffs to be on the lookout for problems so that these demands can be anticipated and evaluated prior to the stress period of actual negotiations.

SOME CONCLUSIONS

The main purpose of this chapter was to review developments in collective bargaining and unionization of employees in hospitals and related health institutions. To date, the number of hospital employees under union contracts is not great. One reason for this was the absence of federal legislation encouraging unionization.

Many labor relations experts are of the opinion that we will see more unionized employees in hospitals and, according to Herman Somers (1974), considerable strife. The reasons cited for unionization include changing attitudes toward unions, which are now seen as serving white-collar as well as blue-collar workers, greater professionalism on the part of union organizers, poor personnel and business practices in some hospitals, racial complications, the increasing conviction on the part of workers that it is no longer possible to "go it alone," and the changing legal environment including the 1974 change in the National Labor Relations Act that removed the exemption of not-for-profit hospitals and eliminated the hodge-podge status of hospital labor laws (Pointer, 1974).

Whether or not a hospital is actually organized, the administrator is constantly engaged in negotiations. In earlier periods, this process was more likely to be on a one-to-one basis. To an increasing extent administrators and other management personnel now find themselves negotiating with groups of employees. This is a natural development as hospitals grow larger and more complex. It is a form of power and must be expected.

In hospitals that are to be organized, the first bargaining session is crucial, since it sets the stage for all others. A key factor is the recognition of the union. This may be done through an election or by management agreement. Key issues to be negotiated are generally wages, hours of working, working conditions, and procedures important to the union such as the place of seniority in promotions or layoffs. The bargaining session itself is sometimes a lesson in frustration, but eventually a contract is developed, and submitted to the union membership for ratification. It is then signed by management and becomes the guide to union-management relations during the contract period.

Contract administration is of equal importance to union-management relationships. It is generally carried out by management with the union playing a watch-dog role. When the contract is violated or management acts unfairly, a grievance is filed. The grievance procedure is an important right in the eyes of the union and must be recognized as such. Of vital importance is the training of department heads so that they understand union procedure and the contract provision.

There can be no question that unions in hospitals will affect employer-employee relationships. Some hospitals with contracts will say that there has been a deterioration in the relationship; others will insist that there has been an improvement. Whatever their attitudes, thousands of managers have learned to live with unions, and many prefer the relationship to one in which employees have no outlet for their expectations, attitudes, and demands.

REFERENCES

Bennett, Addison C.: "Resisting Union Organizing Attempts," *Hospital Topics,* pp. 30-34, Jan. 1972.

Elkin, Randyl: "Recognition and Negotiation under Taft-Hartley," *Hospital Progress,* vol. 55, no. 12, pp. 50ff., Dec. 1974.

Elkin, Randyl D.: "Negotiation and Administering a Union Contract," *Hospital Progress,* vol. 56, no. 1, pp. 40-43, Jan. 1975.

Golodner, Jack: "Unions and Non-Profit Employers," *AFL-CIO American Federationist,* vol. 77, no. 98, pp. 19-24, Aug. 1970.

Goodfellow, Matthew: "How the Union Organizer Rates Your Hospital: A Checklist," *administrative briefs,* American College of Hospital Administrators, Jan. 1973.

Hazard, William R.: "Semantic Gymnastics?" *The Americardion School Board Journal,* Oct. 1967, adapted from National Education Association, *Guidelines for Professional Negotiation* (rev. ed.), Office of Professional Development and Welfare, Washington, D.C., 1965.

Krawleski, John E.: "Collective Bargaining Among Professional Employees," *Hospital Administration,* vol. 19, no. 3, pp. 30-41, Summer 1974.

Kuby, Alma: AHA Research Capsule, No. 6, *Hospitals, J.A.H.A.,* Apr. 1, 1972.

Medical World News: "MD Unions Split Over Issue of Labor Ties," pp. 17-19, Feb. 16, 1973.

Matlock, David R.: "Goals and Trends in the Unionization of Health Professionals," *Hospital Progress,* pp. 40-43, Feb. 1972.

Miller, Ronald L.: "The Hospital-Union Relationship, Part I," *Hospitals,* May 1, 1971.

Mintzberg, Henry: *The Nature of Managerial Work,* Harper and Row, New York, 1973, pp. 90-91.

Nash, Al: "The Hospitals Value System and the Union," *Hospital Administration,* vol. 19, no. 4, pp. 49-64, Fall 1974.

Osterhaus, Leo B.: "The Effect of Unions on Hospital Management, Part I and Part II: Factors Stimulating and Inhibiting Unions," *Hospital Progress,* pp. 68-73, June-July, 1967.

Oswald, Rudy: "A Voice for Hospital Workers," *AFL-CIO American Federationist,* pp. 14-17, Jan. 1975.

Panosh, Michael: "Unionization and Collective Bargaining by Registered Nurses" (unpublished),University of Wisconsin, Madison, 1973.

Pointer, Dennis D.: "Unionization, Collective Bargaining and the Non-Profit Hospital," Monograph Series no. 13, Center for Labor and Management, College of Business Administration, the University of Iowa, Sept. 1969.

Pointer, Dennis D.: "How the 1974 Taft-Hartley Amendments Will Affect Health Care Facilities," *Hospital Progress,* pp. 68-70, Oct. 1974.

Pointer, Dennis D. and Lloyd Cannedy: "Organizing Professionals," *Hospitals, J.A.H.A.,* vol. 46, pp. 70-73, 1972.

Pointer, Dennis D.: "Hospital Labor Relations Legislation: An Examination and Critique of Public Policy," *Hospital Progress,* pp. 71-76, Jan. 1973.

Pointer, Dennis D. and Norman Metzger: "Work Stoppages in the Hospital Industry: A Preliminary Profile and Analysis," *Hospital Administration,* pp. 9-24, Spring 1972.

Somers, Herman: "Effect of Labor Unions on Health Services," Seminar, University of Wisconsin, Madison, Nov. 11, 1974.

West, Allen M.: "Professional Negotiations or Collective Bargaining," *The National Elementary Principal,* Feb. 1963.

Zimmerman, Lettie: "Hospital Unionization: Trends and Implications," unpublished seminar paper, University of Wisconsin, Madison, Nov. 1972.

Chapter 15

External Influences
and Constraints

"No other system of services has come close to equalling the scientific and technological gains, or the assembly of the marvelous resources for implementing those gains, as has been achieved by the health care delivery system. . . . It has been fabulous in its capabilities. So far as lifesaving procedures go, it has been fabulous in its performance" (Brown, 1973, p. 3). On the other side, Brown also notes that the health care system has "serious problems of misutilization and overutilization; suboptional use of facilities and personnel; medical disengagement of substantial segments of the population; quality concerns; and cost effectiveness" (p. 3). It is the latter problems that are calling for increasing regulation of hospitals. Concerns for retaining the strengths of the system present that dilemma to planners and give consternation to health care providers as well as fears for loss of independence.

This book is written at a time of considerable debate when numerous proposals are being made for increased federal financing of health services. We have attempted therefore, to write from the perspective of issues related to controls rather than practices.

This chapter is organized into four sections—Why External Regulation?; Voluntary Regulatory Bodies; Governmental Regulation; and Conclusions.

WHY EXTERNAL REGULATION?

A pattern of increasing regulation of hospitals and health services has developed over the years. Initially regulation was on a voluntary basis. It was sponsored by organized medicine to raise quality through improved education of physicians and improved standards for hospitals through the American College of Surgeons and eventually the Joint Commission on Accreditation of Hospitals (JCAH). Governmental regulations were first imposed at the state level, centering around licensure to protect consumers against untrained and unscrupulous practitioners. Laws and court decisions have also had an important influence on regulating quality and access to care. Space does not permit us to review legal influences, and the reader is referred to Somers' (1969) excellent book on hospital regulations. In recent years regulation has been increasing primarily due to concerns over rising costs of hospital and health care. Those favoring more regulation of hospitals and other health services tend to cite the following reasons (also see Blumstein and Zubkoff, 1973):

Hospital and health service industry is too large and too important to be un-regulated. Health is the second largest industry in the nation in terms of employment and expenditure. What is spent on health is unavailable for other products or services in our economy.

Health care is a right. Only recently has this premise been widely accepted. Even as recently as 1971, there were individuals who argued that health care was not a right (Sade, 1971). To ensure people of this right, many believe there must be regulation and control of the health industry, and even that health care should be provided primarily through the public rather than the private sector, as has been traditional for education and other social services.

The health industry is a classic example of market failure. Economists will point out that the "free enterprise system" is inoperable in health care because:

Externalities are important. This means that health care must be provided to all citizens whether or not they want or deserve it because those who do not receive health care are a loss or hazard to the rest of society.

Consumers are uninformed. Consumers cannot judge the type of service they require nor its quality as they can when it comes to purchasing other goods such as food, housing, automobiles, etc.

Demand in the medical market place is largely determined by the suppliers rather than the users of service. Physicians determine whether or not diagnostic and treatment services are needed and, if so, which ones. Hence it is a sellers' market that seems to require some kind of external regulation.

There is no freedom of entry into the supply market. Supply and demand factors do not operate in the health industry. It functions more as a monopoly. When demand increases it is very difficult and costly to increase the supply of physicians and hospitals. (However, today there is concern that the market does not control for oversupply in relation to need; that is, hospitals continue to expand or retain services in the face of declining need or demand as evidenced by duplicated and unprofitable obstetrical, radiation therapy, and pediatric units.) They conclude that in cases of market failure the industry must be controlled like a public utility, for example.

Current reimbursement plans are based on reimbursement of costs or charges. Consequently, there are no incentives to contain costs; hospitals with higher costs will obtain higher reimbursement.

With centralized financing, controls are more feasible. In the past, with fragmented funding of health care by philanthropists, individual consumers, and a myriad of competing insurance plans, it was difficult to organize financers of health service to exercise controls through the sanction of withholding funds. Now that the government funds more than 37 percent of all health services and more than 53 percent of hospital services, sanctions can be applied.

There are increasing concerns over rising health care costs. Although health and hospital costs have been rising dramatically for decades, consumers were less concerned because increasing portions of health and hospital costs were born by their employers through health insurance benefits. Today, the government and taxpayers are feeling the burdens or rising costs, and as might be expected, they are less tolerant of increases and are seeking methods to control rising costs.

The public is aroused about examples of waste, duplication of expensive services, and high profits in the health industry. Accounts in the press of possible exploitation by a few hospitals, incomes of some physicians exceeding $100,000 annually, and reactionism by health associations have by innuendo implicated all health providers and raised demands for greater external control over the industry.

Those opposed to increased regulation point toward the progress made by the health industry in providing superior quality service and the quality and cost controls being exercised by providers on a voluntary basis. They argue that increased regulation will be no more effective in controlling cost and access, and will result in lower quality. Moreover, when regulations are imposed on everyone, the unique needs and expectations of individuals are compromised. Furthermore, it is pointed out that bureaucratic red tape is expensive, and at times counterproductive to physicians' and hospitals' primary objectives of patient care.

Most of the demands for regulation are based on the need to control rising costs and concern over unavailability of care because of poor allocation of manpower and facilities. Somers (1969) suggests there are two schools of advocates for improved efficiency of hospital operation; one, those who advocate greater public regulation, and two, those who advocate more competitive enterprise. In other words, controls versus incentives. Public utility regulation is an example of the former and prepaid health plans or HMOs an example of the latter.

While there is currently no direct systematic public regulation of hospitals, there is a great deal of piecemeal regulation. Weimer (1968) listed 68 different hospital programs or facilities affected by direct government controls, classified as follows:

Physical plant and equipment	18
Personnel	12
Working conditions	9
Permit to operate	12
Reporting	13
Miscellaneous	4

Weimer listed 16 different federal agencies involved in hospital regulation along with 9 state government bodies, and 12 local government bodies. In addition, many voluntary accrediting agencies such as JCAH exercise some control over hospital operations. One administrator counted over 143 separate required reports including 104 to governmental agencies and 38 to voluntary bodies (Pomrinse, 1969). Somers (1969), in her book on hospital regulation, reports how common, tax, and labor laws affect hospitals. In the next two sections, we will review selected voluntary and governmental regulations.

VOLUNTARY REGULATIONS

Although the Joint Commission on Accreditation of Hospitals has been referred to frequently in this book, it has not been described as an organization. The JCAH has a quasi-governmental role in that it was named in the Medicare Act passed by Congress in 1965 as a benchmark for eligibility for a hospital to participate in the Medicare program. However, the JCAH is a private body, a voluntary not-for-profit corporation that is provider-sponsored and provider-oriented. It was organized in 1951 as an outgrowth of an accreditation program sponsored by the American College of Surgeons started in 1918. Its sponsoring organizations and members on its Board of Commissioners are:

American Medical Association
American Hospital Association
American College of Surgeons
American College of Physicians
American Association of Homes for the Aging
American Nursing Home Association

Its mission is to determine "how health services shall be provided that will make them the best possible quality (Porterfield, 1971b). While it is a voluntary program, it has had a major influence on improving the quality of hospital care in the United States and Canada. Its leverage comes from the influence of sponsoring organizations over providers, its requirement for intern and residency training programs in hospitals, eligibility for 12 of the 74 Blue Cross insurance plans, and a recognition among some consumers that an accredited hospital meets certain minimum standards of quality. Moreover, since 1965, accreditation enables a hospital to be automatically certified as a provider under Medicare if it complies with utilization review requirements. The number of accredited facilities on a bed basis have increased, and at the same time standards for accreditation have risen. Chapters 5 and 11 referred to some of the requirements for accreditation.

Hospitals are surveyed by a team made up of a physician and a hospital administrator that reviews patient charts, quality of care (structure and processes) in the hospital, and the hospital's facilities. Hospitals receiving full accreditation are surveyed every three years and those with provisional accreditation are surveyed annually, but no more than twice on a provisional basis.

The JCAH is not without its critics. On the one hand, some physicians criticize it for overemphasis on minutiae of clinical records and medical staff meetings (Porterfield, 1971a). On the other, consumer advocates criticize it for being a lackey of providers (Porterfield, 1971a). They also charge that it fails to provide standards for outpatient services, does not consider patients' rights (with regard to privacy, participation in teaching, and choice of accommodation), that (until 1975) it failed to consider outcomes (for example, as long as there was a tissue committee it was unconcerned how much normal tissue was removed), and it fails to consider the adequacy of the hospital staff to meet the patient load (Worthington and Silver, 1970). On balance, however, most will agree that the JCAH has had a major influence on improving the quality of hospital care in the nation.

There are other voluntary quality controls on hospitals from external sources although none is as influential as the JCAH. Training programs have certification by the respective professional associations. For example, programs for interns and residents, nurses, x-ray technicians and medical technologists, and other training programs based in hospitals must be certified by appropriate agencies. Training programs themselves and university affiliations also aid in improving quality of care in an institution. The American Society of Clinical Pathologists has a separate accreditation program for clinical laboratories. The American College of Surgeons (ACS) has a Cancer Registry Program that aids in the review of cancer cases in the hospital and brings together physicians from different specialties to consider improved ways of treating cancer.

Professional societies help to regulate quality in a number of ways. For example, medical specialty boards certify competency after a rigorous examination process. Professional associations such as the ACS award fellowships in various specialties upon demonstrated competence as reported by colleagues. Attendance at scientific meetings and contributions to professional journals are examples of other peer pressures for competence. Peer pressure is no small factor, for professionals are usually influenced by peers in their field who may well be outside their local organization (Gouldner, 1957).

Voluntary cost controls are also evident. Blue Cross and Blue Shield plans, which had been provider-sponsored and dominated by hospital and medical associations respectively, have established some regulations over costs. Blue Cross plans in various states have established hospital rate review programs (rate increases must be approved by Blue Cross and hospital-appointed review boards) and prospective reimbursement (i.e., establishing reimbursement formulas in advance of charges, which provides incentives for hospitals to reduce costs and penalizes them if they exceed expected levels). Presumably these efforts have helped to contain rising costs. The Wisconsin Blue Cross rate review program, for example, rejected some proposals and had other proposals withdrawn for rate increases that would have resulted in over $2 million in increased charges in 1972-1973 (Experimental Hospital Rate Review Program, 1973). Moreover, average per diem charges on Wisconsin hospitals increased 4 percent in 1972-1973 compared with 12 to 18 percent in the three years prior to the Economic Stabilization Program (ESP).

Another voluntary cost control is the regulation of demand for hospital services.

Insurance policies with deductible clauses, coinsurance, and prepaid care all place incentives on either the use or nonuse of services. For example, coverage for inpatient care only and duplicate insurance for a service might allow patients to make money by being hospitalized, and thus place incentives on overuse. Prepaid programs, on the other hand, place incentives on keeping patients well and out of the hospital. Co-insurance or no insurance at all, which make it costly for patients to be hospitalized, foster underutilization of service (McNerney, 1962). Voluntary regulations have fostered more effective and efficient hospital services, but apparently the results have been inadequate.

GOVERNMENTAL REGULATION

As noted previously, many laws enacted by legislatures apply to hospitals as well as to other services and organizations; however, in this section we will focus only on those that apply specifically to hospitals. One of the earliest laws covering hospitals was state licensing of health personnel and institutions. However, such controls have been minimal in most states, with only very gross evidence of negligence being cause to revoke a license. Moreover, in most states, it was relatively easy in the past to obtain a license to operate a hospital.

We have already suggested that governmental regulation of hospitals is increasing. In this section we review health planning, hospital franchising, certificate of need legislation, prospective rate review, and federal controls through Medicare and Medicaid. It is important to note that not all of these are governmental programs. Areawide health planning at the local level is usually done by a private nonprofit corporation; however, most are federally funded and have links with state planning agencies; therefore, we included them in this section.

Areawide Health Planning

Planning received its initial impetus from the Hill-Burton legislation of 1946 (federal funds for hospital construction) which provided, among other things, that there be a state survey of the need for health facilities and a state plan for meeting such needs. The state plan was to provide for adequate facilities for all persons in the state and "to furnish needed services for persons unable to pay therefore." In addition, the plan was to assure that the use of all health care facilities would be available to "all persons residing in the geographical area." Hill-Burton has had a major influence on the expansion of hospital facilities in the nation, but it has not assured health services for persons unable to pay. In 1973, federal guidelines were established for hospitals that received Hill-Burton funds requiring "a reasonable volume of services to persons unable to pay." (See the 1973 Hill-Burton Guidelines for requirements and exceptions.)

State planning under Hill-Burton was minimal (Levin, 1972). It provided funds for construction of numerous small hospitals in rural areas and helped to provide hospitals for rapidly growing suburban areas, but neglected needs of many deteriorating inner city facilities.

In 1966, the Partnership for Health Act to accomplish Comprehensive Health Planning (CHP), (P.L. 89-749) was passed. Section 314a of this act provided for state planning agencies, frequently referred to as "a" agencies. Section 314b created "comprehensive regional, metropolitan area, or other local area plans for coordination of existing and planned health services, including facilities and persons required for provision of such services." These local areawide planning agencies were commonly called "b" agencies.

It was the intent of CHP to "focus on all the people's total health needs and all means —services, manpower facilities—to meet these needs" (HEW, 1970). It considered planning as a continuous process of arriving at an agreement of providers and consumers on:

1 Health needs, goals and priorities
2 Resources and measures appropriate to achievement of goals
3 Recommendations of actions by public and private sectors to enhance effectiveness of existing resources and activities and to develop those needed for the future

In the past couple years HEW focused more on the development of state and area plans than on planning as a continuing process. Significant features of CHP were: (1) it involved a highly decentralized process with broadly based participation of providers and consumers of health care, as well as voluntary and governmental agencies aimed at setting goals and establishing priorities; and (2) it attempted to accomplish coordination whenever possible through voluntary cooperation solicited in part by providing better information about potential bottlenecks and shortages to those who are directly responsible for instituting changes, e.g., hospital administrators, physicians, etc. Grants were made available to the approved areawide CHP agency on a basis of 50 to 75 percent federal funds and matching local funds. The law required that a majority of the "b" agency board be consumers of health service and the membership must reflect the geographic, socioeconomic, and ethnic groups of the area.

CHP covered the nation with state "a" agencies, and as of February 1973 federal funding supported nearly 200 areawide "b" agencies covering 70 percent of the nation's population. Most of the "b" agencies were organized as nonprofit private corporations and operated on a voluntary basis. Most of their efforts were used to inventory needs and resources of the area. The concerns of planners have been primarily with duplication of hospital services and overbuilding of facilities. Sanctions of areawide planning agencies were limited in most cases to approving building projects to be funded under the Hill-Burton program. However, most institutions funded their facility additions through long-term financing and/or funded depreciation; consequently, in many cases planning agencies exerted only social pressure on institutions. Indeed the courts ruled in some states, e.g., North Carolina, that a private voluntary hospital cannot be prevented from adding facilities even though there appears to be unnecessary duplication of service if the hospital uses its own resources for construction.

A 1973 amendment to the social Security Act (P.L. 92-603, Section 1122) expands the review and approval authority of areawide comprehensive health planning agencies. It requires that they review all service and bed complement changes in health care institutions, in addition to all capital expenditures in excess of $100,000, and recommend approval or disapproval of such changes or expenditures to the state. Section 1122 provides agencies with substantial authority to impact on health institutional planning undertaken in their area.

Nevertheless, there was widespread agreement that CHP did not live up to its expectations of developing plans and promoting their implementation for more effective and efficient health service. Ardell (1971) in summarizing the literature on deficiencies of health planning councils suggested that:

> A major theme played over and over in the literature is that health planning coordinating councils are restricted purpose organizations without public mandate. Their governing and supporting decision structures are dominated by the interests they represent (i.e., professional leaders), and are thus unrepresentative of the larger community . . . the nonprovider representatives are mostly prestige names from the business sector. The private councils have traditionally lacked power to implement their plans, shown little interest in system changes or experimentation to reshape the status quo, and have long suffered the insecurity of a hesitant and uncertain funding base of volunteer support (p. 30).

Kinzer (1974) feels that the "proper role of consumers is to make demands, and this role is one that should be accomplished *off* planning boards. The health care field must face the fact that planning will be a political process; that planning bores consumers who are interested in having their needs met but not in the mechanics of seeing that such needs are met; and that good or bad planning agencies are also going to have to be policemen if planning is to fly" (p. 124).

Delbecq (1972) suggests that planners lack the knowledge of when, where, and how to involve consumers in the planning process. For example, he suggests using market research as a planning subfunction rather than expecting one or two minority group members to be able to speak for the group as a whole. He also suggests that knowledge of group process techniques be applied to help planning boards or commissions that usually consist of 35 to 50 members and represent diverse interests and have diverse communication skills.

A study by the Comptroller General's office (1974) found problems with CHP services in the following areas:

> Sources of matching funds and difficulties in raising the required amounts [of local money]
> Lack of staff
> Selection and participation of volunteers in planning activities
> Geographic makeup of planning areas
> Proper relationships between state and areawide
> Performance of control functions without sound criteria and systematic procedures

Agencies not being given opportunities to review and comment on proposed
federal health projects
Shortcomings in data bases available to state and areawide agencies
Lack of an implementation process for developed recommendations

This study recommended legislative and administrative action to alleviate these
problems. The result was the 1974 National Health Planning and Resources Development Act (P.L. 93-641), signed into law January 4, 1975, which replaced or revised
the state and areawide CHP "a" and "b" agencies, Hill-Burton Facilities Planning and
Construction, capital expenditure and review under Social Security Administration,
and Regional Medical Programs.[1] The act combined the old agencies into new state
and substate agencies. In addition to congressional dissatisfaction with performance
under CHP, legislators felt that national health insurance was imminent and a unified
planning, resource allocation, and regulatory effort was an essential prerequisite to such
financing. Moreover, they were convinced that functions in this legislation were inter-
related and should therefore be vested in the same agency.

Figure 15-1 describes the organization and responsibilities under P.L. 93-641. This
imposes federal control over local activities. It makes certificate of need (that meets
federal standards) mandatory. It also requires review of all new institutional health
services proposed in a state, and periodic review of all existing institutional health
services in the state, but without federal sanctions. State review and approval of
institutional rates is optional.

This act has important implications for governmental regulation of hospitals
and other health services. Health care leaders are fearful about the centralized, particularly federal, controls included in the act, and about the lack of an appeals
mechanisms and consumer-oriented governing boards. The AMA filed suit in January
1975 contending that the act is unconstitutional and asking that it be struck down
by the courts. However, in spite of these fears, health care leaders see some possible
benefits in that it will cause institutions to relate their plans to community needs and
to other institutions, that the stress on outpatient facilities is desirable, and that the
act eliminates overlapping jurisdictions that were present under CHP, RMP, and
Hill-Burton.

Franchising Hospitals

As far back as 1959, Ray E. Brown stirred the hospital industry when he suggested
that if there were to be public regulation of the community hospital, state franchising
offered the best means of accomplishing this and would do the least damage to the
values of the hospital system. Since then, there has been considerable discussion of
regulating the hospital as a public utility or franchising hospitals. The terms *franchising and public utility* are generally used synonymously. Some appear to prefer

---

[1] Regional medical programs (RMP were established under 1965 legislation for heart,
cancer, and stroke. The objective of these programs was to extend the advanced knowledge and
skills of the medical schools and large medical centers throughout each state and region.

SECRETARY, U.S. DEPARTMENT
HEALTH, EDUCATION AND WELFARE

- Issues guidelines for national health planning policy
- Establishes health areas recommended by governors
- Designates health systems agencies in each area
- Issues regulations governing implementation of the act
- Reviews health plans produced by substate and state agencies
- Administers grant programs to agencies
- Approves most federal assistance plans and project grants

STATE HEALTH COORDINATING
COUNCIL (SHCC)
(a consumer majority council of citizens 60% designated by HSA, 40% designated by the governor)

- Conducts health planning activities for the state
- Implements or supervises implementation of plans
- Prepares preliminary state health plan
- Serves as agency for (S.1122) review
- Administers a state certificate-of-need program
- Reviews and makes findings concerning all new insti-
  tutional health services in the state
- Reviews periodically all health services offered
  in the state
- Coordinates all health data activities in the state
- Assists SHCC in its work
- Administers federally assisted facilities construction
  activities
- Administers optional rate review and approval
  programs

STATE HEALTH PLANNING AND
DEVELOPMENT AGENCY (SPDA)
(a state agency designated by the governor to carry out
activities mandated by the act)

- Reviews and coordinates health planning activities of
  substate agencies
- Prepares and approves state health plan
- Reviews and comments on annual budget of substate
  agencies
- Reviews and comments on annual applications of sub-
  state agencies
- Advises SPDA on its work
- Reviews and approves all state plans and applications
  for funds under federal health legislation

HEALTH SYSTEMS AGENCY (HSA)
(A public or private nonprofit agency with a consumer-majority
board or advisory body which carries out functions mandated
by the act in a defined geographic area. Areas are based on criteria defining minimum population and available health services
to meet the needs of the area's residents.)

- Assembles and analyzes data on health status and health programs in its area
- Prepares and publishes a Health Systems Plan (HSP) and an Annual Implemen-
  tation Plan (AIP) for its area
- Develops specific activities and projects which support plans
- Implements plans through technical assistance and through developmental
  grants to community agencies
- Coordinates activities with other planning bodies and PSROs
- Reviews and approves each use of federal health funds in its area
- Recommends action on each health service offered in area to state
- Reviews and comments to state agency on all capital expenditures and new
  service projects in area institutions
- Recommends health facilities projects to state for funding

COMMUNITY INSTITUTIONS AND ORGANIZATIONS

- Submits all new service and capital expenditure projects for review
- Participates in periodic review of existing services
- Submits all applications for federal support for review
- Conducts special projects under developmental grant authorities

Figure 15-1 Planning Organization and Responsibilities under P.L. 93-641
National Health Planning and Resources Development Act. *(Source:* Adapted
from information provided by the Wisconsin Division of Health Policy and
Planning.)

franchising because it avoids the association that public utilities have with the power and communication industries.

Drake (1973) of the American Hospital Association defines public utility regulation as "a systematic and coordinated administration, probably in a single agency of government, which provides standards for products, pricing, investment, capital financing, public disclosure and for the market structure in which the enterprise operates" (p. 78). He notes that controls currently exist over most of these activities, but on a piecemeal basis without any systematic coordination and without universal application to all of the hospital's patients. Recognizing the inevitability of increasing regulation of hospitals and that hospitals are already highly controlled, the Perloff Committee of the AHA advocated public utility status for hospitals and all health care providers in proposing the establishment of *Health Care Corporations* (AHA, 1970; 1971). The AHA ran into opposition from many of its members and from the AMA; consequently, it dropped official support for Health Care Corporations. However, a bill that generally incorporates the Perloff committee recommendations was submitted to Congress, but so far has received no ground swell support. In a survey of 132 hospital administrators in Minnesota, Whiting (1973) found that less than 17 percent of the administrators thought hospitals should be regulated similarly to public utilities, although "they generally agreed that hospitals should be required to possess a 'certificate of need' before expansion of any service of facility, and that area-wide comprehensive health planning agencies should have formal authority to enforce plans that they develop" (p. 748). Golladay and Smith (1974) note that the "cost of public utilities regulation is staggering" (p. 84). It is estimated that the operation of major federal regulatory agencies alone (e.g., Securities Exchange Commission, Federal Power Commission, Federal Aeronautics Board, Federal Communication Commission) costs over a billion dollars annually.

Somers (1969) initially argued against the public utility model; she felt that it was inappropriate because hospitals are nonprofit with some operating at a loss, the product is highly individualized, the medical staff has a unique role in influencing the hospital, and hospitals have overlapping service areas. She had hoped that the hospital industry would be able, perhaps with the help of the Society Security Administration's incentive reimbursement experiments to devise some effective competitive method of pricing as an alternative to public rate regulation. By 1972, Somers (1973b) recommended an adaptation of the public utility or franchise model—i.e., private ownership and private management within a fairly strictly defined public accountability. She suggested, however, that the approach should be more positive than the traditional utility regulation, with much greater emphasis on explicitly mandated responsibilities and on professional and institutional self-regulation rather than on limited earnings. Somers believes that the hospital is most likely to provide a viable base for effective self-regulation within a framework of public accountability. One can assume that therein lies organized medicine's opposition to this model.

Certificate of Need

As of September, 1973, some 22 states had adopted certificate-of-need legislation that supposedly prevents hospitals from expanding or developing facilities where the planning agency says there is no need for such facilities. Certificate of need is now required under P.L. 93-641. Moreover, states must follow federal standards. This CHP certification program disapproved $10.8 million and effected a modification in another $129.3 million in previously approved plans from July 1970 through November 1972 (Comptroller General, 1974). Apparently such programs can influence hospital construction and presumably limit some "unnecessary" facilities, however defined. Broader issues of proper spatial distribution facilities and service are for the most part untouched by certificate-of-need-type activities because of large investments in existing unplanned facilities, or those whose plans are obsolete. Moreover, certificate-of-need-type regulation usually does not cover physician service facilities, which have a major influence on the spatial distribution of medical care services.

Prospective Rate Review

A number of states have attempted to regulate hospital rates by reviewing and approving rate increases in Blue Cross plans, which in turn provide a significant portion of hospital income. Blue Cross plans were established by hospitals in the thirties and forties as prepaid hospital plans to provide full coverage of specified hospital services such as semiprivate room rates for a given number of days. Many commercial hospital insurance plans are indemnity plans that pay so much per day for a hospital room and other services; therefore, as hospital rates increased, the patient rather than the carrier paid the increased hospital costs until the insurance coverage and premiums were adjusted. Because it was limited by some state insurance commissioners in what it could charge its customers, Blue Cross was forced to try to limit hospital cost increases. This method of approving premium costs of Blue Cross subscribers had the effect of driving a number of Blue Cross plans to near bankruptcy until they had approval to raise their rates. Predictably, however, such a passive approach has had no discernible effect on hospital costs.

Blue Cross and commercial carriers that attempt to provide for nearly full coverage of hospital costs have been the target of consumer complaints over rising costs rather than the hospitals, because patients have paid a declining portion of hospital costs directly. In 1966, individuals paid, on the average, $94 for health care out of their own pocket, which represented 51 percent of their total health care bill. By 1972 they paid $119, which was only 35 percent of the bill (DHEW, 1973). In 1972 only 8 percent of the hospital care bill came from the patient's pocket with most of the rest coming from health insurance and the government.

To help place more of the burden on hospitals, a number of Blue Cross plans inaugurated prospective rather than retrospective rate review. That is, hospitals had to submit their budgets to Blue Cross for review and approval in advance of any increases in rates. The ability of Blue Cross to take a hard line in prospective rate review is limited because its relationship to hospitals is voluntary; a number of hospitals resigned their membership as participating hospitals when they believed Blue Cross took too hard a line. Even though Blue Cross has been separated from the American Hospital Association, appearances of collusion between hospitals and Blue Cross may limit public acceptance of these controls. By August 1973, only 10 states had prospective rate review controlled by a state agency.

Prospective rate review provides some incentives that retrospective rates do not.

Medicare-Medicaid and most private insurers have a modified retrospective rate review. Retrospective rates allow customary charges and reimbursement on the basis of historical costs, and sometimes adjustments to cover losses incurred by the institution. However, prospective rate review also has some characteristics that reduce incentives to control rising costs. For example, input costs of wages and supplies are usually indexed for current prices; therefore, institutions usually have no incentives to resist demands for salary and price increases from employees and suppliers (Golladay and Smith, 1974). Moreover, rate review must be coupled with utilization review or be based on a total budget or capitation prospective reimbursement as discussed in the previous chapter if it is to have any significant effect. Golladay and Smith also note problems in determination of hospital rates due to:

Variations in quality of services available
Effects of occupancy rates and volume of services
Scope of services
Prices of inputs such as wages and salaries
Funding of charity patients and uncollectables
Availability of philanthropy to some institutions

Nevertheless, prospective rate review coupled with utilization review appears to be a more effective method of equitable cost containment incentives than many other approaches.

Medicare and Medicaid

Medicare and Medicaid (Title XVIII and Title XIX of Social Security legislation) were passed and signed into federal law in 1966, and have had a significant impact on hospitals as well as on the financing and delivery of health care in the United States. Medicare provides health insurance for persons over 65 who participate in the Social Security program. Title A of Medicare provides for nearly full coverage of hospital and nursing home costs for a specified period of time. Premiums are included in Social Security payments. Title B is voluntary and requires the individual to pay a portion of the insurance for physicians' services.

Medicaid was intended to provide health care for the indigent and the medically indigent (those who can cover normal living costs but not medical care costs). It was expected to provide a means for the poor to enter the "mainstream" of health services; that is, it was supposed to give health care funds for the poor to purchase services in the private sector. Medicaid, unlike Medicare, is administered on the state and not the federal level with matching state and federal monies. In attempting to implement the program, a number of states found their health and welfare funds near bankruptcy. As a result, most cut back their services for the indigent and today there are wide discrepancies in the various state Medicaid programs.

Medicare and Medicaid have affected hospitals in a number of ways:

The increased demands for health services, particularly physician services, severely strained the supply and no doubt contributed to rising costs.

The programs resulted in a centralization of the financing of health services, which in turn led to increased controls over costs and services. In 1966, 36 percent of hospital costs were met by governmental funds; this rose to 53 percent by 1972.

The programs brought the controversy of reimbursement of hospital-based specialists to a head (Somers and Somers, 1967).

The programs increased demands for extension of federal funding and controls for hospitals and other health services.

As noted previously, P.L. 93-641 places increasing controls over hospitals. The 1973 amendments to Social Security (P.L. 92-603) are also resulting in further changes and controls over hospitals. For example, they call for Professional Standards Review Organizations (PSROs) which have been mentioned previously. Section 1122 of the law imposes controls on capital expenditures by hospitals that are in excess of $100,000, and on any changes in service or bed capacity. Section 234 requires formal plans and budgets.

CONCLUSIONS: VOLUNTARY OR COMPULSORY REGULATION—LOCAL, STATE, OR FEDERAL?

Clearly, regulation over hospitals is large and still increasing. Moreover, with a national health insurance program impending, mechanisms are being developed for further regulation and controls. The current literature indicates that most scholars of the American health care system support the continuation of the so-called pluralistic system in preference to a single, nationwide system. On the other hand, public funding of the system almost by definition calls for public accountability. It seems likely, therefore, that hospitals will be regulated even more in the future.

If compulsory regulation should increase still more, should it be at the local, state, or federal level? Ideally, one might argue for consumer control over health services. Each consumer has his own needs and expectations and an informed consumer in a free market has the most effective control. However, we currently have neither informed consumers nor a free market, particularly in urban and rural poverty areas.

Consumer control over provider services is being attempted on a broad scale, but results to date are by and large not encouraging. Nevertheless, consumer groups who bargain collectively with professionals for provision of service, as in some of the prepaid health plans, do seem to provide an effective control mechanism particularly when individual consumers have alternatives to choose from, for example, the Federal Employee Benefit Plan.

Historically most controls over health services have been exercised at the state level through licensing mechanisms. States such as New York, Illinois, California, and Connecticut are taking an increasingly active role in the regulation of health services through regulatory commissions, rate reviews, hospital admission and surveillance programs, and so forth. Problems with state regulation center on the wide variation in regulation, or the lack of it, among different states, limited financial resources, problems in attracting competent individuals to regulatory services, and the conservatism of many states in the face of rapidly changing needs and expectations.

Federal regulation, on the other hand, has inherent problems of inflexibility, competing and unwieldy bureaucracies, unresponsiveness to differing local and state needs, and diseconomies of scale. Current difficulties in government, and uncertainties in funding are evidence of such problems.

The scope of this book does not permit us to evaluate the many proposals for regulation and the arguments against it. However, we are concerned with the administration of hospitals, and implications of increased regulation are clear. While external regulation limits the independence of institutions and may also limit chances for individual success, it does not diminish the need for good administration. Indeed, it forces hospitals to apply modern management practices in order to cope with regulatory agencies. Some of the recommendations we have suggested previously with regard to defining objectives, improving information systems, personnel practices, and systems designs become critical for demonstrating needs and marshaling limited resources under a regulated system.

REFERENCES

American Hospital Association: *Report of a Special Committee on Provision of Health Services,* Chicago, 1970.

American Hospital Association: *Policy Statement on Provision of Health Services,* approved by House of Delegates of AHA, Aug. 24, 1971.

Ardell, Donald B.: "CHP, Regional Councils and the Public Interest: A Case for New Leadership," *Inquiry,* pp. 27-35, Dec. 1971.

The Blue Sheet: "HEW Proposal, Rogers Bill to Clash on State Health Powers," Drug Research Reports, p. 3-4, Jan. 30, 1974.

Blumstein, James P. and Michael Zubkoff: "Perspectives on Government Policy in the Health Sector," *Milbank Memorial Quarterly,* pp. 395-431, Summer 1973.

Brown, Ray E.: "Rationale for Regulation," *Regulating the Hospital,* a report of the 1972 National Forum on Hospital and Health Affairs, Duke University, Department of Health Administration, Durham, N.C., 1973, pp. 3-8.

Comptroller General of the United States: *Report to Congress: Comprehensive Health Planning as Carried Out by State and Areawide Agencies in Three States,* 1974.

Delbecq, Andre L.: "Critical Problems in Health Planning," a paper presented at the 32d Annual Meeting of the Academy of Management, Aug. 13-16, 1972.

Drake, David: "The Hospital as a Public Utility," *Regulating the Hospital,* a report of the 1972 National Forum on Hospital and Health Affairs, Department of Health Administration, Duke University, Durham, N.C., 1973.

Experimental Hospital Rate Review Program: Report on First Years Activities: Wisconsin Hospital Association, Madison, Oct. 24, 1973.

Golladay, Frederick and Kenneth Smith: *Regulating the Health Industry: A Study Prepared for the Health Planning Council* (of Wisconsin), Wisconsin Regional Medical Program, Madison, 1974.

Gouldner, A. W.: "Cosmopolitans and Locals: Toward an Analysis of Latent Social Roles—I and II," *Administrative Sciences Quarterly,* vol. 2, nos. 3 & 4, pp. 281-306, 1957.

Kinzer, David: "Planning Fallacy Cited," *Hospitals, J.A.H.A.,* vol. 48, p. 124, June 1, 1974.

Levin, A. L.: "Health Planning and the U.S. Federal Government," *International Journal of Health Services,* vol. 2, no. 3, pp. 367-376, 1972.

McNerney, Walter J., et al.: *Hospital and Medical Economics,* vol. 2, Hospital Research and Educational Trust, Chicago, 1962.

Pomrinse, S. David: "To What Degree Are Hospitals Publicly Accountable?" *Hospitals, J.A.H.A.,* p. 42, Feb. 16, 1969.

Porterfield, John: "A Brief Discourse on the Current States and Future Anticipation of the Joint Commission," *Bulletin,* American College of Surgeons, pp. 13ff., Dec. 1971*a.*

Porterfield, John: "What Is the J.C.A.H.?" *Hospital Management,* p. 17, Aug. 1971*b.*

Sade, Robert: "Medical Care as a Right: A Reputation," *New England Journal of Medicine,* vol. 285, no. 23, pp. 1288-1292, Dec. 2, 1971.

Somers, Anne and Herman Somers: *Medicare and the Hospitals,* The Brookings Institution, Washington, D.C., 1967.

Somers, Anne: *Hospital Regulation: The Dilemma of Public Policy,* Industrial Relations Section, Princeton University, Princeton, N.J., 1969.

Somers, Anne: "Toward a Rational Community Health Care System: The Hunterdon Model," *Hospital Progress,* pp. 46-54, Apr. 1973*a.*

Somers, Anne: "The Public Policy Rationale for Regulation and Control," in *Management Memorandum on Hospital Franchising,* Booz Allen and Hamilton, Chicago, 1973*b.*

U.S. Department of Health, Education and Welfare: *Project Guide for Areawide Comprehensive Health Planning,* issued by U.S.D.H.E.W., H.S.M.H.S., C.H.S., D.C.H.P., Rockville, Md., 1970.

U.S. Department of Health, Education and Welfare: *The Size and Shape of the Medical Care Dollar: Chart Book 1972,* Social Security Administration, DHEW PUB. No. (SSA) 73-11910, Washington, D.C., 1973.

Weimer, Edward W.: "Controls for Regulation of Hospitals," unpublished material, Aug. 9, 1968, as reported in Somers (1969) op. cit., p. 16.

Whiting, Roger N.: "Suggested Organizational Changes for the Hospital Industry," *Health Services Reports,* vol. 88, no. 8, pp. 743-749, Oct. 1973.

Worthington, William and Laurens Silver: "Regulation of Quality of Care in Hospitals: The Need for Change," *Law and Contemporary Problems,* Law School, Duke University, vol. 35, no. 2, pp. 304-333, Spring 1970.

Chapter 16

Trends and Perspectives

Students who are in health services administration graduate programs today are likely to be practicing well into the twenty-first century. Health services themselves as well as their administration will be very different in the future. External influences and constraints such as collective bargaining and hospital regulation are merely manifestations of changes in society, which include changing values and expectations, advancing technology, and population growth. In this chapter, we will review historical developments, current trends, and possible changes that could substantially affect the delivery of health services. This chapter is divided into four sections. The first reviews historical developments in the delivery of health care. The second reviews the current issues and trends that we have already described as well as some we have not. In the third section, we engage in speculating on the future, drawing on forecasts of futurologists, and in conclusion we review some implications.

HISTORICAL PERSPECTIVE

Many administrators still practicing today have seen transportation technology advance from the horse to space travel. They have seen personal health care advance just as dramatically. A recently retired administrator of a small but modern facility in northern Wisconsin reports being administrator of a community hospital in the late 1930s in which water was carried from a town pump to surgery on the second floor of the house that served as the hospital. While such primitive conditions are unthinkable in the United States today, in a large part of the world they continue to exist.

Advances in health in the United States are evidenced by the decline in death rates since 1900. Death rates have, however, leveled off since about 1954. Most will agree that the dramatic decline in the death rate in this century is primarily the result of advances in public health and improvement in other environmental factors described in Chapter 1.

Looking at some of these changes in more detail, Walsh McDermott (1969) suggests there have been four stages of medicine:

Stage 1: Impersonal measures that result in better health such as eating off a table instead of a dirty floor, improvements in roads and other means of transportation and communication, etc.

Stage 2: Environmental health measures such as safe water supply use of insecticides for control of malaria, etc.

Stage 3: Public health measures such as immunization programs.

Stage 4: Personal health measures such as physician-patient-related health care programs.

Each of these stages has been grafted on to the next. Stages 1, 2, and 3 are still important today, since we recognize the influence of transportation, pollution, measles and polio vaccinations, etc., on health. Stage 4 measures became really effective only in the mid-twenties and thirties; it is the stage in which modern medical technology became decisive. Prior to Stage 4, according to McDermott, physicians provided only human comfort. It is interesting to note that it is the decline in human comfort services from providers that is disturbing the public today. McDermott suggests that Stage 4 coincides with the introduction of antimicrobial drugs—sulfonamides. Drug therapy, and its success with TB, pneumonia, scarlet fever, and streptococcal infections, was a major factor in reducing death rates between the 1930s and 1954.

Risse (1974) suggests that the 10 major events in American medicine from 1900 to 1972 were as follows:

Modern public health and preventive medicine measures.

Reform in medical education as noted in the often-quoted Flexner Report of 1910 which called for the end of proprietary medical schools and the establishment of university- and labor-based medical education (Flexner, 1910).

Medical specialization, which has continued and has had a profound affect on the organization and delivery of health services.

Rise of modern surgery—anesthesia and aseptic techniques were developed in the nineteenth century but really applied only in the twentieth.

Development of laboratory medicine—rise of biochemistry and other basic sciences has been a major factor in improving diagnosis and some aspects of treatment.

Progress in therapeutics—the availability of modern chemotherapy, antibiotics, and hormones.

Development of immunization against polio. This put virology to use and was the beginning of targeted research.

Development of modern diagnostic techniques in radiology, electrocardiography, and electroencephalography.

Use of isotopes in medical research and treatment—this came after World War II with progress in application of nuclear technology.

Organ transplants and immunology—surgical and immunological breakthroughs permitted kidney transplants beginning in the late 1950s and heart transplants as of the late 1960s.

These advances in the health sciences have resulted in the development of large and complex medical care delivery institutions, particularly hospitals. Other technological changes that have contributed to these developments are improved transportation, communication, and information systems. Social changes have also contributed to the development of hospitals and other health institutions through a rise in standards of living, improved education, higher expectations and demands, and a growth in population.

Along with these pressures, which resulted in larger, more sophisticated, and more complex hospitals, came the need for professionally trained hospital administrators. Programs in hospital and health services administration developed. The first program was founded at Marquette University in 1924, but it was discontinued after a couple of years. The University of Chicago is the oldest program active today having been founded in 1934. The major development of graduate programs in hospital and health services administration has been in the past twenty-five years.

CURRENT TRENDS

Role of the Hospital in the Health System

In Chapter 1 we suggested that medical care, that is, the diagnosis and *treatment* of accidents and illness, is only one portion of the total health system. Assuming that an ultimate objective for society is improved health, we noted that genetic and environmental characteristics, including demographic, behavioral, and physical factors, have a major influence on health. In the area of personal health care, promotion of health, prevention of disease, and rehabilitation have a major influence. Nevertheless, most of society's health care efforts and expenditures are directed toward medical treatment. Although widely accepted indicators of health stature are not as yet available, it does not appear that increasing expenditures for medical care are producing a marked improvement in health. For example, the death rate has been relatively stable in recent years in the United States, even though medical care expenditures and medical services have increased dramatically. Life span has increased in the past 50 years because infant mortality has been reduced primarily due to public health and environmental factors. But life expectancy for men who reach 50 years of age has not changed for a half-century in the United States.

After reviewing a number of studies, Haggerty (1972) concludes that there is not much evidence that illness care (which is what most medical care consists of) reduces mortality or morbidity very much. Winkelstein and French (1970) suggest that "medical care is largely unrelated to health status of population," but that "ecology is the primary determinant of the health status of a population" (p. 7). Thomas (1972) suggests that the bulk of current medical services are either nontechnological, or only partly so, and urges policy makers to give high priority to more basic research in biological sciences. Fuchs (1974) suggests that demand for life—not medical care nor income—is a primary determinant in an advanced society and Kish (1974) in a rather strong indictment suggests . . . "the time has come to focus attention on the fact [that] in the absence of at least some resolution (and a clearer mandate from society), the nation's second largest industry [i.e., health care] is expending vast national wealth while responding in a large measure to its own vested interest" (p. 271).

The current emphasis on health maintenance organizations is also an indication of the reordering of priorities away from expensive hospital services toward keeping people well. While the general public still appears to be primarily concerned with medical services, health services researchers and the policy makers are beginning to look in other directions in order to improve health. There could well be a Stage 5 grafted onto McDermott's (1969) four stages of medicine. The fifth stage would appropriately be a focus on health in its broadest sense, with emphasis on the promotion of health through the types of efforts suggested throughout this book (particularly in Chapters 1 and 7).

We suggested in Chapter 2 and elsewhere that medical care systems are in a period of transition. For example, the development of HMO group practices around physician services and outside the hospital setting could change the role of the hospital as a unifying core for comprehensive medical care services in a continuum. Currently, in the solo practice fee-for-service model the hospital serves this function. We also suggested in Chapter 9 and elsewhere that there could be a further separation of medical staffs and hospital administration, leading to relationships through negotiation rather than an integrated organization. This, too, could diminish the role of the hospital as a unifying core for medical care systems. There are a number of issues for the future role of hospitals:

What would a shift in priorities from medical care to health care mean to the role of hospitals other than leaving fewer resources available for traditional hospital diagnostic and treatment services?

Can hospitals have a meaningful role in the broader services for improving the health of a community? Will they take a proactive role in health—e.g., promoting legislation, occupational health, health education, and other programs aimed at improving the health of a community?

How might hospital, medical staff, and physician services be effectively integrated? What are the implications of not integrating them? What sort of organizational and administrative changes would have to take place in order to integrate them?

We have suggested throughout this book that the hospital can and should have a larger role as a unifying core to meet broad community health care needs. As stated by

Wade Mountz, Chairman of AHA's Board of Trustees (*Hospital Week,* 1975) ... "the test of a hospital's viability today and in the future, is how well it can provide care that is best for the community and its patients within the community's resources. . . . We have to start paying more attention to developing the necessary range of health services for our citizens, not within a single institution, but within the framework of the community as a whole" (pp. 1-2).

Hospital Combination and Regionalization

In recent years, there has been a trend toward combining hospitals and other health facilities on a regional basis. This can have an important influence on the roles of individual hospitals. There are many good reasons for combining facilities, including:

Emphasis on comprehensive health services in a continuum.

Financial pressures of low-volume services such as obstetrical or emergency services, and potential economies of scale from combined facilities and services.

Small hospitals and independent physicians cannot afford specialized personnel or the scope of services large institutions can provide.

Obsolete facilities, e.g., a laundry, can be replaced, so that several institutions could support a central laundry at less capital cost.

An institution in an inner city could meet objectives of growth by developing satellite operations.

Medical procedures such as reading electrocardiograms can be done remotely with telecommunication devices.

Regional planning has expedited combinations, e.g., categorization of hospitals for emergency services.

Starkweather (1971) suggests seven dimensions of facility combinations in a range from pluralism to fusion (Table 16-1). Many types of combinations between hospitals are possible, from referral of patients by medical staff members of a small hospital to a medical center (informal pluralism) to shared services on a purchased or joint venture basis (e.g., laboratory or laundry services), to an outright merger (fusion). Medical schools may affiliate with hospitals; group practices might share ancillary services with a hospital or another group. In their survey of hospital-shared services, Astolfi and Matti (1972) found that two-thirds of the nearly 4,700 hospitals responding reported sharing 1 to 73 services with other hospitals on a variety of purchased or joint venture bases.

It is likely that combinations will continue to increase for the reasons cited above. In addition, expansion of certificate-of-need legislation, Medicare controls, and other pressures should result in new combinations. For example, the head of the (Wisconsin) Governor's Health Task Force stated that over one-third of that state's hospitals should be closed. These are small institutions, some of which should probably combine with larger hospitals rather than close their doors. A number of mergers have been aborted. Baydin and Sheldon (1975) suggest the following as internal potential problems:

1 Loyality of trustees, auxiliaries and other volunteers
2 Personal autonomy and security of existing medical staffs
3 Job security sought by employees

Table 16-1 Seven Dimensions of Health Facility Combination on a Scale of Pluralism to Fusion

Pluralism			Fusion
Informal (preformal)		Informal (latent)	
	Shared services, joint undertakings, cooperatives, affiliations	Consolidations, multiple units under single mgt., satellites, branches, chains	Mergers
Dimension			
I Organizational pattern	Informal relationships, complete formal integrity	Voluntary subscriptions, joint development of support services	Tradeoff agreements Common delegation of authority to outside agency	Absorbtion Fusion
II Legal bonds	Preformal relationships, formal independence	Implied agreements Contracts Formal agreements with escape provisions	Formal agreements, permanent, which preserve self-sufficiency of prior organizations	Formal agreements, permanent, which prohibit independent operation Replacement agreements
III Nature of combined services	Informal arrangements, no formally shared services	Support and administrative services only	Professional services	Direct patient care services ambulatory inpatient both
IV Stages and forms of production	Natural exchanges formal separation	Affiliations	Vertical combinations	Horizontal combinations, transformations
V Geography of population served	Natural regionalization and localization	Dispersed populations	Common geographic population, partial services	Common geographic population, all types of services Geographic expansion
VI Facility location	Distant	Same community	Approximate, adjacent	Contiguous, integrated
VII Organizational impact	Unofficial relationships, status quo	Minimal to changes of tasks, jobs, rules	Substantial —new function, reorganization of departments	Evolutionary—system-wide changes, deliberate restructuring Spontaneous —sudden impact, unpredictable consequences

Source: David Starkweather, "Health Facility Mergers: Some Conceptualizations," *Medical Care,* vol. 9, no. 6, p. 473, Nov.-Dec. 1971.

4 Disruption of existing management system and its ability to be integrated

5 Initial costs of merger with regard to losses of medical staff patients and key personnel

6 Overextension of management resources

7 Overestimation of ability of existing hospitals to provide expanded services

8 Underestimating the difficulties of integrating basically incompatible institutions

For at least the last quarter-century there have been efforts to rationalize hospital services on a regional basis. An expected outcome of the 1946 Hill-Burton legislation was that state plans would support new hospitals on the basis of regional needs for primary, secondary, and tertiary services that they called area, regional, and base hospitals respectively. Because of pressures for hospitals in rural areas, population growth, and shifts to suburban areas planning along the basis of primary, secondary and tertiary care needs did not really develop. There have been examples of regionalization and sharing of services, among them the pioneering programs in the Rochester, New York hospitals. However, the independence of hospitals, the relative ease of raising capital funds, and institutional and community goals for growth and prestige have generally thwarted such efforts until recently.

Figure 16-1 portrays three general models for combining and/or regionalizing hospital services on a vertical, horizontal, or regional basis. They are based on scope and depth of services and referral patterns. There can be modifications or combinations of these models and within each one the arrangements can vary from informal pluralism to fusion.

In the vertical model, a primary care, small rural, or suburban hospital might have an informal or fused relationship with a larger community secondary care hospital. The primary care hospital might treat patients who require less specialized and sophisticated services. Professional pathology, radiology, and pharmacy services might be supplied by the secondary hospital as might some of the management support services. The tertiary university or major referral hospital would provide sophisticated heart surgery, neonatal services for high-risk infants, and other tertiary care services. The tertiary hospital would probably also provide teaching programs in primary care hospitals for family practice clinical experiences, and in secondary hospitals for general medicine, surgery, ob-gyn., and pediatrics. The tertiary hospital should also be able to provide management consultation to secondary and primary hospitals in areas such as medical records, nursing, and systems engineering. A number of university hospitals are moving in such directions out of their need for stronger ties with other hospitals, and for more and broader teaching experiences, and because of mandates from the states. Area Health Education Center (AHEC) proposals by the Carnegie Commission (1970) for such regional arrangements fit into this model. While there are a few examples of rather strong AHEC (AHECs), a lack of funding and other incentives have handicapped their development in most areas.

In the horizontal model, services would be shared more evenly among hospitals. For example, one hospital might have a neonatal center for the area, another a trauma center, another a cardiac center, and so forth. Management and support services such as data processing and laundry might be shared as well. Primary care

Vertical

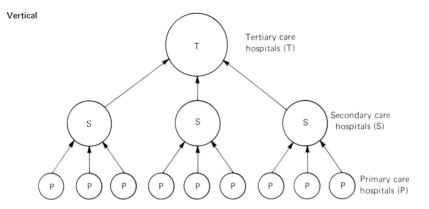

Horizontal

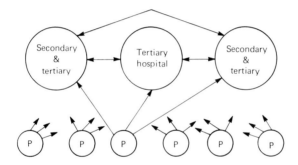

Chains

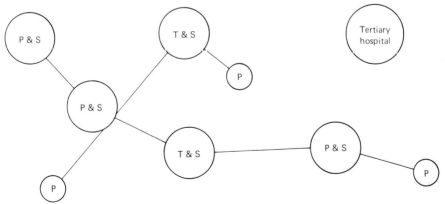

Figure 16-1 General models of hospital combinations

hospitals would then use a variety of secondary-tertiary hospital combinations for specialized services. While hospitals are generally eager to develop a specialized service for the area, few are willing to give up a service to another hospital unless forced to. Consequently, little progress has been made toward wide application of this model.

The third model is a chain-type operation, which is usually associated with a fused arrangement. Proprietary chains are examples of this, as are Catholic hospitals and prepaid group hospitals such as the Kaiser Hospitals. Centralized management services such as purchasing, data processing, and systems engineering can be found in the majority of not-for-profit and profit chains. Diagnostic and treatment services are frequently shared along the lines described in the horizontal model when medical staffs are affiliated as in the Kaiser-Permanente System. When medical staffs are not affiliated, there are usually major problems in sharing medical services.

In most cases, insufficient time has elapsed to study the effects of combinations. A preliminary evaluation of the Samaritan Health Service in Phoenix, Arizona (HRET, 1972), a chain-type operation, suggested that the merger of those hospitals achieved major gains in comprehensiveness, quality and availability of care. A financial analysis of the Samaritan Health Service indicated that this merger was helpful in containing costs relative to the services provided (Neumann, 1974).

Again, these trends have important implications for individual hospitals. If hospital governing boards and administrators wish to have maximum control over the destinies of their institutions, they should examine opportunities for associations with other services in order to meet community needs more efficiently and effectively. The logic of combinations and regionalization suggests that governmental policy will move in that direction. Two key questions hospital managers should ask themselves are:

Can the hospital associate, in one or more ways, with another or other hospitals to deliver medical and health care more effectively and efficiently?

Can the hospital associate, in one or more ways, with other types of health services such as mental, dental, public, preventive, rehabilitative and/or custodial services to deliver comprehensive services in a continuum more effectively and efficiently?

Governance and Control of Hospitals

In Chapter 4 we noted that control over hospitals changed from board dominance, when hospitals were founded by wealthy donors many years ago, to medical staff dominance as expertise and specialization evolved, to increasing influence of the administrator as negotiations with third-party payers became increasingly important. In recent years there have been demands for consumer controls over hospitals, in recognition of the fact that many hospital boards are dominated by economically influential persons in the community. Consumer representatives as governing board members have not been particularly successful from most points of view.

As noted in Chapters 4 and 15, the autonomy of nonprofit hospitals has been further eroded by governmental regulation. Areawide health planning has influenced hospitals to coordinate their plans with other health institutions and services.

Functions of the board, as defined in Chapter 4, are controlling and maintaining organizational effectiveness, representing the region and subgroups, and obtaining resources from the hospital's environment. With increasing externally imposed constraints, the role of the governing board is changing.

There have also been increasing pressures for boards to include internal representation, e.g., having the administrator and medical staff members as voting members of the board. Traditionally, many Catholic hospitals have had internal boards consisting of members of the religious community, who also work in the hospital. Currently, however, while non-Catholic hospitals may be moving toward more internal representation, Catholic hospitals are moving toward external representation.

These trends raise a number of issues for hospital governance and control:

How do these changes affect the roles of the governing board, administrator, and medical staff?

What composition of board members, e.g., internal versus external, consumer versus community leaders, is most effective in linking the hospital with its changing external and internal environments?

With increasing controls, what can hospitals do to: (1) correct problems causing pressures for more control, (2) promote the type of controls it believes to be best for that community under current and anticipated circumstances, and (3) effectively cope with increasing controls?

Health Team

In previous chapters it was noted that the health team has increased greatly in both size and scope. From the 1940s through the 1960s the United States went through a period of population growth, increasing demands for health services, and severe shortages of health personnel. Today, in the middle 1970s we are beginning to see, or project surpluses in many of the health professions.

The growth in number of different health specialties and occupations has helped to apply the explosion of knowledge to the diagnosis and treatment of patients. It has also contributed to problems of role definition, status, coordination, and rapidly rising costs. There is conflict within the medical profession. The patient is at times caught between differences of opinion between specialists. There is maldistribution of physicians geographically and also among specialties. For example, surpluses of general surgeons and shortages of primary care physicians are reported. The debate regarding family practitioner generalists versus primary care specialists continues. We also suggested earlier in this chapter that problems exist with regard to integrating physician and hospital services and as to where the unifying core for comprehensive services in a continuum should be located.

Nursing, pharmacy, and other health professions appear to be going through identity crises as they strive for expanded roles and greater professionalism. New health professions such as physicians' assistants show promise of improving the utilization and productivity of physicians, but their mobility and relationships with other health professionals also complicate the health team concept.

Assuming it requires a broad scope of specialists to learn and apply all the knowledge available today to meet the medical care needs of the individual, these specialists should be working as a team focusing on individual patients. We have reviewed a number of proposals designed to coordinate the team more effectively such as service unit management, management team concept, matrix organizations, and educational changes to develop team concepts early in career development. Issues surrounding a team approach to medical and health service remain:

What is the role of the hospital in improving coordination of the health team both internally and externally?

How can the needs and fears of individual health professionals as well as the needs of individual consumers for a coordinated health team effort be met more effectively?

How might the conflict between *administrative authority,* directed toward public accountability, and *professional authority,* often preoccupied with professional prerogatives be resolved? Austin (1975, p. 142) identifies this as the single most important challenge facing the health system today.

Hospital Administration

Hospital administration, including functional specialists, physician, nursing, and other health professionals in managerial roles in addition to the hospital administrator, are faced with the major issues described in this book. Management has become a much more critical function as institutions have increased in size and complexity. Administrators have multiple roles, and these roles have changed over the years and are still in the process of change. Knowledge related to management has advanced greatly as have the tools to aid management. Yet they have not been effectively applied to hospital management. External pressures are forcing administration to document the needs, plans, and resource expectations of hospitals. Operations research, systems analysis, financial management, and other knowledge sources offer advanced information systems to help in problem solving, decision making, documentation of needs, and evaluation of operations.

As suggested in other chapters, the hospital administrator appears to be concerned about his status and role as are other members of the health team. Just as we suggested that institutions look to community needs above their own, so, too, should administrators try to look at their roles in relationship to what will help the institution meet its objectives most effectively. In that way administrators will be able to develop a role model that will be best not only for the institution, but also for themselves in the long run. In this process the administrator and board might want to examine alternatives in the perspective of the following questions:

How can advanced managerial knowledge and techniques be applied more effectively in hospitals that have diverse goals and with professionals who are not oriented in such directions?

What role and qualifications would enable hospital administrators and others in administration to create a unified health team responsive to needs and expectations for medical and health care?

What management development and continuing education efforts would be most appropriate to meet the increasing challenges faced by administration and governance of the hospital?

Information Systems in Managing Quality, Cost, and External Influences

Information systems are becoming more important to the administration of hospitals. With increasing regulation, it is reasonable to expect that measures of costs and quality of service will be used. At the present time almost everyone will agree that effective measures of cost and quality do not exist. As we suggested in Chapter 10, structure and process are generally used as indicators of quality, but more effective measures of outcome and links to process measures are needed. Moreover, assuming the ultimate objective is to improve health, better measures of health status need to be developed. Current available data on mortality and morbidity are insufficient measures in view of the many demographic, environmental, and health service factors to be considered. A number of researchers are working on developing appropriate health status indicators, and within the next decade we may have more effective measures. In the meantime, primitive surrogate measures will be used since the allocation of federal resources will have to be based on some sort of service and/or health status indicators.

Current comparative cost measurements are also inadequate. Cost per patient-day is most frequently used, but it is ineffective for a number of reasons; for example, patient-days are not appropriate measures of hospital products; moreover, there are many service and treatment variables between hospitals.

A lack of measures makes it difficult for hospital managers to establish explicit objectives and to develop operative comparisons with other hospitals. It is much easier to develop measures in for-profit, tangible-product companies. However, improved measures are likely to be developed in the years ahead in the nonprofit sector because institutions will need them in order to successfully manage and obtain necessary resources within increasing federal, state, and local regulations.

Information systems should be designed to measure hospital effectiveness. Effectiveness may be defined as the hospital's ability to (1) meet community needs, (2) provide high-quality service, (3) minimize cost of inputs needed to produce such service, and (4) achieve institutional objectives. Measures should be devised to answer the following questions:

What are the community needs the hospital can and should serve and how can the hospital know how well it is meeting them?

What are structure, process, and outcome indicators of quality, and at what level should the hospital be for each of the important indicators?

What are appropriate output indicators and levels for the hospital, and how can it be determined that the hospital is providing the output at least cost?

What explicit targets of achievement should the hospital set up, and how can the hospital know how well it is meeting them?

THE FUTURE

We have suggested that most of the historical changes in hospitals came as a result of economic, social, and technologic changes. Change will continue to occur at an accelerating rate (Toffler, 1970). For example, during the 1960s and early 1970s there was a dramatic rise in the standard of living in many nations, and particularly in those that, in the preceding 25 years or so, had been devastated by war, e.g., West Germany, Japan, and the Peoples Republic of China. We are beginning to see a trend in the economies of the Western World away from rapid growth and toward conservation and contraction largely because of a belatedly acknowledged energy crisis. In the months and years ahead there may be further unforeseen economic changes that could have dramatic effects on hospital governance and administration.

Social changes in recent years have been equally dramatic. In the 1960s we experienced the civil rights movement, the sexual "revolution," campus riots, and, in our field, the development of health care rights. Technological advances of the sixties such as successful space programs, the application of computer technology, and organ transplants were events few had anticipated 10 to 15 years earlier. Fabun (1967), in underscoring the accelerating rate of change, suggests that in the next 20 years the rate of changes will not be similar to that of the past 20, but more like the rate of change between the Civil War and today.

Using a Delphi technique (Helmer, 1966), a number of studies have been done to project the future of health care. Selected projections from three Delphi studies— Gordon and Helmer (1969), which used 83 scientists, Bender et al. (1969), which used 33 experts, and a Smith, Kline and French (SK&F) study that used 196 members of that company's R and D staff—are summarized in Table 16-2. These projections, which may become realities within the lifetime of today's students, have almost inconceivable implications for society and, of course, for health administration.

McLaughlin and Sheldon (1974) did a Delphi study on the future of medical care using about 100 panelists representing basic sciences, political medicine, social science, legal and administrative health, and futurologists. Starkweather et al. (1973) conducted a Delphi study among 24 "prominent" experts, six from each of four groups representing (1) hospital and health services administrators and planners, (2) physicians, (3) community service professionals (i.e., consumer advocacy and voluntary health and welfare agency executives), and (4) health care financing, both private and government. Table 16-3 reports the results of this study as it relates to medical service organizational patterns and their effect on hospitals. The table shows the proportion of panelists (in percentages rounded to nearest 5 percent) who estimated the 90, 50, and 10 percent likelihood that the conditions paraphrased by each statement would occur in the 5 to 10 years following mid-1973. Rectangles and squares are used to graphically indicate consensus attainment for each statement.

Results indicate that a majority of the panel predicted a 50 percent or better likelihood that hospitals would assume the status of "quasi-public utilities" and become federated into some sort of central sponsorship. They saw increasing public accountability for hospitals and increasing relationships between hospitals. The panel

Table 16-2   Projection of Changes from Three Delphi Studies

Projection	Median date of achievement		
	Bender et al.	Helmer & Gordon	SK & F
Implanted artificial organs made of plastic and/or electronic components	1983	1982	1985
Chemical alleviation of serious mental disorders	1993	1992	1985
Chemical control over hereditary defects	1998	2000	2009
Chemical synthesis of protein for food	1978	1990	1985
Use of personality control drugs	1983	1983	1995
Worldwide immunization against bacterial and viral diseases	1993	1994	2009
Simulation of new organ growth	1988	2007	>2017
Ability to control aging process permitting significant extension of life span	1993	2023	>2017
Use of drugs to raise intelligence level	1978	1989	>2017
Creation of primitive life form	1978	1989	>2017
Use of telephathy and ESP in communications	Never	Never	>2017

Source: A. Douglas Bender et al., *A Delphic Study of the Future of Medicine* (monograph), Research and Development Division, Smith, Kline and French Laboratories, Philadelphia, 1969.

did not predict important new relationships among different medical staffs, but they did foresee stronger relationships between each medical staff and its hospital, and especially, greater physician responsibility for hospital operations.

IMPLICATIONS

What might these accelerating changes mean to administrators, governing boards, physicians, and others? Possibly nothing. After all, most of the issues have been apparent for some time and hospitals are generally getting along quite well. Moreover, even if major changes occur people will always require medical care services and the industry will be supported. Hospitals are necessary, and the skills and services of health professionals and administrators will always be needed. Even in totalitarian societies a major emphasis is placed on health care, and there is usually little interference with what physicians think is best for their patients.

Nevertheless, governmental regulation of hospitals is likely to increase. Organized medicine and hospital administration may continue their attempts to thwart any steps toward more regulation, which has generally been the AMA role. Or they may attempt

Table 16-3 Medical Service Organizational Patterns and Their Effect on Hospitals

Question	Percent of panelists indicating likelihood of occurrence in next ten years		
	90%	50%	10%
Hospitals in respect to sponsorship			
a Little or no change	20	20	60
b More profit-oriented ownership	0	35	65
c Government-run hospitals will convert to private nonprofit status	15	45	40
d Hospitals will assume status of quasi-public utilities	45	50	5
e Federation of hospitals into central sponsorship/ ownership	20	45	35
Hospitals in respect to public accountability			
f Little or no change	5	5	90
g More voluntary public responsiveness in terms of types of services, financial accounting, expansion, etc.	35	55	10
h More representation of the underserved public on hospital boards	55	45	0
i Public disclosure of hospital income, expenses, and plans	95	5	0
j Officially authorized agency review of performance in fiscal management and of service quality	55	45	0
k Greater commission-type regulation of services, expansion, and rates	80	20	0
Hospitals in respect to relationship with other hospitals			
l Little or no change	5	20	75
m Continued voluntary development of shared services not involving patient contact	35	55	10
n Greater voluntary coordination, cooperation, and functional specialization among hospitals regarding all services, research, and education	65	30	5

Table 16-3 (continued)

Question	Percent of panelists indicating likelihood of occurrence in next ten years		
	90%	50%	10%
o Stronger management alliances	55	35	10
p Formation of consortia of hospitals which will jointly assume financial risk	35	40	25
q Physical consolidations and complete organizational merger	15	40	45
Hospitals in respect to medical staff organization			
r Physicians will be required to admit all of their cases to one hospital rather than to several	0	35	65
s Hospitals will continue to have their own medical staff and will continue to be closed to nonstaff physicians	50	25	25
t Hospitals will no longer have their own medical staff, physicians will become members of a common staff sponsored by a federated organization such as a health care corporation	10	20	70
u Staff privileges among hospitals will be interchangeable	20	40	40
v Hospitals will contract with medical care foundation for medical staff	5	55	40
w One medical staff for two or more hospitals	45	40	15
x Greater physician participation in hospital affairs, including direct operating responsibilities	40	45	15
y Doctors will be closer to their principal hospital, having an interlocking incentive and penalty system linked to the hospital	10	80	10
z Medical staff will be more oriented into health teams coordinated with neighborhood clinics in addition to hospitals	30	50	20

Source: David Starkweather et al., *Delphi Forecasting of Health Care Organization,* paper no. 1, Occasional papers in Hospital and Health Administration, School of Public Health, University of California, Berkeley, 1973.

to influence the direction regulation takes, as the AHA has done in some cases (but not always with the support of its membership, as in the case of the health care corporations proposal reported in the previous chapter).

We believe there are many opportunities for individual hospitals to solve problems and prepare for accelerating changes. This means planning for change rather than reacting to it. Change can be accomplished in a number of ways. It can be imposed by regulation. It can also result from the tension created by confrontation tactics, including strikes or even violence. We have repeatedly suggested throughout this book that change is best brought about by a positive approach, one that systematically and carefully examines changing needs, defines explicit objectives, and designs programs to fulfill these objectives.

We have also suggested that in a complex open system such as a hospital this process should be conducted with broad participation. With heterogeneous groups focusing on purposes, needs, and objectives, a positive framework can be established rather than a negative one in which the emphasis is on problems and who's at fault. A positive goal-oriented approach helps to cope with the insecurity that comes with most changes, and to promote creativity.

In conclusion, we are firmly convinced that, while hospitals face serious challenges, they also have exciting opportunities to help improve the health of society to an even greater extent than in the past. We appeal to those responsible for the governance and administration of hospitals to take the initiative in finding and demonstrating better ways of meeting the health needs of the community and in managing institutions with greater efficiency and effectiveness.

REFERENCES

Astolf, Adrienne and Leo B. Matti: "Survey Profiles Shared Services," *Hospitals, J.A.H.A.,* vol. 46, pp. 61-63, Sept. 16, 1972.

Austin, Charles J.: "Emerging Roles and Responsibilities in Health Administration," in *Education for Health Administration,* vol. I, Report of the Commission in Education for Health Administration, Health Administration Press, Ann Arbor, Mich., pp. 137-155, 1975.

Bender, A. Douglas et al.: *A Delphic Study of the Future of Medicine* (monograph), Research and Development Division, Smith, Kline and French Laboratories, Philadelphia, 1969.

Carnegie Commission on Higher Education: *Higher Education and the Nation's Health,* Berkeley, Calif., 1970.

Fabun, Don: *The Dynamics of Change,* Prentice-Hall, Englewood Cliffs, N.J., 1967.

Flexner, Abraham: *Medical Education in the United States and Canada,* Carnegie Foundation for the Advancement of Teaching (reprinted by Science and Health Publications, Washington, D.C.), 1910.

Fuchs, Victor R.: Presentation, University of Wisconsin, July 22, 1974 (unpublished).

Gordon, Theodore and Olaf Helmer: "Report of a Long-Range Forecasting Study," *Social Technology,* parts I and II, Rand Corp., Santa Monica, Calif., 1966.

Haggerty, Robert J.: "Boundaries of Health Care," *Pharos,* pp. 106-111, July 1972.

Helmer, Olaf: *Social Technology,* Basic Books, New York, 1965.

Hospital Week: American Hospital Association, Chicago, Feb. 14, 1975.

HRET: *Demonstration and Evaluation of Integrated Health Care Facilities, Samaritan Health Service, Phoenix, Arizona,* Health Services Research Center of the Hospital Research and Education Trust, Final Report, vol. IV (technical version), for period June 1970-June 1972, Chicago, 1972.

Kish, Arnold I.: "The Health Care System and Health: Some Thoughts on a Famous Misalliance," *Inquiry,* vol. II, pp. 269-275, Dec. 1974.

McDermott, Walsh: "Demography, Culture, and Economics in the Evolutionary Stages of Medicine," in Edwin D. Kilbourne and Wilson G. Smillie (eds.), *Human Ecology and Public Health,* Macmillan, Toronto, Canada, 1969, pp. 7-28.

McLaughlin, Curtis P. and Alan Sheldon: *The Future and Medical Care,* Ballinger, Cambridge, Mass., 1974.

Neumann, Bruce: "A Financial Analysis of a Hospital Merger: Samaritan Health Service," *Medical Care,* vol. 12, no. 12, pp. 983-998, Dec. 1974.

Risse, Guenter, B., Associate Professor, History of Medicine, University of Wisconsin, Madison, personal communications, 1974.

Starkweather, David B.: "Health Facility Mergers: Some Conceptualizations," *Medical Care,* vol. 9, no. 6, pp. 468-478, Nov.-Dec. 1971.

Starkweather, David, Louis Gelwicks, and Robert Newcomer: *Delphi Forecasting of Health Care Organization,* paper no. 1, Occasional papers in Hospital and Health Administration, School of Public Health, University of California, Berkeley, 1973.

Thomas, Lewis: "Aspects of Biomedical Science Policy," an address to the Institute of Medicine, Washington, D.C. Fall meeting, Nov. 9, 1972.

Toffler, Alvin: *Future Shock,* Random House, New York, 1970.

Winkelstein, Warren Jr. and Fern E. French: "The Role of Ecology in the Design of a Health Care System," *California Medicine,* vol. 113, no. 5, pp. 7-12, Nov. 1970.

Subject Index

Name Index

Hazard, William R., 248
Health Insurance Institute, 90
Hedgepeth, Jay H., 186
Helmer, Olaf, 187, 284
Hemmelgard, Ronald, 51, 52, 54
Hemphill, J.R., 56
Henshaw, Stanley, 131, 133, 157
Hershey, Nathan, 125
Hetherington, Robert W., 25
Heydebrand, Wolf U., 122
Hickey, W.J., 49, 50
Highriter, M.E., 92
Hill, Lawrence, A., 215
Hoke, Bob, 12
Holloway, R.G., 58
Hopkins, Carl E., 25
Horn, J.S., 8
Hospital Financial Management Association, 169
Hospital Statistics, 203
Hospital Week, 104, 203, 276
Hospitals, 33, 101, 105, 208
House, Robert J., 58, 157, 225, 226
Howes, Nancy J., 162, 165, 170, 171, 187
188, 209, 210, 217
Hrebiniak, Lawrence, 92
Hummel, Patricia, 102
Hurtado, Arnold V., 121
Hutts, Joseph C., 130-132, 148
Hynnimann, Clifford E., 114

Illinois Study Commission on Nursing, 97, 104, 105, 159, 161, 209
Ingbar, M.L., 208

Jaco, E. Gartly, 40
Jameson, J., 94
Janeway, Charles, 71
Jehring, J.J., 217
Jelinek, Richard, 124
Johnsen, Gordon, 207
Johnson, Alton C., 139, 158, 207, 223
Joint Commission on Accreditation of Hospitals, 75, 192
Journal of the American Pharmaceutical Association, 114
Jydstrup, Ronald A., 172

Kahn, Robert L., 34, 148, 224, 225
Kaluzny, Arnold D., 49, 51
Kast, Fremont E., 34
Katz, Daniel, 34, 148, 149, 225

Katz, Delores, 82
Kerr, Lorin, 120
Kessel, Ruben, 73
Kinzer, David, 263
Kish, Arnold I., 275
Klarman, Herbert E., 25, 209
Knowles, John, 68, 72, 74, 82, 161, 209, 218
Kovner, Anthony R., 50, 51, 165, 203
Kovner, Joel, 23
Kralewski, John Edward, 138, 240
Kuby, Alma, 244

Lambertson, Eleanor, 101, 117
Lamy, Peter P., 114
Lanser, Ross E., 50, 62
Lattin, Norman D., 48
Laur, Robert, 50
Leavell, H.R., 12
Lefcowitz, Myron L., 5
Lentz, Edith, 49
Levey, Samuel, 165
Levin, A.L., 261
Levine, Peter, 120
Levit, Edith J., 71
Lewin, Kurt, 232
Lewis, Charles E., 72, 101
Likert, Rensis, 158, 232
Lipzin, Benjamin, 209
Little, D., 103
Logan, James P., 135, 136
Loomba, N. Paul, 165
Lumpp, Sister M. Francesca, 104
Lusk, Edward J., 165, 203
Lysaught, Jerome P., 95, 96, 98, 101

McCleary, Robert, 186
McDermott, Walsh, 38, 273
MacEachern, Malcolm, 60
McGregor, Douglas, 232
McLaughlin, Curtis P., 284
McNamara, Mary, 19, 21
McNerney, Walter J., 261
Maier, Norman F., 144, 231
Maiman, Lois, 20
Mali, Paul, 231
Mann, Floyd C., 58, 83, 224, 227
Mariner, E.T., 172
Markgren, Paul, 121
Mather, H.G., 218
Matlock, David R., 240
Matti, Leo B., 276
Mauksch, Hans O., 101